The Politics
of Care
Work

The Politics of Care Work

PUERTO RICAN
WOMEN ORGANIZING
FOR SOCIAL JUSTICE
Emma Amador

DUKE UNIVERSITY PRESS   *Durham and London*   2025

© 2025 Duke University Press
All rights reserved
Project Editor: Livia Tenzer
Designed by Courtney Leigh Richardson
Typeset in Minion Pro and IBM Plex Sans
by Westchester Publishing Services

Library of Congress Cataloging-in-Publication Data
Names: Amador, Emma, [date] author.
Title: The politics of care work : Puerto Rican women organizing
for social justice / Emma Amador.
Description: Durham : Duke University Press, 2025. | Includes
bibliographical references and index.
Identifiers: LCCN 2024038457 (print)
LCCN 2024038458 (ebook)
ISBN 9781478031833 (paperback)
ISBN 9781478028598 (hardcover)
ISBN 9781478060819 (ebook)
Subjects: LCSH: Puerto Rican women—Political activity. | Women
caregivers—Political activity—Puerto Rico. | Women caregivers—
Political activity—United States. | Women political activists—
Puerto Rico. | Women political activists—United States. | Social
justice—United States. | Social justice—Puerto Rico.
Classification: LCC RA645.35 .A396 2025 (print) |
LCC RA645.35 (ebook) | DDC 362/.0425—dc23/eng/20250218
LC record available at https://lccn.loc.gov/2024038457
LC ebook record available at https://lccn.loc.gov/2024038458

Cover art: Yolanda Sánchez, from *Women Making History:
Conversations with Fifteen New Yorkers*, ed. Maxine Gold
(New York: New York City Commission on the Status of Women,
1985).

For my parents and teachers, Salvador and Deborah.
For my loves, Kyle and Luna.

Contents

Acknowledgments

When I was twenty years old, I interviewed my grandmother, Formeria Jiménez Amador, using a tape recorder that produced a scratchy recording of her life story. After I asked her about her life, she spent hours telling me about growing up in rural Puerto Rico and her later migration to the United States. She also recounted the difficulties and joys she experienced as a seamstress, domestic worker, and mother. Over two decades later, long after she passed away, I revisited these recordings while completing this book. Listening, I laughed as I heard roosters crowing, a chorus of coquí frogs, and my grandmother's constant side conversations with her beloved dog Bingo. I regretted that when I conducted the interview I had not yet studied much Puerto Rican and Latina history and hadn't asked relevant follow-up questions. However, I was also struck by the beauty of this recording precisely because I didn't know how to ask the "right" research questions. The interview is now a record of my grandmother teaching me about her history, my history, and the broader history of Puerto Ricans. The lessons she taught me about women's history and the importance of care work in Puerto Rican migrant communities have profoundly shaped my work and this book. Thank you, *abuelita*.

At the University of Michigan, I began this project among a vibrant community of scholars exploring US Latinx, Caribbean, United States, and Latin American history. Thank you to Jesse Hoffnung-Garskof, Richard Turits, María Cotera, Sueann Caulfield, Paulina Alberto, Matthew Countryman, Hannah Rosen, Mary Kelly, Rebecca Scott, and Jean Hébrard. I am incredibly grateful to Jesse for his constant encouragement to pursue my research interests and his careful mentorship. Thank you to María for inspiring me and modeling how to be a feminist scholar. Thanks also to my fellow graduate students Christine Walker, Kara French, Cookie Woolner, Minayo Nasiali, Colleen Woods, Sarah Hamilton, Christina Abreu, Iván Chaar López, and Francheska Alers-Rojas. Thanks also to Margaret Chowning for her support during my time as a visiting student researcher at the University of California, Berkeley.

I was also very fortunate to have received my master's degree at the University of Connecticut, where I studied with the trailblazing historian of Puerto Rico Blanca Silvestrini. I am forever grateful to Blanca for lighting a fire in me that has only grown over the years. Thanks also to my fellow students Jessica Xiomara García, Kerry Stefancyk, and Christine Walker. I am also thankful to the faculty at Sarah Lawrence College who inspired me as an undergraduate, especially Isabel de Sena, Shahnaz Rouse, Eduardo Lago, and María Elena García.

As a junior scholar, I was lucky to receive support from several institutions that made this book possible. I am grateful to have spent my first year as a history professor at Goucher College with Matthew Hale, James Dator, and Evan Dawley. The Summer Institute on Tenure and Professional Advancement, run by Duke University and the Mellon Foundation, provided critical support during this period, and I am very thankful to my SITPA mentor Mérida Rúa. As a Presidential Postdoctoral Fellow at Brown University, I found community at the Center for the Study of Race and Ethnicity in America and the Department of History. I am particularly grateful for the support of Tricia Rose, Robert Self, Naoko Shibusawa, Kevin Escudero, Emily Owens, Daniel Rodríguez, Maríaelena Huambachano, Yalidy Matos, Nicole Burrowes, Amanda Boston, and Stephanie Larriuex.

As a faculty member in the Department of History at the University of Connecticut, I have been incredibly lucky to join a wonderful community. Thank you to my UConn colleagues, Mark Healey, Melina Pappademos, Mark Overmyer-Velázquez, Jason Chang, Fiona Vernal, Sarah Silverstein, Ariel Lambe, Cornelia Dayton, Micki McEyla, Christopher Clark, Nancy Shoemaker, Melanie Newport, Nu-Anh Tran, Manisha Sinha, Jeffrey Ogbar Hana Maryuama, Dierdre Cooper Owens, Katerina González Seligmann, Samuel Martínez, Rodolfo Fernández, and Anne Gebelein. My research has also been generously supported by the Humanities Institute at the University of Connecticut, which provided a Humanities Faculty Research Fellowship, a Felberbaum Family Faculty Award, and a Humanities Book Support Award that made completing this book possible. I am also thankful to my department for organizing a manuscript workshop and to all the participants, including the invited outside readers, Lara Putnam and Laura Briggs, for their excellent comments, which helped shape the project.

While conducting research in Puerto Rico, I received encouragement and generous guidance from María del Carmen Baerga, Jorge Duany, and Nilsa

Burgos Ortiz. Thank you to Humberto García Muñiz for helping me arrange a visiting position and library access at the Instituto de Estudios del Caribe at the University of Puerto Rico, Río Piedras. Thanks to María E. Ordóñez Mercado at the Colección Puertorriqueña at the University of Puerto Rico, Río Piedras, and to Julio Quirós Alcalá at the Fundación Luis Muñoz Marín. At the Archivo General de Puerto Rico in San Juan, I am grateful to numerous archivists who guided me along the way, and especially to Hilda T. Ayala González and María I. Rodríguez Matos for helping me include images from the archive in this book. In New York City, at the Center for Puerto Rican Studies at CUNY, Hunter, I am grateful for the early support for this project provided by Edwin Meléndez, Pedro Juan Hernández, and Yosenex Orengo. More recently, I thank Aníbal Arocho and Cristina Fontánez Rodríguez for their help in completing research for this project and including images from CENTRO's collections.

This book has been profoundly shaped by so many fellow scholars interested in Puerto Rican, Latin American, and Latinx studies and the history of migration with whom I have shared the ideas in this book on conference panels, in paper workshops, and over too many cups of coffee. I am particularly grateful to Eileen Findlay, whose work constantly inspires me and who guided me toward many of the archives explored in this project. Thanks also to Sandy Plácido, Carmen Whalen, Takkara Brunson, Genevieve Carpio, Olga Jiménez de Wagenheim, Lisa Materson, Natanya Duncan, Sara Awartani, Reena Goldthree, Delia Fernández-Jones, Petra Rivera-Rideau, Vanessa Díaz, Mónica Jiménez, Margaret Power, Jorell Meléndez-Badillo, Aimee Loiselle, Joanna Camacho, María Canino, Aldo Lauria-Santiago, Ismael García-Cólon, Ileana Rodríguez-Silva, Solsiree del Moral, Melli Velázquez, Isabel Córdova, Aura Jirau Arroyo, Rhadhika Natarajan, Marisol LeBrón, Aurora Santiago Ortiz, Marisol Negrón, Shakti Castro, Michael Staudenmaier, Kaysha Corinealdi, Vanessa Rosa, Zaire Dinzey-Flores, Ginetta Candelario, Arlene Torres, Maura Toro-Morn, Frances Aparicio, Lorgia García-Peña, Arlene Dávila, Yomaira Figueroa-Vásquez, Amanda Guzmán, Karianne Soto Vega, Elena Rosario, Adrianne Francisco, Melisa Galván, Alyssa Ribeiro, Tatiana M.F. Cruz, and Llana Barber.

My work has also been deeply shaped by dialogues with a feminist community of scholars interested in the history of care work, domestic work, welfare, and social reproduction. I am particularly thankful to Eileen Boris for her enthusiastic support of this project and dedication to mentoring junior scholars. Thank you also to Premilla Nadasen and Annelise Orleck for their mentorship. Thank you to Kitty Kish Sklar, Jessica Wilkerson, LaKisha

Simmons, and Alina Méndez for our reading group on social reproduction theory. Thanks also to Felicia Kornbluh, Robyn Muncy, Julie Greene, Jocelyn Olcott, Keona Irvin, Anasa Hicks, Rhacel Salazar Parreñas, Joan Flores-Villalobos, Alison Parker, Tamar Carroll, Catherine Ceniza Choy, Kirsten Swinth, and Sarah Knott. Thanks to the Labor and Working-Class History Association for providing an intellectual home and space to share ideas.

I am also grateful to my fellow scholars of Latina history in the United States who have gathered with me over the past few years to discuss the writing of Latina history and biography. Thank you to our mentor, Vicki L. Ruiz, for lighting the way and encouraging our research. Thank you to Sarah McNamara for helping me dream about future projects. Thanks also to Sandy Plácido, Lori Flores, Yuridia Ramírez, and Tiffany González.

Thank you to my editor at Duke University Press, Gisela Fosado, who has championed this project from the very start and whose steadfast support over many years made this book possible. I am also very grateful for the careful guidance of Alejandra Mejía and Livia Tenzer, who helped me navigate the process of preparing the manuscript for publication. The book was greatly improved because of Duke University Press's anonymous reviewers' careful and deep engagement with my manuscript. Thanks to Jessica Newman, who stepped in at a crucial moment and helped me finish revisions. Thank you also to every person over the years who provided copyediting and comments on drafts and presentations, and helped shape the words and ideas on these pages.

I am grateful for the funding that I received from numerous institutions, including the Rackham Graduate School of the University of Michigan; the Center for the Education of Women at the University of Michigan; the Institute for Research and Women at the University of Michigan; the Center for Latin American and Caribbean Studies at the University of Michigan; the Ford Foundation and the National Research Council of the National Academies; the Center for Puerto Rican Studies, Hunter College, CUNY; the Summer Institute on Tenure and Professional Advancement funded by Duke University and the Mellon Foundation; the Center in the Study of Race and Ethnicity and the Department of History at Brown University; the College of Liberal Arts and Sciences at the University of Connecticut; and the Humanities Institute of the University of Connecticut.

My work on this project would not have been possible without the support of friends and loved ones over many years and in many places. Thanks to Paula Booten and Don Booten for welcoming me into their family and for their love and support. Thanks to Pace Kendall, Cora Brooks, Wanda

Knudsen, Amelia Gardner, Holly McCreary, Nana Dakin, Mia Gomez, Xochitl Vinaja, and Jessica Xiomara García. Thanks also to my Puerto Rican, Norwegian, and Pennsylvanian family members who have shaped my life and work. Thanks to the ancestors for their love and care. As I have already noted, this book honors my grandmother Formeria Jiménez Amador and was shaped by our conversations and the histories she shared with me. It has also been made possible by my mother, Marit Synnøve Stumo, who passed away when I was two years old but who is undoubtedly my guardian angel.

This book was written because of the unconditional love I received from my wonderful parents Salvador Amador and Deborah Reger. My father, Salvador, made my life a great adventure full of love. His passion for history inspired my own, and I miss him tremendously. Deborah is my mother, teacher, and role model. She came into my life when I was seven and has lovingly taken care of me every single second since. She never let me give up. I have been truly blessed to learn how to be a mother from her. Thank you, Deborah, for everything.

Most of all, thank you to my great loves, Kyle Booten and Luna Booten-Amador. There is not enough room here to properly thank my husband, Kyle. He has made completing this book possible by traveling with me to archives, reading last-minute drafts, and photographing documents. He has also cooked countless meals, kept me laughing with his mischievous wit, and been my best friend. I love you, Kyle. And, finally, thank you to my curious, beautiful, and bright daughter, Luna. I am so grateful you have arrived and made this whole world sparkle.

Introduction

Yolanda Sánchez, a social worker and community organizer born in Harlem in 1932, was a child of the Puerto Rican diaspora. Sánchez was part of a community that formed after millions of islanders migrated to the United States following the turn of the twentieth century. She was an activist who dedicated her life to public service and helping her community. As a Puerto Rican, a Black woman, a feminist, and a civil rights leader, she inflected her community organizing with the perspectives and concerns of multiple social movements. Her work was also grounded in day-to-day efforts as a social service provider, educator, and advocate to ensure the civil, political, and economic rights of Puerto Ricans. When she was asked how she wanted to be remembered, she said she hoped "that people will remember me as a person who cared for her community, who cared for people, and who attempted to use her life and her energies to improve conditions."[1] This book tells the history of the caring labor of Puerto Ricans like Sánchez. It is a story about care work as a space of politics—a story that maps an intergenerational legacy of political activism demanding dignity for Puerto Ricans on the archipelago and in the diaspora.

In the case of Sánchez, her own experiences growing up poor in New York City shaped her later efforts as an activist. Her parents had migrated to the United States from Puerto Rico to make new lives in the city and ran upon difficult times. After her father left the family, her mother applied for public assistance benefits in the South Bronx to support her six children. Sánchez later reflected, "Sometimes I look back and say, 'My God, the little Puerto Rican girl who started out on welfare, look where she wound up.'"[2] Soon after she graduated from the City College of New York in 1954, she became a caseworker for the New York City Department of Welfare (figure I.1). She brought her perspective of having been a welfare recipient to her new job and soon began meeting with other Puerto Rican youth and social workers to discuss how they could use their professional status to develop new ways of helping their communities. These collaborations would result

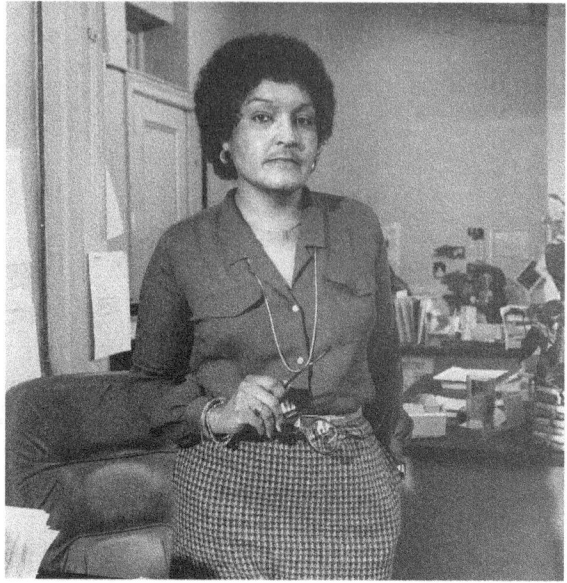

FIGURE I.1. Yolanda Sánchez. Photograph by Adál Alberto Maldonado. Source: Louis Reyes Rivera and Julio Rodríguez, eds., *Portraits of the Puerto Rican Experience* (New York: Institute for Puerto Rican Urban Studies–IPRUS, 1984), 78.

in the flourishing of community-organizing approaches in social work and bind together their efforts with grassroots movements for civil rights in New York.

Alongside other Puerto Rican social worker activists of this period, like Antonia Pantoja and Marta Valle, Sánchez helped create foundational Puerto Rican-led social service institutions. The story of this group of activists illuminates how social work evolved into a dynamic space for political action in 1960s New York. They built on the achievements of previous generations of social work activists while also fighting to transform the profession by making it more accountable to the community.[3] For example, Sánchez became the first social worker hired by the activist educational organization ASPIRA of New York, which advocated on behalf of Puerto Rican youth and organized for bilingual education.[4] Institutions like ASPIRA ("aspire," in Spanish) played crucial roles in addressing the needs of the Puerto Rican community in the United States in the wake of mass displacement and migration. Sánchez's work brought her into conversation and collaboration with like-minded organizers agitating more broadly for the equal rights and care of Puerto Ricans, African Americans, Latinos/as/xs, and women.

While Sánchez's activism was rooted in the community in New York City where she was born, it was also connected to her commitment to Puerto

Rico and the ongoing struggle of its people for self-determination. In 1962 when Sánchez was working for ASPIRA, she helped bring groups of Puerto Rican youth in New York City on trips to Puerto Rico. These were her first visits to Puerto Rico, and they further connected her work to communities on the archipelago.[5] She also became involved in discussions about the political future of Puerto Rico, and this work became increasingly intertwined with her ongoing activism in New York City. Alongside other activists, she argued that Puerto Ricans should have a political voice beyond organizations managed by the Puerto Rican government—in fact, at times she joined criticisms of their work in the United States. Her activism illuminates the interconnections between political organizing in New York City's Puerto Rican community with that in Puerto Rico as well as the continued political significance of the migration of Puerto Ricans to the United States.

In the years that followed, Sánchez became an increasingly important figure in New York City politics. She held directorship positions in ASPIRA, the Puerto Rican Association for Community Affairs (PRACA), and the East Harlem Council for Human Services.[6] In each of these roles she helped lead the charge for accountable and community-oriented social and economic programs for Puerto Ricans in New York City. After receiving her master's degree at Columbia University, she also worked in higher education, and, in her role as a staff member at City College, she helped develop one of the first Puerto Rican studies programs in the United States.[7] Her work within these organizations was linked to her feminist activism, and she also assisted in the development of both the National Conference of Puerto Rican Women and the National Puerto Rican Women's Caucus.[8] In the 1980s, she said, "I think we have a long way to go, not only as Americans, but specifically within the Puerto Rican community, before we really accept women as equals," and she noted that she wanted her daughter "to feel that she has options that [she herself] didn't have as a Puerto Rican woman."[9] As an institution builder and feminist organizer, Sánchez continued to care for her community.

The political path that Sánchez followed was made possible in large part by her work and training as a social worker. The social work profession created opportunities for Puerto Rican women to professionalize and organize with those who shared their concerns and political goals. In fact, in this book I show how the occupation had already served as a space of vibrant political organizing for over fifty years.[10] This activism was a part of broader struggles for Puerto Rican rights in the wake of US colonialism, displacement, and migration to the United States in the twentieth century. I explore how social work became one site of this activism, specifically around citizenship rights and care. As Sánchez and her cohort became community organizers, they forged new paths within the profession that connected back to a long intergenerational history of social worker activism in Puerto Rico and the United States. These forms of activism continue to have lasting impacts in Puerto Rican communities today.

This book considers the story of Sánchez alongside other Puerto Ricans as they fought to survive and help their communities in the face of massive political, economic, and social upheavals. I look in particular at the stories of social worker activists alongside the stories of working-class women who became clients of social welfare programs in Puerto Rico and the Puerto Rican diaspora. Many of these working-class women were also care workers, providing reproductive labor in their own homes and working in the homes of others. This includes women like Sánchez's mother, who migrated to the United States and raised six children while receiving welfare benefits. This book considers the everyday resistance of applicants at the welfare office who pushed back against cuts to benefits as they sought to care for their families. It connects such stories to those of migrant domestic workers who organized alongside professional women social workers to demand labor standards to protect care workers. There is a common thread in each of these moments: Puerto Rican women organized around the politics of care.

I explore the history of the politics of care work through an examination of social work and social welfare. This approach reveals how Puerto Ricans were involved in building and navigating social welfare programs and policies in Puerto Rico and the Puerto Rican diaspora and how these efforts were inherently political. Within the creation of social welfare programs, Puerto Ricans negotiated the terms of their US citizenship, which had been imposed in 1917 but remained colonial and second class. Despite these restrictions, Puerto Ricans fought for equal rights as citizens and contested their colonial citizenship. This struggle played out on the archipelago and in the growing Puerto Rican migrant community that formed in the United States over the course of the twentieth century. Through their engagement with social welfare policies, Puerto Ricans also found an important avenue to demand care for their communities. Therefore, the history of social welfare and social work can serve as a fulcrum for rethinking US colonialism and citizenship in Puerto Rico and the Puerto Rican diaspora, with a focus on Puerto Rican activism.

At the heart of this book are stories of women like Sánchez whose lives were defined by relentless efforts to care for their communities. For Sánchez this meant working tirelessly to build organizations that helped Puerto Ricans on both the archipelago and in the diaspora. Later in life she had a home in Puerto Rico, continued her work as a community organizer, and supported the independence of the archipelago from US colonialism. After she passed away in 2012, the community organizing efforts that she helped develop would continue as numerous other activists followed in her foot-steps. Indeed, women care workers, some of whom are social workers, have been at the forefront of recent Puerto Rican struggles for citizenship rights and care. Some of these activists protested contemporary austerity measures and led relief efforts in the wake of natural disasters like Hurricane Maria in 2017 and the social and political uprisings in Puerto Rico in the twenty-first century. Others have been at the forefront of creating new initiatives to ad-dress the needs of recently displaced, migrant, and diasporic Puerto Ricans in the United States. This work remains vital as the archipelago grapples with out-migration to the United States. This book aims to provide some historical context for these continued political mobilizations. Each chapter centers on the lives and work of women like Sánchez. The stories of these activists reveal the often-untold centrality of Puerto Rican women to the political history of Puerto Rico and its diaspora.

Puerto Ricans, Citizenship, and Social Welfare

Puerto Rico was colonized by the United States in 1898, and since 1917 its people have held a form of colonial and territorial US citizenship that remains unequal to that in the continental United States. This book considers how, despite these restrictions, the granting of symbolic US citizenship has nonetheless had the effect of opening up a discursive space for Puerto Ricans to make political claims to the rights and benefits of full US citizenship. Throughout the twen-tieth century, Puerto Ricans on the archipelago continuously lobbied and argued for access to protection, coverage, and rights as US citizens.[11] In a parallel and sometimes overlapping struggle to lay claim to US citizenship rights, Puerto Rican migrants in the United States, who are legally entitled to full citizenship rights, have also fought for access to these rights because of racial exclusions they faced in the United States. I consider how demands for full coverage under federal social welfare policy and the social provi-sions provided by US citizenship became an important arena of political action in Puerto Rican communities. While Puerto Ricans were often un-successful in negotiating change to their formal political status, organizing around social welfare policy was sometimes more fruitful. In fact, over the decades covered in this book, these social welfare programs in Puerto Rico expanded from serving hundreds of people to nearly half the population.[12] Therefore, studying the political mobilization that resulted in changes to social policy can shed new light on the history of Puerto Rican citizenship, US colonialism, and the politics of social welfare.

The history of social welfare policy and programs has long been considered important to understanding citizenship in both the United States and Latin America. Previous studies have shown that the creation of social welfare programs in the twentieth century shaped social inequalities and led to differential access to rights based on gender and race.[13] However, the development of social welfare programs and social policy in Puerto Rico has remained underexamined in historical scholarship, as have the ways these programs have impacted how Puerto Ricans have experienced US citizenship.[14] Moreover, Puerto Rico has been glaringly absent from histories of US social welfare, despite the central role US colonial administrators played in the territories.[15] The history of social welfare has either been overlooked or cast as a realm of colonial domination in which political agency was largely absent. While this study recognizes social welfare as a place of state control and regulation, it also draws on histories of the state and social welfare that have called for deep investigation of social welfare formation as a space of social struggle over class, race, and gender.[16] This includes critical studies of the history of social welfare in Latin America and the United States, as well as within colonial and imperial projects more broadly.[17] It also builds upon Puerto Rican feminist social scientific scholarship on social welfare policies in Puerto Rico, which has long emphasized the need to recognize social welfare policies as central to Puerto Rican society.[18] This approach allows me to grapple with the history of the Puerto Rican state as a colonial institution that is raced and gendered and that was built, reworked, and contested over the course of the twentieth century by Puerto Rican actors and the political projects they developed.

This book explores the history of social welfare in Puerto Rico by mapping the colonial contours of US social welfare provisions in Puerto Rico. It considers how Puerto Rican officials shaped the colonial state alongside how clients of social welfare programs experienced differences in colonial citizenship as a result of new social welfare policies and benefits. This approach draws on historian Donna Guy's insight that the development of social welfare programs must be considered as a process rather than a product, something that is built and reworked by state officials, administrators, and clients.[19] Guy also notes that the history of welfare is often women's history and that overlooking women's stories in history has resulted in an analysis of the state that has often erased women and gender from the story of state formation. In this book, I put the history of women and gender fully into the frame of the history of the state. Thus, this is a story about Puerto Ricans and the history of social welfare programs in which these terms are understood to be categories in flux, whose definitions have changed over time and across contexts.

In order to tell the interconnected history of Puerto Rican citizenship and social welfare over the past century, this book draws on archives in both Puerto Rico and the United States. In doing so, it sheds light on the creation of US colonial bureaucracies and the colonial officials who managed them. However, its main focus is on Puerto Ricans who participated in creating or navigating these institutions and their political work. Part of this research included examining the records of the massive bureaucratic archive in the Archivo General de Puerto Rico that resulted from the creation of social welfare programs in the mid-twentieth century.[20] These social welfare archives, largely untouched by researchers, document the formation of social welfare programs as well as the work of those who built and managed these programs. These social welfare records also reveal that from the beginning social welfare bureaucracies were concerned with Puerto Rican migration. Additionally, the Puerto Rican state circulated information about migrant clients between its offices on the archipelago and the offices that it created in the continental United States. Therefore, this book also draws on social welfare records located in the collections of the Archives of the Puerto Rican Diaspora at Hunter College in New York City.[21]

My use of these social welfare records allows me to explore histories of displacement, migration, and mobility over the course of the twentieth century, a period when nearly a third of the population of Puerto Rico migrated to the continental United States.[22] The impact of these migrations touched every aspect of Puerto Rican society, both on the archipelago as well as in the growing diasporic community in the United States. Building on historical research focused on migration and transnational communities, this book covers both Puerto Ricans on the archipelago and in the United States.[23] It moves between archipelagic and stateside communities, crossing boundaries that can be seen simultaneously as national and colonial. For the purposes of this study, the emphasis is on an integrated history of Puerto Ricans in both locations.

Over the course of the twentieth century, Puerto Rico remained a colony of the United States. This colonial relationship has afforded its population limited self-government but no voice in the government of the United States.

US officials explained the takeover of Puerto Rico to constituents in the United States and to Puerto Ricans alike by describing the legacy of Spanish rule as chaotic and backward and the local population as racially inferior to that of the United States. Puerto Rico needed, the argument went, the tutelage of the US government before it would be able to exercise its own sovereignty.[24]

Within the US empire, the construction of Puerto Rican difference was also profoundly shaped by US beliefs about Puerto Ricans' gender and sexuality. As historian Eileen Findlay has shown, US colonists defined Puerto Ricans as hypersexualized, inherently immoral, and often feminized.[25] They believed that US colonialism would "civilize" and "modernize" Puerto Rico through a campaign of moral reform that would regulate the wayward sexuality of its people. Therefore, from the start, the paternalistic US colonial project emphasized state-sponsored regulations that centered on the regulation of sexuality, such as reforms that promoted marriage and policed prostitution. Historian Laura Briggs has also emphasized how the US empire in Puerto Rico specifically focused on eugenics through the promotion of birth control and sterilization programs.[26] The various types of reform that colonial officials enacted would significantly impact the lives of working-class women, who were the main targets of many of these colonial policies.

Some Puerto Ricans hoped that the territory might eventually become a full part of the United States, while others struggled for independence that would not arrive. In 1900, the United States formalized its colonial relationship with Puerto Rico via the Foraker Act, which determined that the archipelago's residents were "Puerto Rican citizens" and not US citizens. It also outlined that the US government had the right to apply US laws and policies at its own discretion without affording Puerto Ricans voting representation in the US Congress.[27] Shortly afterward, the US Supreme Court case *Downes v. Bidwell* excluded Puerto Ricans from US citizenship, making Puerto Rico a "non-incorporated territory," which meant it would remain a possession without being annexed. This distinction marked the archipelago as "foreign in a domestic sense," a territory of the United States, under the legislative oversight of Congress.[28]

Change came in 1917 when Congress made Puerto Ricans "United States citizens" with the signing of the Jones-Shafroth Act. However, Puerto Rico's status as a non-incorporated territory still restricted this version of US citizenship. Puerto Ricans remained without voting representation in the US Congress or entitlement to the rights mandated to US citizens living in the United States. Despite these restrictions on Puerto Rican citizenship, some heralded its imposition as a decisive step toward permanent incorporation and full citizenship rights. However, the territorial differences inherent to Puerto Ricans' US citizenship were further inscribed in 1922 with the US Supreme Court case *Balzac v. People of Porto Rico*. In its ruling, the Court officially determined that the US Constitution did not cover Puerto Rico and that, in turn, the Bill of Rights did not apply to the people of Puerto Rico.[29] Puerto Ricans were citizens in name but this citizenship lacked political substance. This ruling was a blow to Puerto Ricans who hoped that the archipelago was going to eventually be incorporated into the United States as well as to those who sought independence.

While the US citizenship that Puerto Ricans held after 1917 remained second class, the creation of social welfare programs during and after World War I would provoke discussion about extending social benefits to Puerto Rico. In fact, this book shows that from the very first moments when social reformers and activists in the United States worked to create social welfare legislation and programs that would develop new rights and benefits for US citizens, Puerto Ricans were actively lobbying for Puerto Rico and other territories to be included under these provisions. While the inclusion of Puerto Rico under the titles of federally mandated child and maternal health programs mainly only had symbolic effect (because only a small population were the beneficiaries of these programs), the inclusion began to set a new precedent that the archipelago could be covered under social policy. This suggested to Puerto Rican reformers and US colonial administrators on the archipelago that, while formal citizenship rights remained elusive, they could successfully advocate for benefits for Puerto Ricans.

This political organizing would only gain steam when the Great Depression of 1929 hit Puerto Rico with ferocity. While the archipelago's political status remained unchanged, the decade was nonetheless marked by increasing political mobilization. When social reforms in the United States were passed to alleviate the ongoing impact of the Depression, Puerto Ricans also called for parallel relief to help workers and their families. Eventually, Puerto Rico was partially included under federal social programs created during the New Deal. Most notably, this included the development in 1933 of the Puerto Rico Emergency Relief Administration (PRERA) and in 1935 of the Puerto Rico Reconstruction Administration (PRRA).[30] Within a year of the creation of PRERA, over 33 percent of the Puerto Rican population was relying on some form of assistance from the organization. This marked a massive change in the relationship between the colonial state and the Puerto Rican population; suddenly relief administrators and social workers were in the position of forging new forms of governance. The expansion of social programs, paired with a developmentalist discourse, resulted in growing support for continued economic and social reform.

During the 1930s, Puerto Ricans also fought for coverage under the newly created titles of the US Social Security Act of 1935, which initially did not include provisions for Puerto Rico. The passage of the Social Security Act created sweeping new forms of social provisions in the United States, including old age assistance, unemployment insurance, and social welfare programs for the poor, women, and children. In the US context, its passage transformed the nature of US citizenship by allocating benefits according to new gendered and raced divisions. In particular, it defined only certain groups as "workers" and some as "dependents"—while leaving others unprotected. As historian Linda Gordon has shown, the outcome of these policies was that certain programs of social provision (particularly those for single mothers) were defined as "welfare," a term that became stigmatized and set them apart from other benefits for retired or elderly workers.[31] This book shows how in Puerto Rico the fight for coverage under Social Security reflected the colonial history of this policy and decades of struggle by Puerto Ricans to seek equal coverage under its provisions.[32] Over these decades, Puerto Ricans were able to secure partial and provisional coverage under these policies, though their administration in the territories remained at the discretion of the US Congress. And while this coverage was limited, it nevertheless did reshape Puerto Ricans' colonial citizenship by providing access to some federal social welfare benefits and by binding together social welfare agencies in Puerto Rico and the United States.

The impacts of the New Deal in Puerto Rico would also result in new debates over Puerto Rico's political status and the rise of a new political party, the Partido Popular Democrático (Popular Democratic Party; PPD). PPD leaders worked with liberal US reformers and New Deal policymakers and promised a populist transformation in Puerto Rico through economic and social reform.[33] Its leader, Luis Muñoz Marín, had lived in both Puerto Rico and the United States and had previously supported the archipelago's independence. After 1938 the party he led would denounce the need for political independence and promote a continued but reformed union between the United States and Puerto Rico. When Muñoz Marín became leader of the Puerto Rican Senate in 1940, this paved the way for a consolidation of the PPD agenda. The PPD's populist and reformist political platform was closely tied to discussions of social justice that included the promise of social services. During the 1940s this led to the creation of new social welfare organizations, including the first island-wide Department of Public Welfare in 1943.[34] While often severely limited by a lack of funds, these new social programs and policies led to growing expectations among the Puerto Rican population that the state should be attentive to its citizens. In 1948, when the US Congress allowed Puerto Ricans to elect their own governor, the population chose Muñoz Marín, and a formal reworking of Puerto Rico's status began.

The economic and political changes under PPD leadership culminated in the 1952 creation of the Estado Libre Asociado de Puerto Rico (ELA), or the Free Associated State of Puerto Rico. Effectively, the development of the ELA defined Puerto Rico as a "commonwealth," whose change in status was meant to appease concerns about the continuation of the archipelago's colonial status during a period when the decolonization of European colonial possessions was demanded globally. Some heralded this change as a "peaceful revolution" that illustrated the superiority of Puerto Rican and US handling of decolonization.[35] Opponents, however, argued that as an *estado libre asociado* the archipelago legally remained a colony of the United States because of the continuation of US congressional oversight, lack of coverage under the US Constitution or Bill of Rights, and, therefore, the limited and contingent variant of territorial citizenship held by Puerto Ricans.[36] Puerto Ricans across the political spectrum (among them supporters of statehood, continued affiliation, or independence) remained frustrated by the lack of full representation and citizenship provided to the ELA. However, this book reveals how this moment of stagnation in the political status of Puerto Rico was also a moment of change, as debates about decolonization led to demands for more extensive coverage under federal social policy. Subsequently, amendments to the US Social Security Act were passed that provided more coverage to Puerto Rico and federal assistance to growing numbers of its people. Concurrently, as debates over social policy continued, they became intertwined with concerns about Puerto Rican migration and the growing diasporic community in the United States. These changes further provided populist social welfare programs in Puerto Rico with increased, albeit still second-class, federal funding. Thus, while the terms of colonial governance were renegotiated, the underlying system was maintained.

During the same period, a growing diaspora of Puerto Rican migrants in the United States formed due to colonialism on the archipelago, US labor recruitment, and state-sponsored labor migration.[37] One of the particularities of US colonial and territorial citizenship was that, while it had not afforded Puerto Ricans on the archipelago equal citizenship to those in the United States, it did allow Puerto Ricans to migrate to the United States without being subject to immigration restrictions. Moreover, when Puerto Ricans migrated to the United States, they formally had access to full citizenship rights while living in the United States. However, when Puerto Ricans arrived in the United States, they discovered that these rights were often curtailed locally by systems of racist and xenophobic discrimination.[38] Despite this, Puerto Rican migrants did gain access to a broader range of citizenship rights, which created an inequality in the value of Puerto Rican citizenship based on location. When living in the United States, Puerto Ricans legally had voting representation in the US Congress and access to the rights and services allocated to all US citizens. Over time, the Puerto Rican migrant population, mobilizing the fuller citizenship rights available to them in the United States, would begin attempting to exert influence on US politics in ways unavailable to them on the archipelago.[39]

After the 1940s, migration from Puerto Rico to the United States would also transform dialogues about Puerto Ricans, social welfare, and citizenship rights. During this period, the Puerto Rican government directed a program of state-sponsored labor migration to the United States, catalyzing mass migration and the formation of Puerto Rican communities in the United States.[40] The combined results of these programs and subsequent migrations over the next fifty years resulted in nearly half of Puerto Rico's population relocating to the United States. Through these changes, Puerto Rico became a community with a population that increasingly circulated between the archipelago and the United States. The Puerto Rican government also expanded its work in the United States by creating a Migration Division of the Puerto Rican Department of Labor to sponsor and direct Puerto Rican labor migration.[41] Over time, representatives of this agency also came to work on behalf of Puerto Rican migrants who faced racist exclusions from exercising their US citizenship. This book shows how the Migration Division also addressed the social service needs of migrants and how over time it wove together social welfare programs in Puerto Rico with those in the United States.

Puerto Ricans in the United States also developed their own struggles to extend social welfare provisions to provide coverage and care for their communities. Activists and grassroots organizations increasingly contested the racial and ethnic discrimination Puerto Ricans faced as well as their limited citizenship. I show how Puerto Ricans who joined the US civil rights movement at this time found new ways to demand equal rights, including coverage under social welfare policies. Their political organizing included mobilization for access to social services, health care, and education. Some activists were critical of the role of the Puerto Rican government in sponsoring migration, and they worked to create Puerto Rican-led social service organizations in the United States that were not government affiliated. This book shows how, as the Puerto Rican community continued to migrate back and forth between the archipelago and the United States, these movements bound together in organizing for Puerto Rican rights. It concludes by considering the enduring legacy of struggles over social welfare in both Puerto Rico and its diaspora.

Throughout each of these moments in the history of social welfare, this book traces how, even though the US citizenship of Puerto Ricans was severely restricted, Puerto Ricans nevertheless mobilized around this citizenship to demand better coverage under US social policy. While at first US social welfare programs only provided services to small groups of Puerto Ricans, this would change with the partial extension of New Deal programs and the Social Security Act to Puerto Rico. These changes would result in increasingly larger groups of Puerto Ricans being eligible for social welfare provisions from both the Puerto Rican and US governments over the twentieth century. At the same time, the growing population of Puerto Rican migrants in the United States would campaign for equality under social welfare policy. In this book I consider how these two interconnected struggles reveal a long history of Puerto Rican political organizing around the terms and meaning of Puerto Rican citizenship since US colonization.

The Politics of Care Work in Puerto Rican Communities

The stories of social worker activists like Yolanda Sánchez reveal how Puerto Rican women took on the expansion of social welfare benefits as a key political struggle. By focusing on the lives and work of both social workers and working-class women (some of whom were on welfare), I also show how for many women caring labor and political work were entangled. Furthermore, I argue that centering social welfare in labor history can offer a productive vantage point from which to investigate the history of women's work and the production of gendered divisions of labor in both professional and working-class groups. This history reveals how the creation of social policy and the development of social welfare programs have been influenced in powerful ways by the organizing and activism of generations of women whose own gendered labor has been largely missing from the historical record.

The political history of care and social welfare policies in this book builds on labor history scholarship about Puerto Rico, the United States, and Latin

America that has examined the history of women and gender. In particular, it draws on the rich tradition of labor histories written by scholars of Puerto Rico and the Puerto Rican diaspora who have investigated the history of US colonialism, labor, and migration with a focus on gender and race.[42] This work also has suggested the importance of reproductive and caring labor in these communities, which I investigate further in this book. In doing so, my research is also in dialogue with scholarship on care labor, domestic work, and the history of social welfare in both the United States and Latin America.[43] This study is also in conversation with the vibrant and growing field of feminist scholarship on care work, caregiving, and the politics of social reproduction.[44] The growing literature on the history of care work in both regions has focused on the intersection of race and gender as well as on the significance of migration, immigration, and the formation of transnational communities. This book contributes a history of Puerto Rican caring labor in the twentieth century—as it took various forms across the archipelago and diaspora—to this dialogue.

This book examines the history of Puerto Rican women's care work and social reproduction by building, in particular, on scholarship that has documented how care work has been shaped by systems of exploitation under capitalism and colonialism. As Evelyn Nakano Glenn has shown, the "social organization of care" in US society and under US empire has relied on coercion that has often "forced" women into positions as care workers, especially those that are immigrants, migrants, or racial minorities.[45] Glenn emphasizes how the power relationships produced under capitalism and colonialism create labor systems that result in "racialized gendered servitude." Historical scholarship on care workers who were paid domestic workers and household workers has demonstrated how there has been a long and painful legacy of these workers being excluded from labor protections and exploited. As Eileen Boris and Jennifer Klein have shown, transformations in US social policy have also served to push poor and immigrant women into positions as care workers who are sometimes paid by the state.[46] Like Boris and Klein, I aim to "rethink the history of the American welfare state from the perspective of care work" through telling a story that also centers on the history of these policies in Puerto Rico.[47]

This book also builds on Premilla Nadasen's insight that discourses about "care work" in recent years have often obscured the power hierarchies and forms of exploitation that take shape in the organization of reproductive labor.[48] For Nadasen, using the term *social reproduction* can more fully capture these power relationships by building on Marxist feminist and Black/

feminist of color scholarship, both of which have long traditions of critically examining social reproduction within the history of capitalism. In this book, I use the terms *care work, reproductive labor,* and *social reproduction,* and my study aims to think critically about these forms of labor and the politics of defining their meaning and value in different moments in Puerto Rican history. I locate my investigation of care work and reproductive labor within broader histories of what Eileen Boris calls the "racialized and gendered state," and particularly consider the creation of social welfare policies as locations of struggle over these forms of labor.[49] In this project, my analysis of care work considers a variety of forms of reproductive labor and also explores forms of collective care that emerged within Puerto Rican communities and social movements.

In addition, this book centers specifically on Puerto Rican women's political activism focused around care work and social reproduction. I build on feminist scholarship and social reproduction theory that have argued that political struggles over social reproduction have long raged under capitalism and colonialism and that overlooking these histories of political mobilization has often served to erase women's activism from history. As Cinzia Arruzza, Tithi Bhattacharya, and Nancy Fraser have argued, "class struggle includes struggles over social reproduction," which cover a wide range of battles, including those for health care, education, and women's liberation.[50] I also on build on Jessica Wilkerson's argument that an examination of "caring labor is fundamental to understanding the limitations and successes of social and political movements that sought to expand democracy and citizenship rights."[51] In her work on US women's political activism, she underscores how their politicization of "caregiving labor" offered powerful "critiques of capitalist logics."[52] This book also emphasizes that examining Puerto Rican women's activism around care work and social reproduction can shed new light on class struggles and fights for social justice.

This book shows how in Puerto Rican history the development of welfare programs is integral to a broader labor history and histories of care, as some women emerged as state agents and architects of the state and others became targets of both government labor recruitment and management schemes and clients of social welfare programs.[53] This labor history is twofold. On the one hand, it shows how the creation of social welfare programs required a massive amount of work. Over the course of the twentieth century, a group of women became professionalized as social workers and, in turn, played a large role in building welfare programs in Puerto Rico. These professional care workers crafted social welfare programs in ways that reflected their political agendas and that conditioned the political aspirations of Puerto Rican communities throughout the twentieth century. On the other hand, this is also a labor history of women on welfare. It argues that clients of welfare programs were mainly working-class women, many of whom were care workers, who provided essential productive and reproductive labor in their communities.[54] When these women became clients of social welfare programs, they entered new roles and were cast in new relationships to state institutions. The book traces the emergence of these two groups of care workers and the interactions between them and the larger communities in which they lived.

The book also traces how the profession of social work changed over time and became more community oriented. As growing numbers of working-class women entered its ranks, they brought their own ideas and concerns into the profession. They advocated for the creation of social welfare programs that responded to the needs of welfare recipients and that were accountable to local communities. An early move toward more community-oriented work can be seen in the 1930s with the training of social workers (and social work aides) within New Deal programs. However, the community input in these moments was limited as the expansion of state-run social welfare programs emphasized a top-down structure within social welfare projects, which came to rely heavily on means-testing that often alienated local communities. The more revolutionary moment of transformation in the social work field came in the 1960s when the mass migration of Puerto Ricans to the United States opened a new space for social workers to become advocates for Puerto Rican communities. This advocacy would begin in the 1940s and would deepen as social workers increasingly connected their work to their involvement in civil rights and feminist organizing and struggles for civil rights, women's rights, and independence. Puerto Rican social workers became deeply involved with the expansion of the rise of a community-organizing approach in social work, which resulted in an even deeper commitment to working in collaboration with the communities they served. By the 1970s, the social work profession had become an important space of political organization for Puerto Rican women.

As I mentioned previously, I piece together the history of Puerto Ricans and social welfare programs by drawing on archives from social welfare agencies in Puerto Rico and the United States. These sources shed light on the history of Puerto Rican women, who were everywhere, busy shaping politics and history. From social workers navigating the highest levels of politics (lobbying Congress for the extension of federal social provisions) to working-class clients demanding access to social provisions, women emerged as political actors in varied and complex ways. I also use the case file archives of Puerto Rican social welfare agencies to track the new interactions between Puerto Ricans and the state that resulted from the creation of social welfare programs. One of these archives is the massive bureaucratic archive of the Department of Social Welfare in Puerto Rico, whose records provide fleeting glimpses into a history of massive social transformation. Its files contain stories about the Puerto Rican government's interventions in the lives of working-class Puerto Ricans. The files also reveal how the creation of social welfare programs impacted Puerto Ricans and how they laid claim to new social provisions. I use my exploration of these files as a way to trace major social changes while also focusing on specific political histories of women's lives and work.

An examination of the lives and work of Puerto Rican social workers, this book offers a unique window into the history of Puerto Rican organizing. At the start of the twentieth century, women's professionalization in care work occupations such as social work and nursing opened up new opportunities to build and shape both state and private institutions.[55] Scholars have demonstrated that the work of professional care workers was particularly important to the development of imperial projects globally and to the expansion of US empire specifically. For example, historian Catherine Ceniza Choy has highlighted how training women to be nurses in the Philippines advanced US imperial goals while laying the foundation for labor recruitment to the metropole and thus paving the way for future migrations.[56] I show how, in Puerto Rico, women were also called on to be agents of transformation under US imperial projects and were sometimes later recruited to the United States to further these projects. I also highlight how, in the Puerto Rican diaspora and the United States, professional women played an important role in organizing institutions that served migrant communities.[57] Social work and political activism were far from separate.

The histories of social workers in this book also specifically focus on their political work, centering them in political history, which has often overlooked women in favor of the activism of male leaders and political parties. This book shows how social workers were leaders in a wide range of political organizations and moments of political mobilization. They were active in the Puerto Rican movements for independence, commonwealth, and statehood as well as within labor and feminist groups. I also suggest that social workers' stories reveal some significant particularities about Puerto Rican women's political organizing. First, I show how social workers balanced their work seeking larger political outcomes (including participation in political organizations and parties) with their day-to-day efforts to care for other people, a type of praxis that was often grounded in their work in local communities. Second, these histories show how social workers oftentimes worked together across divides in political beliefs and ideologies toward common goals. Through collaborating in their jobs and professional organizations, they sometimes built surprising allegiances that allowed them to advance their broader agenda. By excavating the forms of political organization developed by these women and considering the implications of the political collaborations they forged, I hope to shed new light on Puerto Rican politics.

By focusing on biographies of social worker activists whose work was also linked to social movements and community organizing, I emphasize women whose work would likely have been defined as radical in their time. My use of biography and prosopography to explore the history of social movements draws on feminist scholarship on Latina and African American women that has examined individual life histories to make sense of major social changes.[58] While the histories they reveal are not comprehensive, they shed light on social work as a complex terrain of politics in which women shaped history. For Puerto Rican women, this included participating in early efforts to create labor standards and protections for women and child workers, advocating for the independence and the decolonization of Puerto Rico and participating in the US civil rights movement. These efforts share similarities with those developed by other colonized women and women of color in the United States, who have sometimes used professional care work as an avenue through which to contest violence and oppression in their communities. My research is particularly in dialogue with histories of social work that have highlighted the intersection of social worker activism with movements for social justice and labor, as well as civil and economic rights.[59]

This book also grapples with the painful repercussions of practices developed by social workers in Puerto Rican communities. It is important to note that not all social workers were heroes and that their actions sometimes resulted in long-lasting difficulties for poor people, especially when the discourse and rhetoric they deployed emphasized that people were in poverty because of individual failures rather than broader social and economic structures or when they suggested that people needed to change to be deserving of benefits. They also administered casework and means-testing practices that were invasive and sometimes discriminatory against clients. In particular, the book explores the treatment of working-class women as they applied for social welfare programs as well as how regulatory, invasive, and punitive practices of means-testing were created as a part of social welfare programs. The production of social welfare projects was plagued by the damaging consequences of the deployment of Americanization and modernization discourse, the separation of families under the guise of child saving, and the role of social workers in eugenics and sterilization projects that led to reproductive injustice in working-class communities. More generally, adverse outcomes often resulted from trying to adjust individuals to the conditions they faced rather than pushing for broader societal and economic transformations that could result in better living conditions for all people.[60] Telling these difficult stories works to restore Puerto Rican women to history as political figures with complex and sometimes troubling legacies.

This book also tells the stories of Puerto Rican women and girls who became clients of social welfare programs. I include the experiences of mothers, daughters, children, and elders who made a life and a living in Puerto Rico and its diaspora during a period of great social transformation. Many of these individuals were also care workers—in their own homes and in the homes of others, of whom some were paid and others unpaid. These caring occupations were segregated by both gender and race, and many of these workers were given little or no choice in becoming care workers.[61] Scholars of women and gender in the United States and Latin America have emphasized the importance of care work, domestic work, and household labor to the history of women's labor in both regions. For example, historians of care work and domestic labor have demonstrated how working-class women of color's experience of being "forced to care" has shaped their experience of citizenship and belonging in the United States and within the US empire. This book is in dialogue with scholars who have examined how working-class women of color's participation in caring labor has shaped their lives and how they have struggled for social change.[62]

By focusing on the history of Puerto Rican women's labor as care workers, this book emphasizes the importance of race in Puerto Rican labor history as well as the persistence of discrimination against women of African descent.[63] Scholars of the history of care labor and domestic work have shown that racial hierarchies and discrimination have often been enacted through labor systems that have relegated African American, Indigenous, and Latina women into low-wage and precarious caring occupations. In this book, I consider how, in Puerto Rico, women and girls of African descent often made up much of the domestic work labor force and how occupational segregation in the mid-twentieth century remained connected to the legacy of slavery on the archipelago. I also show how, after the US colonization of Puerto Rico, Puerto Rican women were recruited to work as domestic workers in the United States specifically because they were seen as racially inferior to US colonists and as well-suited for caring labor. Moreover, I show how Puerto Rican government agencies trained and placed Puerto Rican women as domestic workers in the United States as a part of state-sponsored labor migration schemes. When these workers arrived in the United States and became migrant workers, they were further racialized as nonwhite and faced rampant discrimination.[64] These examples show how caring labor was racialized and how working-class women, particularly those of African descent, experienced being funneled into care work positions in both Puerto Rico and the United States.

My investigation of the case files of social work programs also considers how working-class women and girls who performed domestic, service, and care work became a key demographic applying for social welfare benefits. Using the case files of social welfare agencies, I explore social workers' interventions in the lives and work of the working-class Puerto Ricans who became their clients, observing how state programs regulated Puerto Rican lives in particularly gendered and raced ways that often made them targets of regulation. Poor women and women of African descent became the primary targets of reform policies.[65] This book shows how social workers investigated women and children's caring labor in early studies of maternal health, managed work-relief programs for women during the New Deal, and developed casework processes that recorded women's labor in the first island-wide social welfare programs. Social workers were also instrumental in regulating the migration of Puerto Rican women to become domestic workers in the United States, and as agents of Puerto Rican government and US social welfare agencies in the United States, they came to work with migrant care workers in the United States.

Social work interviews were sites of struggle both among social workers and between social workers and clients over how benefits would be administered. Through a close reading of case files, I examine how clients negotiated the contents of their benefits with social workers in the intimate and often invasive process of social casework. Every individual applying for benefits underwent interviews with social workers in which the new roles of social worker and client were constructed and performed. Examining case files from social welfare offices, I show that social workers manifested the abstract political ideologies of the state into concrete social policy, in turn locating their clients within categories of gender, class, and race. Placement into these categories had tangible material consequences for those seeking food, shelter, and care. Combined, these stories interrogate how clients were produced within the textual practices of casework and provide a glimpse of how the formation of social welfare programs and the meaning of women's labor were negotiated in interactions between state officials and citizens.

The records of social welfare agencies also offer a window into how social work practices developed and changed over the twentieth century as some forms of social work became more community oriented. While this book shows that this change over time was not always a linear or progressive narrative, and there were many moments of tension and solidarity between social workers and working-class clients, it demonstrates that community-oriented work has grown and developed as a part of the profession. This book reveals how, when social work practices were first developed in Puerto Rico in the 1920s, maternalist social reformers were mainly focused on reforming local populations and regulating forms of child labor within local communities. These maternalists cast themselves as more enlightened than the women they worked with. However, as increasing numbers of working-class women became a part of the profession, including those who had received social welfare benefits, growing numbers saw themselves as joining a struggle with their "clients" for social and economic rights for all people. The history of the development of more community-oriented social work as a part of the story of the profession is traced throughout this book, even though it was not always the path taken.

The history of Puerto Rican social workers of African descent is also a crucial part of the story about care work and social work told in this book. The stories told here often focus on the outsized role of Puerto Ricans of African descent in transforming the social work profession, making it more centered on community-engaged methods. In writing about these stories, I build on scholarship on the history of Afro-Puerto Rican participation in the history of social movements and in the civil rights movement in the United States in particular.[66] In the earlier chapters of the book, Puerto Rican women of African descent who had access to social work education like Beatriz Lassalle del Valle and Felicia Boria may have identified as white or as racially different than the working-class women of African descent who were their clients. However, the forms of social work they engaged in also reveal deep connections to social justice activism, socialist feminism, labor organizing, and broader agitation for social rights that may have been in part shaped by their own experiences of racialized social marginalization either in Puerto Rico or in relationship to Americans in the United States.

In the final chapter, the book centers fully on the work of social workers of African descent like Antonia Pantoja, Yolanda Sánchez, and Esperanza Martell, whose identifications as Afro-Puerto Rican and Black Puerto Rican were essential to their political work. These women were part of a broader group of Afro-Puerto Rican civil rights activists who used careers in social work to advance broader struggles against racism and for social justice.

The social welfare archives I examine in this book also provide a unique resource for considering how Puerto Ricans navigated displacement and migration over the twentieth century. Among other things, the archives reveal how migration was influenced by day-to-day interactions between Puerto Ricans and the state as well as by state-sponsored labor migration schemes. I trace the movements of state agents, migrant workers, and clients of social welfare programs between Puerto Rico and the United States by using social welfare records from both locations. These movements reveal how the Puerto Rican government increasingly served as an intermediary between thousands of migrant Puerto Ricans and US government agencies, both federal and local. I also examined bundles of documents that were mailed between these offices and that contained case file information about Puerto Rican clients. These archives reveal how a colonial state organized and circulated information about its citizens over decades. They also shed light on how individuals navigated these dramatic social changes and how some went on to build lives and communities in the United States.

THIS BOOK IS ORGANIZED chronologically and thematically, focusing on the care work and political activism of Puerto Rican social workers and working-class women care workers between 1917 and the 1970s. Each chapter considers Puerto Rican histories on the archipelago and the United States, following protagonists on the move and emphasizing the impact of displacement and migration on Puerto Rican communities. Part 1 of the book, "Making Care Count in Puerto Rico," focuses on the US colonization of Puerto Rico and the history of the construction of social welfare programs on the archipelago. Part 2, "Care Work and Women's Activism in the Puerto Rican Diaspora," centers on Puerto Rican migration to the United States and highlights the ways that Puerto Rican social welfare agencies, policies, and programs were instrumental in shaping labor migration and the integration of migrants into US communities after 1940. The book concludes by emphasizing the development of Puerto Rican forms of community-oriented social work practice in the United States, practices that were connected to earlier struggles over social and economic rights but that also sought new ways to make social welfare provisions better serve their communities.

The book begins by examining the creation of social welfare programs in Puerto Rico under US colonial rule, paying particular attention to Puerto Rican women social workers and the working-class women and children who became targets of their reforms. The first chapter, "Women Building Social Welfare Programs in Puerto Rico after 1917," argues that social workers used their professional occupations as care workers to organize politically for the extension of social policy to Puerto Rico despite the continued restrictions on citizenship imposed by US colonialism. It shows how they worked alongside US reformers of the US Children's Bureau to conduct a study of maternal and child welfare in Puerto Rico that was used as evidence to support their advocacy for the extension of US social welfare provisions like those created by the Sheppard-Towner Maternity and Infancy Protection Act. Questions about Puerto Rican citizenship and belonging were paramount in these debates. I show how the extension of partial and provisional funding under these policies resulted from political organizing, setting a precedent for a century of struggle over the form that social policies would take. While the number of people covered under these social welfare programs remained small, these nascent programs would rapidly expand in the following years.

In Puerto Rico, political organizing for social welfare would come to a head after the Great Depression with the extension of specific reforms administered under the New Deal. These reforms would transform the relationship between the US government and Puerto Rico by reworking and reinforcing the colonial status of the archipelago. In Chapter 2, "Labor, Welfare, and Gendered Citizenship in New Deal Puerto Rico," I show how Puerto Rican women (both social workers and working-class women) were instrumental in demanding and shaping social welfare policy and programs. By examining debates over the extension of the Social Security Act of 1935 to Puerto Rico, I highlight how Puerto Ricans waged a long struggle led by activists and workers to have the archipelago included under this legislation. This organizing led to the gradual and constrained incorporation of Puerto Rico under the act. In part, this coverage resulted from the organizing of women activists who advocated for labor standards and protections for women workers and demanded social provisions for women who provided caring and reproductive labor in their homes. However, this moment was also one in which working-class Puerto Rican women became prime targets of state interventions through labor reforms and eugenics policies that were propelled by the expansion of social welfare agencies. The New Deal, therefore, resulted in more intrusion by the state into the private lives of Puerto Rican citizens.

In the 1940s and 1950s, social welfare programs continued to expand, and these programs transformed the relationship between the state and society by bringing more social workers into the homes of Puerto Rican families and communities. As working-class people claimed benefits, they also articulated demands for state support and care that they increasingly perceived as their rights as Puerto Rican citizens. Chapter 3, "Working-Class Women, Claims for Benefits, and the Politics of Deservingness under the Puerto Rican Populist State," focuses on the experiences of working-class women care workers who became clients within these programs. These women applied for assistance from the newly minted Department of Public Welfare created by the populist programs of the PPD, which would further expand with the creation of the ELA in 1952. Through a focus on the case file records of working-class women care workers who sought assistance, this chapter shows how clients struggled over these benefits with social workers. The chapter examines how clients contested how information about their labor and income was recorded and sought to shape the outcome of their petitions. At the same time, social welfare programs became increasingly regulatory as they focused on means-testing and separating out clients who they deemed deserving of benefits from those they believed were not. The outcome of tense struggles between social workers and clients that took shape in this moment was that working-class women's reproductive labor was minimized and devalued. Moreover, clients of social welfare programs were increasingly cast in broader social and political discourses as nonproductive and undeserving citizens.

During the same period, Puerto Rican communities were deeply impacted by migration to the United States, some of which resulted from state-sponsored labor migration schemes. Both Puerto Rican social workers and working-class women care workers became essential participants in these efforts, and their work was instrumental in establishing new and expanding Puerto Rican communities in the United States. Chapter 4, "Care Workers, Household Labor Organizing, and Puerto Rican Migration after 1944," examines the history of a group of Puerto Rican domestic workers in a contract-labor program in Chicago who ended up at the center of a storm of labor activism, reform, and regulation. When these migrant domestic workers faced terrible conditions in the United States, they organized protests and soon found support from US women reformers who were already fighting for labor standards for household workers. Their activism also drew the attention of Puerto Rican social workers and students studying in Chicago. These professional women became intermediaries between the workers and the Puerto Rican state, and eventually the tensions over the labor issues in Chicago put pressure on the government to reform its migrant labor programs. These actions contributed to the formalization of this oversight of state-sponsored migration with the creation of a new regulatory agency, the Migration Division of the Puerto Rican Department of Labor. As a result, the Puerto Rican government also realized that the expertise Puerto Rican social workers had developed while studying and working in social welfare programs in the United States could provide a crucial bridge between the Puerto Rican government and local agencies in US cities.

As representatives of the Puerto Rican government operating in the United States, Puerto Rican social workers took up new roles working in the United States as advocates for migrant clients. In Chapter 5, "Women's Leadership in Struggles over Welfare, Citizenship Rights, and Decolonization in the Puerto Rican Diaspora," I highlight the role of two groups of women: first, Puerto Rican women who became migrant advocates and the architects of state agencies that regulated migration and, second, working-class migrant women who became their clients. This chapter considers how these groups interacted within the Migration Division's offices throughout the United States. The Migration Division also created a Social Service Section, managed by social workers whose case files I use to trace the development of new casework practices for migrant clients. In these offices, social workers served as intermediaries between migrant clients and US social welfare agencies and bound together the work of Puerto Rican and US social welfare programs. As migration experts, these social workers also worked on behalf of Puerto Rican citizens and successfully advocated for broader coverage of Puerto Rico under US social policy. At the same time, the Puerto Rican migrants who became their clients demanded that the agency take up a more robust role in advocating for their civil and economic rights. As a result, some social workers connected to the Migration Division also began challenging the Puerto Rican government's agenda and imagining new ways of doing Puerto Rican–led social justice work in the United States.

The 1960s ushered in a new period in Puerto Rican social work history in the United States focused on community organizing. During this time, many more poor and working-class women (including some who had received welfare benefits themselves) trained to become social workers and entered the profession. Some of these social workers would turn away from traditional social work practices and instead build service programs and institutions that were more focused on accountability within local communities. The final chapter, "Community Organizers, Civil Rights Activism, and Demands for Care in Puerto Rican Communities in the United States," examines how some of these social workers developed Puerto Rican forms of community-oriented work in New York City. It particularly looks at the life history of Antonia Pantoja, an Afro-Puerto Rican social worker and civil rights activist who migrated from Puerto Rico to the United States and worked tirelessly to create Puerto Rican–serving social and educational programs. Pantoja was a member of a cohort of like-minded activists, including the already-mentioned Yolanda Sánchez. The work of these activists was also deeply connected to contemporary grassroots social movements, and the chapter tracks how social workers used their professional work as a platform to advocate for social justice. Their work as educators would also have lasting impacts; they trained a new generation of community organizers who would soon emerge as leaders in the Puerto Rican community. This chapter concludes by considering the broader intellectual and political legacy of this generation of social workers as they helped found departments of Puerto Rican and ethnic studies in US educational institutions.

The form of activism that emerged around access to social welfare provisions and benefits in Puerto Rican communities on the archipelago and the United States continued in the following decades. An epilogue, "Envisioning Caring Futures," provides a final analysis of how considering the long history of Puerto Rican struggles for access to social welfare and care—with Puerto Rican women at the center—can shed light on how Puerto Ricans have defined citizenship and contested colonialism in the twentieth century. It shows the enduring relevance of the history of social welfare more broadly by documenting connections to contemporary struggles over the extension of social policy, particularly the Social Security Act. This book makes the case that curtailments to Puerto Rican citizenship inscribed into early forms of social policy on the archipelago still provide a foundation for contemporary inequalities with deeply troubling legacies. The US Congress continues to decide on a case-by-case basis what parts of social legislation will be applied to Puerto Rico without Puerto Rican input. Furthermore, colonial restrictions on social welfare benefits continue to be fiercely contested and debated by Puerto Ricans on the archipelago and in the diaspora. However, despite this struggle, colonialism remains in Puerto Rico, and the citizenship rights of Puerto Ricans continue to be provisional, tenuous, and fragile.

It is my hope that this book contributes to ongoing dialogues about Puerto Rican history, citizenship, and community formation by offering a story of the politics of care work that is rooted in the lives and experiences of Puerto Rican women. The life histories and biographies of women at the heart of this book are meant to breathe life into political history—from which they have often been missing. These stories aim to shed light on the complex forms of political mobilization that emerged from Puerto Rican women's day-to-day experiences and led to lasting changes in their communities. The political action of these women was remarkable; it crossed national boundaries, challenged colonial governance, and imagined new futures for their communities. Moreover, contemporary struggles over Puerto Rican citizenship continue to be both led and supported by Puerto Rican women care workers despite the enduring colonial exclusions and marginalization that such women face. In the future, I hope that the stories of women like these will be considered key parts of the history of Puerto Rican struggles for social justice and also help to historicize ongoing political organization for care.

Part I

MAKING CARE COUNT
IN PUERTO RICO

Women Building Social Welfare Programs in Puerto Rico after 1917

In 1921, Beatriz Lassalle del Valle, a Puerto Rican social worker, joined Helen Bary, a social worker from the United States, in producing a study of maternal and child welfare in Puerto Rico. The study was conducted as a part of a collaboration between Puerto Rican government officials and the Children's Bureau of the US Department of Labor, which had recently begun expanding its work to the colonized archipelago.[1] The study focused on "abandoned mothers" and "homeless children" living in urban regions. It centered on working-class women and children, the majority of whom were care workers, performing domestic labor and care work in their employers' homes. This included working-class women weaving in and out of waged work for US industries, washing laundry for pay, and caring for their own children. It also included child servants who worked and lived in families' homes in exchange for room and board. The report shed light on the often-underreported importance of reproductive labor in Puerto Rican society, labor often done by women and children. It showed not only that private homes were often workplaces but also underscored the deeply entrenched social hierarchies of gender and race in Puerto Rican society that had created conditions in which working-class women and children were often forced into unremunerated care work.

In the Children's Bureau report, Lassalle and Bary argued that if the Puerto Rican and US governments invested in creating new social welfare programs, it might put an end to the systems of racialized and gendered servitude commonplace on the archipelago. The study noted that many child workers were of African descent and that racialized occupational segregation had persisted on the archipelago in the wake of slavery.[2] Its authors also emphasized the inability of working-class women to take care of their children as they entered waged work in increased numbers as the Puerto Rican economy transformed under US capitalism and colonialism. As liberal reformers, Lassalle and Bary believed that social welfare programs for women and children could curtail colonial capitalism's destabilizing impact on working-class people's lives without upending the larger economic or political system.[3] They believed that the state should support some aspects of women's labor in the home and advocated for the idea of a protected childhood. They cast themselves, and other professional women, as the ideal candidates to oversee new state-managed social welfare programs, including public health clinics and social welfare clinics that would distribute monetary assistance to working-class families.

The Children's Bureau study represented one of many investigations of social conditions in Puerto Rico that resulted from exchanges between US social welfare and sociological institutions in the wake of US intervention in Puerto Rico. Scholars have documented how social scientific studies during the period became arenas where US reformers engaged in colonial knowledge production.[4] The Children's Bureau study also provides a window into the work of Puerto Rican reformers during the period, women like Lassalle, who was one of the first Puerto Rican professional social workers.[5] As women like Lassalle found opportunities to professionalize, they also brought their own concerns and political agendas to their work. In Lassalle's case, her work was deeply shaped by her own experiences and identity as an educator and an ardent women's rights advocate. Lassalle likely identified as white and was considered white in Puerto Rican society, but historical records also suggest she was of African descent. She was categorized racially in different ways in both Puerto Rico and the United States throughout her life.[6] For Lassalle, social work also became an avenue to organize politically, and she argued that "someone that receives the benefits of a good education and academic preparation has the obligation to help better the welfare of the community in which they live."[7]

Of course, the working-class women and children who became the targets of social workers' interventions had their own agendas and concerns. Within early records of social welfare officials and the fragments of reports on their casework that remain, the voices of these actors are often submerged beneath the narratives of reformers. Nevertheless, these women and children had ways of seeing and experiencing their lives and work as they negotiated often-tense encounters with state officials. After over twenty years of US colonial rule on the archipelago, those in both rural and urban communities also faced dire levels of poverty.[8] At the time, the consolidation of corporate agriculture had forced many rural workers into metropolitan areas, and other workers began migrating out of Puerto Rico in search of new opportunities. The economic results of US colonialism also further entrenched raced and gendered inequalities, leaving many poor women and children toiling in difficult occupations that were often low paying, if they paid at all.[9] As these workers encountered social workers who came armed with questionnaires and ideas about what was best for poor people and their families, we can imagine their new "clients" were rightfully trepidatious about what would come. This moment of encounter between reformers and working-class people, and the desire of social workers to speak on behalf of the poor, would have lasting implications in the lives of both groups traced throughout this book.

After 1917, the extension of US citizenship to Puerto Rico sparked debates about whether nascent US social welfare policies would also be extended to the archipelago.[10] In Puerto Rico, where colonialism limited the meaning of US citizenship, debates over the extension of social policy soon became important arenas for women reformers to participate in larger political debates. The work of Puerto Rican and US reformers on the Children's Bureau's studies, which were composed of multiple surveys, shows the central role of women's work and activism in shaping conversations about Puerto Rican citizenship. However, the political work of Puerto Rican women reformers has often been overlooked in the literature on the history of struggles over citizenship in Puerto Rico. This is partly because social policy has not always been considered an arena of politics and neither have struggles over colonial variants of social programs. This oversight has often erased Puerto Rican women's maternalist activism from narratives of the period and failed to capture the way that these reformers pressured the state to support specific aspects of social reproduction in society, particularly through social welfare funding for single mothers and their children.

The social scientific knowledge produced by Puerto Rican women reformers also played a significant role in political debates around Puerto Rican citizenship. For example, during hearings over the possible extension of the Sheppard-Towner Maternity and Infancy Protection Act to Puerto Rico in 1924, Puerto Rican and US politicians referred to a Children's Bureau report by Bary and Lassalle.[11] Santiago Iglesias, the leader of the Socialist Party and a member of the Senate of Puerto Rico, described the study as a "profound and deep study of the conditions of maternity and the children in Puerto Rico" that "gives everything that you need to know" about "the true condition of children in Puerto Rico."[12] Although male politicians presented the proposal to Congress, the political activism of women from Puerto Rico and the United States played a significant role in pushing for the bill's extension. This was just one moment in a long history of women's participation in political debates over how social policy would be developed in the colonial context of Puerto Rico.

The most lasting import of the Children's Bureau produced by Lassalle and US Children's Bureau reformers was their use as justification for creating new social welfare provisions in Puerto Rico. Over time, these social welfare studies also served as evidence of the need for creating social welfare agencies in Puerto Rico to be staffed by a growing number of professional women social workers. The knowledge they produced was later taken up in larger debates and discourses between officials from Puerto Rico and the United States over how Puerto Rico was to be included under new federal social provisions created for women and children. In the years that followed the publication of the Children's Bureau report, Puerto Ricans would become increasingly active in these debates, calling on the US government to extend new social welfare programs and protections to the archipelago. However, the continued colonial status of Puerto Rico would limit the outcome of these claims, as a growing number of US officials reached a consensus that Puerto Rico would not be fully incorporated into the United States.[13] In the end, Puerto Rico was partially included under US social policies, which opened the possibility that Puerto Rican advocacy for inclusion under social provisions might be fruitful in the following years.

This chapter maps the creation of social welfare programs in Puerto Rico by examining the history of the early development of social work and studies of child welfare. It begins by focusing on the political organizing and activism of Puerto Rican women reformers, particularly looking at the life and work of Beatriz Lassalle del Valle. Lassalle's story offers a window into the complex legacy of such women who were at once agents of empire and also brought their political desires and advocacy to the stage. In short, it shows how social work became an arena of political action for some Puerto Rican women. Next, it takes a closer look at the Children's Bureau report of the early 1920s and the studies—or "surveys"—that were described in the report, which included conducting a "homeless" child survey, to consider how Puerto Rican and US reformers undertook their work with working-class communities. In doing so, it suggests some of the ways that raced and gendered divisions in labor and care work done by working-class women and children became central concerns of reformers of the period. These stories reveal how the creation of social welfare programs provided some forms of assistance and relief to poor communities while simultaneously creating new forms of regulation and control. Finally, the chapter shows how the resulting interactions and reports became part of larger state discourses and debates over social welfare and the rights and benefits of Puerto Rican citizenship within the US empire.

Social Welfare and Political Organizing in Puerto Rico after 1917

The political organizing of women activists, such as Lassalle, played a significant role in shaping the colonial state of Puerto Rico under US rule. For professional women who had become agents of the colonial state, debates over US citizenship became an arena to advance their political agendas. These agendas were often framed by social feminism and maternalism and were centered on advocating for the rights of women and the "protection" of children.[14] In some cases the activism of this generation of women was also connected to earlier histories of charity and benevolent organizations in Puerto Rico, many of which had often centered on targeting working-class communities and people of African descent for reform.[15] The activism of women reformers after 1917 was also closely linked to their work and leadership in the suffrage movement. Scholars have shown how Puerto Rican suffrage organizing was plagued by division over class and race, which often hindered the movement.[16] During this period, elite women often advocated for their rights at the expense of working-class women. Therefore, as professional women entered new roles as political actors, they did so in ways that sometimes conflicted with working-class communities.

This chapter traces the activism of Puerto Rican women during a period of massive political transformation that followed the colonization of Puerto Rico by the United States. After the Spanish–American War in 1898, Puerto Rico was ceded to the United States, which led to the expansion of US corporations, particularly US-owned sugar trusts.[17] This domination of the local economy resulted in more workers becoming wage laborers and established an extractive economy where the profits were primarily directed at US stockholders. Moreover, the consolidation of land previously used for subsistence agriculture led to the displacement of rural people who began migrating to urban areas. These changes resulted in growing dissatisfaction with US management and the extraction of profits from the archipelago by working-class and elite Puerto Ricans. During this same period, Puerto Rican politicians, who were excluded from representation in the US Congress, attempted to influence US politicians to advocate on their behalf. In 1917, Puerto Ricans were granted US citizenship under the Jones-Shafroth Act, but this citizenship was limited by the US government's decision to maintain the archipelago as a territory and colony. This status of Puerto Rico disappointed both working-class and elite Puerto Ricans, and the following years were marked by political unrest and mobilization.

During this period of mass political mobilization and social transformation, elite liberal feminists emerged as prominent political leaders who utilized their roles as professional care workers on social reform projects to further their political agendas. Scholarship on the history of gender, sexuality, and race in Puerto Rico has shown that, after the US takeover of Puerto Rico, the new colonial government worked to advance social reform programs that aimed to Americanize, "modernize," and "civilize" Puerto Rico.[18] As historian Eileen Findlay has shown, the United States administered a form of "benevolent colonialism" in Puerto Rico that, while cloaked in humanitarian language, was still an extractive system that often reified social hierarchies based on gender and race.[19] This chapter reveals how women who became agents of the colonial state were also deeply involved in statecraft through their work on social welfare programs. These Puerto Rican women played an active role in what historian Donna Guy has called "building the welfare state."[20] Their ideas on maternalism, eugenics, and women's and children's rights shaped the social welfare institutions they created. In Puerto Rico, these institutions would also be deeply influenced by the ongoing colonial context in which they were developed.

The story of Beatriz Lassalle del Valle (figure 1.1) provides one demonstrative example of how elite Puerto Rican women became professional care workers while promoting liberal feminist politics and ideals. It also highlights how their new roles were influenced by their position within Puerto

Rican and US social hierarchies of gender, race, and class. Born in Ponce in 1882, her family moved to the capital city of San Juan soon after, where she later witnessed the United States invade and take over the island.[21] Francisco Lassalle Doval, her father, was a lawyer who worked for the Catholic Church and later became a judge. Historical documents from the period suggest that Francisco Lassalle Doval was of African descent, and he is sometimes described as "mulatto," including on the US Census of 1910, where both he and Beatriz Lassalle are listed as "mulatto."[22] While the family seems to have amassed enough class privilege and status to be generally understood as white in Puerto Rican society, this whiteness may have been more tenuous within the racial hierarchies they encountered under US rule.[23] Notwithstanding, Lassalle's high social and racial status within Puerto Rican society provided her with excellent educational opportunities, and she was able to join a new cadre of professional women who would become key figures in island politics.

Like many other elite Puerto Rican women of her time, Lassalle started her career as a teacher before becoming a professional care worker on US reform projects. Lassalle graduated from the Normal School in San Juan, which would later become the University of Puerto Rico. In 1898, she boarded a steamship for the United States, where she attended a summer program at Harvard University alongside numerous other Puerto Rican and Cuban students.[24] The educational program she participated in sought to prepare students to become agents of "Americanization" in their homelands; therefore, they were taught about US institutions and culture so that they could disseminate them back home.[25] When Lassalle returned to Puerto Rico, she began working for the public education system as a teacher. She soon became a leader and administrator, teaching pedagogy at the Normal School and becoming the first woman principal and school inspector for the new Department of Education.[26] As a school inspector, Lassalle traveled throughout the archipelago, evaluating the work of other teachers and developing school curriculum and teaching materials.[27] Women teachers like Lassalle were seen as particularly important to the US colonial project because they were believed to be naturally suited to maternal and caring labor due to their gender and capable of playing a domesticating role within the US empire.

Lassalle's work as a teacher was also deeply interconnected with her feminist activism and participation in the Puerto Rican suffrage movement. As scholars have shown, this movement was a vibrant space where both elite and working-class women from across Puerto Rico demanded rights for women and children.[28] Lassalle became a leader in the movement, and she

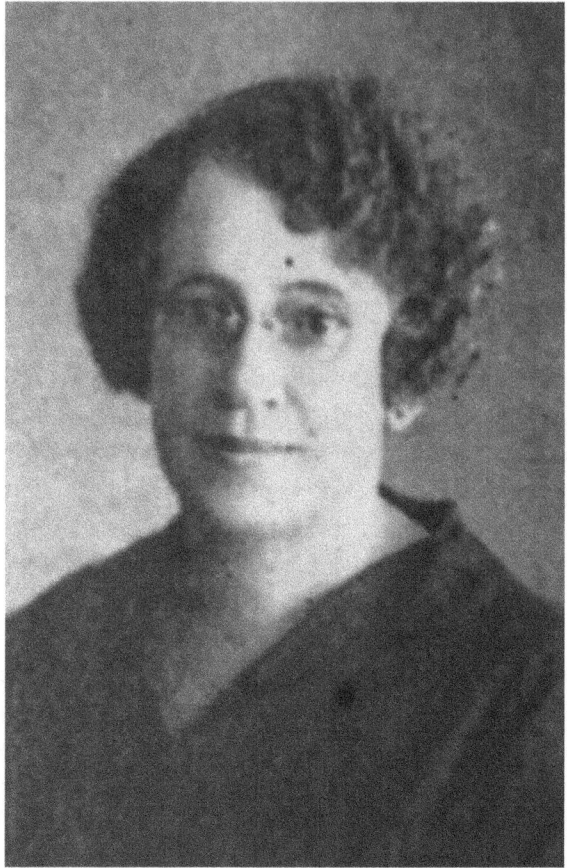

FIGURE 1.1. Beatriz Lassalle del Valle. Source: Angela Negrón Muñoz, *Mujeres de Puerto Rico: Desde el período de colonización hasta el primer tercio del siglo XX* (San Juan: Imprenta Venezuela, 1935), 170.

helped found the Liga Femínea Puertorriqueña (Puerto Rican Women's League) and the Liga Social Sufragista (Suffragist Social League). Historian Gladys M. Jiménez-Muñoz has documented how Lassalle's friend and fellow feminist Angela Negrón Muñoz wrote that Lassalle was a shining example of "spiritual motherhood."[29] According to Jiménez-Muñoz, Lassalle was seen as embodying the highest ideals of the women's movement during the 1920s, which included their new role as guides in the "modernization" of the archipelago. Lassalle also worked closely with socialist feminist leaders, including her friend Ricarda López de Ramos Casellas, and according to one source, agitated for the feminist cause "on the porches of the working-class."[30] However, when tensions emerged in the suffrage movement that broke down along class and racial lines, and some suffragettes proposed extending suffrage at first to only literate women, Lassalle sided with the elite group.

While Lassalle did break with working-class women over literacy requirements for voting, her larger political legacy was firmly rooted in broader
Latin American feminist advocacy for social change that would specifically
address economic inequality. As historian Katherine Marino has shown,
the feminist politics articulated by Latin American feminists during this
period often emphasized social and economic inequality within broader
Pan-American discourses.[31] Lassalle was an active participant in these Pan-
American gatherings, and her understanding of feminism was deeply shaped
by socialist feminist thought in both Latin America and the United States.
Like many other social feminist reformers of her time, she was particularly
inspired by reading socialist feminist social workers. This included women
like Florence Kelly, who had helped create the US settlement house movement and advocated for what historian Kathryn Kish Sklar called "social
justice feminism."[32] Like other social feminist reformers of her time, Lassalle
believed that the state should provide for all its citizens and rein in capitalism to ensure that the economy served society.

During World War I, Lassalle joined the expanding social reform projects
by creating a Junior Red Cross (JRC) branch in Puerto Rico. The JRC programs reflected a new dedication to the ideas of child welfare and "hygiene" as
a part of the public education curriculum and a broader understanding that
cultivating a protected childhood could benefit society.[33] These ideas were
also closely linked to popular understandings of eugenics and puericulture,
which stressed that social change could manifest in society through regulating public health, reproduction, and childcare. In Puerto Rico, the agency
took on a more expansive role as a public health agency than in the continental United States, and officials referred to using the "machinery" of the
public school system to administer a host of new reforms and regulations.
The local directors were home economics teachers who emphasized providing vocational education to girls and instructing them in "scientific forms of
motherhood" because they were seen as future mothers and workers.[34] In addition, the JRC raised funds, often from selling goods produced by vocational
education students, to distribute to needy families. In this way, the programs
began to provide a new form of social service in the community.

During the war, Lassalle also began collaborating more closely with American Red Cross officials in Puerto Rico, and the work of the agency brought
together Puerto Rican and US social feminists in various social reform projects that centered broadly on public health.[35] Scholarship on Puerto Rican
history during WWI has shown how Red Cross workers directed "hygiene"
and antiprostitution campaigns that became collaborations between public

health officials and the insular police force that targeted working-class women as sexual deviants and in need of reform. These histories reveal how elite women's groups such as the Woman's Christian Temperance Union sought to define a reformist, maternalist identity in juxtaposition to the wartime perception of working-class women as sexually deviant.[36] The programs they created primarily targeted urban women, some of whom were of African descent, but all of whom were imagined as racially "other" by reformers. In developing these programs, reformers shaped ideas about race in local and imperial discourse.

The work of social reformers also included elite women's participation in the less-documented development of Red Cross relief projects that allocated financial assistance through payments to military families and the poor. During the war, a series of natural disasters, including a hurricane and a fire, left hundreds homeless and in need of help.[37] Red Cross workers were trained in disaster relief, and the agency was reworking itself as a global humanitarian organization.[38] In response to the Puerto Rican disasters, the agency began operating a tent city for over five hundred individuals and providing some financial relief for its residents. Around the same time, the agency experimented with creating a Puerto Rican branch of Home Services, a program that provided economic support to families of soldiers. The Puerto Rican branch received most of its referrals from public school teachers and health clinics in the San Juan area. Small stipends were distributed to soldiers' wives, whom social workers evaluated for financial need. During this period, Beatriz Lassalle helped organize work alongside other Puerto Rican women reformers, including Rosario Belleber González, Olimpia Torres Zeno, Catalina Homer, and Hortensia Calderón.[39] These programs spread through the archipelago throughout the war and were precursors to developing more formal social services.[40] When the American Red Cross sought to create "peacetime" variants of these programs, they called on local social reformers like Lassalle to help them envision this transformation.

In 1920, Lassalle traveled to the New York School of Social Work (NYSW) to be trained as a social case worker and to gain hands-on experience working for US social service agencies. While in the United States, she also began working with working-class Puerto Rican migrants settling in the city.[41] She received a scholarship from the Department of Education and the American Red Cross to fund her studies, joining numerous other Puerto Rican women who traveled to the United States to receive professional training in caring professions. While at the NYSW, she would have encountered a student body mainly composed of white American women but also international students from Cuba and Japan and a small group of African American students.[42] At the school, she met numerous faculty members with imperial ties, including Walter Pettit, a colonial administrator in the Philippines who became a close friend. She also joined a group of women laying claim to new professional identities and was trained in "casework"—a form of allocating relief based on interviewing clients and analyzing cases using specific methods and protocols.[43] Lassalle also joined her fellow students in following seasoned caseworkers into the field by completing an apprenticeship.

During her training to become a social worker in the United States, Lassalle worked with migrant communities from Puerto Rico and Latin America. Her experience is a clear example of the unique aspects of colonial social work in Puerto Rico, where most professionals were integrated into the field by attending US universities and working with migrant communities. While at the NYSW, Lassalle gained practical experience in charity organizations and settlement houses that aimed to assimilate and Americanize immigrant and migrant communities.[44] Her fluency in Spanish made her a welcome expert on Latin Americans in these agencies, and she volunteered at the Brooklyn Board of Charities and the Associated Charities in New York for a few months.[45] Here, she witnessed the class and racial divides within the migrant Puerto Rican community, and this "allowed [her] to see how Puerto Ricans in the United States live and the indifference with which they are treated by their countrymen, who have come to occupy advantageous positions and looked down on them."[46] Lassalle criticized wealthy Puerto Ricans for turning their backs on those in the community who were less fortunate. Her experience working with migrants in the United States would later influence her work back on the archipelago.

Following her return to Puerto Rico in 1920, Lassalle embarked on a project reorganizing the Junior Red Cross agencies after being appointed its executive secretary. She utilized the knowledge and skills she gained while training at the NYSW to redefine the JRC's function in the public education system, helping the organization extend its child welfare and public health activities. Additionally, she began providing social work training to Puerto Rican students, teaching them the techniques she had learned in the United States. Some of these social workers later worked on child health-related projects for the Department of Education while others focused on state-sponsored public health initiatives. The social welfare techniques that Lassalle and her students developed expanded the role of social workers and public health nurses beyond the boundaries of schools, clinics, and hospitals into the homes and communities of their working-class clients and patients.

Professional women, such as Lassalle, came to play a significant role in Puerto Rican politics by designing social welfare programs and serving as social workers. They presented themselves as professionals with the necessary expertise to establish a more robust colonial state. Their political agenda focused on advocating for women's and children's rights as part of broader initiatives for social reform. However, their approach was maternalistic and influenced by their essentialist views on gender and their own class and racial prejudices. Overwhelmingly, they depicted themselves as professional "managers" of working-class women and their children. This perspective would create tensions between social workers and the working-class communities they claimed to serve. Nonetheless, their politicization of professional care work provided them with a crucial opportunity to participate in broader political discussions of the time.

The Children's Bureau in Puerto Rico

After the extension of US citizenship to Puerto Rico in 1917, there was debate and dialogue between Puerto Rican and US reformers over what parts of social welfare policy might be extended to Puerto Rico. In 1912, the United States made a decisive move toward institutionalizing progressive reform by creating the Children's Bureau of the Department of Labor, which resulted from decades of child welfare activism led by Progressive Era social reformers in the United States who also created the settlement house movement.[47] The agency's leaders advocated for the regulation of children's labor as well as for the creation of state-sponsored social welfare programs. In the 1920s, the Children's Bureau also became involved in debates about extending social rights to the US territories and possessions, and they forged connections with Puerto Rican reformers.[48] Together, US and Puerto Rican social welfare advocates would become involved in debates about extending social rights to the US territories and colonies of the period and advocate for extended programs to Puerto Rico. However, the production of the Children's Bureau report on Puerto Rico also reveals how those involved in creating the surveys that made up the report grappled with ideas of "modernity" and racial differences in Puerto Rico. In the end, the Puerto Rican Children's Bureau report showed how the agency's work took on new meaning in a colonial context.

The Children's Bureau conducted a report on maternal and child welfare in Puerto Rico based on similar reports they had previously conducted in the United States. The reformers who created the surveys that made up this report drew on Progressive Era maternalism and ideas about how immigrants needed to be "Americanized" and to be taught how to adopt middle-class Anglo-Saxon family structures.[49] They combined their maternalism with modernization ideology in Puerto Rico, arguing that US colonial institutions could bring "civilization" to Puerto Rico. Their belief that Puerto Ricans were uncivilized was rooted in their acceptance of the racist idea that Puerto Ricans constituted a racially inferior population to that of white US communities. Many Children's Bureau reformers also believed they could improve and reform the colonial institutions created by earlier US colonists, which had failed to modernize Puerto Rico adequately. Some also believed that the United States had a responsibility to ensure the welfare of Puerto Ricans within the US empire, and they thought the best way to do this was through their reform projects. Therefore, the entire Children's Bureau project in Puerto Rico was framed by the basic understanding that Puerto Ricans needed the guidance of US officials and institutions.

During their time in Puerto Rico, the agents of the Children's Bureau collaborated with local reformers who shared their views on modernization. These reformers were interested in regulating the gender roles of women and girls and promoting caregiving as a crucial aspect of these roles.[50] They believed that the caregiving labor of women as mothers sustained families, communities, and nations, and that proper education was necessary to carry out these responsibilities. By training Puerto Rican women in "scientific forms of motherhood," they hoped to produce healthier and more productive citizens (figure 1.2).[51] The reformers also believed that educating women and girls in these modern methods of motherhood would transform Puerto Rican society and push it toward modernization.[52] To achieve this goal, they focused on developing programs that educated women and girls to be care workers, either directing them toward positions in the home as mothers or as professional care workers in fields such as education, nursing, and social work.

The Children's Bureau activities in Puerto Rico relied on close collaborations with Puerto Rican reformers. In 1920, the director of the Puerto Rican Department of Education, Paul G. Miller, requested Julia Lathrop, the director of the Children's Bureau, to produce a report about child welfare in Puerto Rico.[53] Estelle B. Hunter, a seasoned social worker, was sent to investigate and suggested that Lassalle, who had training in social work, should direct the Puerto Rican side of the investigation. Lassalle traveled to Washington, DC, to study the Children's Bureau's social investigation methods and to prepare a Puerto Rican study.[54] In Washington, DC, Lassalle worked with

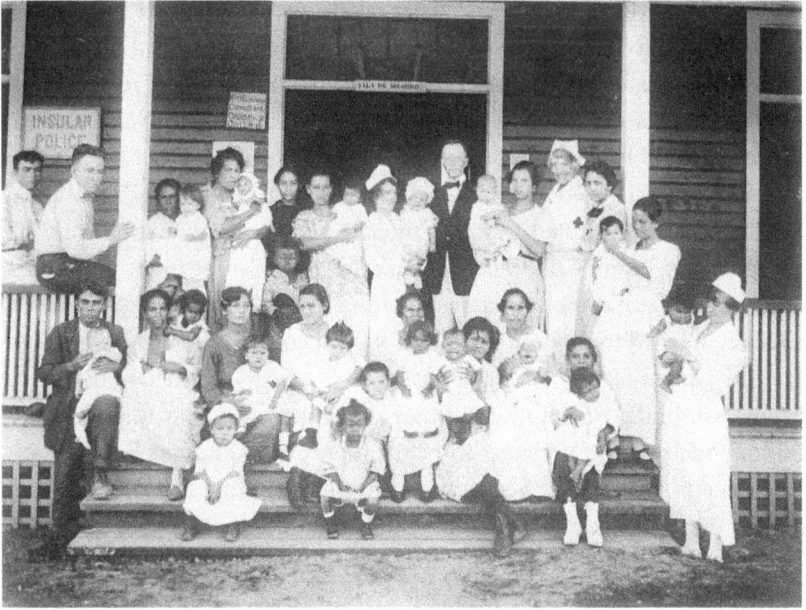

FIGURE 1.2. Baby clinic in Barrio Obrero, Puerto Rico, 1922. Courtesy of the American National Red Cross photograph collection, Library of Congress, Washington, DC.

Children's Bureau representatives and participated in their daily activities. Over multiple stays, she took part in the daily activities of Children's Bureau representatives, including those of Julia Lathrop, Grace Abbott, Emma Lundberg, and Katherine Lenroot.[55] While Lassalle was seen as the leading Puerto Rican participant in the study, Helen Bary, the agency's director of publications, was selected to oversee the entire project and to produce the final report.[56]

Helen Bary was a feminist, former suffrage leader, and writer who documented her experiences in Puerto Rico in the Children's Bureau report on maternal and child welfare about the archipelago. She traveled with Lassalle to Puerto Rico and met with colonial officials to discuss developing a child welfare survey program in Puerto Rico.[57] Under her pen name, Valeska Bari, she also wrote a series of articles about her experiences in Puerto Rico in the *Atlantic* that dramatized her understanding of the social transformations underway on the archipelago due to US intervention in the 1920s. In one of them, Lassalle surfaces as a partially fictionalized character.[58] The story focuses on a "modern" and "Americanized" Puerto Rican woman who works in her community to build better roads to help develop the rural area.

Her work faces significant barriers and challenges because of corrupt and inefficient local male political leaders. She can finally overcome these obstacles with the help of a handsome young "modern" man she marries. The story's protagonist is named Beatriz; it seems likely that the modern woman Bary centers in this narrative is modeled on Lassalle. However, the story's romantic aspect seems to be embellished, as Lassalle, like many other contemporary social welfare leaders, never married. In the end, the Children's Bureau study that Bary authored was shaped by her views about US institutions bringing modernization to Puerto Rico and her close collaboration with Puerto Rican reformers like Lassalle.

While working together on a Children's Bureau study in Puerto Rico, Lassalle and Bary's relationship was also shaped by racial politics and racism in both the United States and Puerto Rican communities. In an oral history later in her life, Bary revealed how race impacted the study. She mentioned that Lassalle had spent time in the United States and had connections to US social welfare agencies. She also noted that Lassalle "had a touch of colored blood" and "apparently in the States she had met with prejudice on that account, which made her highly sensitive on any possible topic that would reflect on race prejudice," which "created situations that were a bit difficult." When asked if this was also the case in Puerto Rico, Bary said it was in "connection with some North Americans."[59] It is likely that Lassalle was displeased with her North American colleague's ideas about the race of Puerto Ricans. She may have disapproved of how they defined all Puerto Ricans as nonwhite or had specific frustration with how they racially identified her as nonwhite. However, it is also possible that Lassalle was more broadly concerned with racial discrimination in Puerto Rican society. Her family's previous experience being racially categorized as nonwhite in Puerto Rico may have shaped her understanding of race and made her more broadly concerned about racial discrimination in society.

After discussing Lassalle's supposed "sensitivity" to race, Bary emphasized that in Puerto Rico, some people of African descent held positions of power that they would normally not hold in the United States. She stated, "Puerto Rico is fairly oblivious to the color line." She said that "the mayor of San Juan was a black man; the principals of most of the schools were colored; the population of the island had a large admixture of colored blood."[60] Furthermore, she noted that "the census figures were not indicative of the color line as we would draw it in the North." Moreover, she said, "Some families had the tradition of being white, and maybe they had chocolate-colored members; some families were considered colored who had members that could pass as white." It is noteworthy that she provided a detailed explanation of Puerto Rican racial hierarchies immediately after her discussion of Lassalle. This implies that she may have perceived Lassalle as someone of mixed racial heritage who held a position of power that would have been less attainable for her in the United States.

The Children's Bureau also decided that its investigation would be coupled with the administration of a "Children's Year" in Puerto Rico. In the United States, the Children's Year program began in 1918 during the war as a way of "stimulating and coordinating public and volunteer effort for child welfare."[61] Its main goal was to advocate for "public protection of maternity and infancy," "mother's care for older children," "enforcement of child-labor laws and free schooling for all children of school age," "recreation for children and youth, abundant, decent, protected from all form of exploitation."[62] Among the activities conducted during the Children's Year were weighing and measuring children, creating recreation activities, and doctor and dentist visits in local schools and newly formed public health centers. The agency also distributed large amounts of educational literature and "inaugurated a correspondence extension course on scientific motherhood."[63] The goal of these projects in the United States and Puerto Rico was to lay the foundation for separate state-sponsored institutions dedicated to child health and hygiene.

The Children's Bureau linked their Children's Year activities to the peacetime program of the Red Cross. They selected Red Cross worker Knowlton Mixer to direct the Puerto Rican program; he was accompanied by his wife, Margaret, a trained social worker. Mixer went on to document his Puerto Rican experiences in a book about the social conditions of the archipelago.[64] In addition to Mixer, the Red Cross assigned Kathleen D'Olier, a nurse who had worked in a reconstruction program creating child welfare programs in Greece after the war.[65] Lassalle was the leading intermediary between these agents and the offices of the Children's Bureau, the Red Cross, and the Junior Red Cross. She also worked to link the activities of these agencies to local charitable work Puerto Rican women were already conducting. The goal of these agencies' collaborative efforts was for Bary to write up a final report for the Children's Bureau and the US government in the hopes that more funding and programs for children would be administered to the archipelago.

The Children's Year initiative aimed to coordinate the charitable work of women already involved in such activities under the state's supervision. The project was carried out by volunteer groups trained by Lassalle, who worked on various individual projects. The initiative's overarching goal was to introduce and promote the idea that charity was a science, and volunteers were encouraged to take on new professional caregiving roles as they participated in the Children's Year programs. Lassalle's training program emphasized the importance of casework and scientific record-keeping, which she believed could provide more efficient services through individual diagnosis and treatment rather than a one-size-fits-all approach. These activities also showcased the potential of this type of social work in the community to the insular government.[66] The Children's Year program led to an increase in women entering caregiving careers while simultaneously advocating for government agencies to hire professional women to develop social service programs. As these women took on new roles as professional care workers, they soon used these positions within the state government to promote their political agendas.

Working-Class Women and Children, Social Welfare, and the Politics of Care Work

In 1920, the Children's Bureau began conducting surveys of maternal and child welfare in Puerto Rico that would shed light on broader societal perceptions about caring labor and social reproduction in Puerto Rican communities. These studies would later be included in the Children Bureau's published report on Puerto Rico. The researchers began their work by examining a neighborhood called Puerta de Tierra, located outside the urban center of San Juan.[67] This neighborhood was primarily made up of working families, many of whom were of African descent. The working-class women from this community provided much of the service and caring labor that sustained the capital city of San Juan.[68] The Children's Bureau study focused on women and children who were care workers and criticized the commonplace labor arrangements in this community. Its authors argued that social welfare reformers should intervene in these social and labor systems, creating new programs and institutions to reform child labor and to end child servitude.

After the Children's Bureau study, working-class women and girls, many of whom were care workers and servants, became the targets of social reforms and policies proposed by the agency. While the Children's Bureau aimed to restrict child labor practices, they mainly focused on training girls and women in "scientific motherhood" through home economics programs.[69] This reinforced the traditional role of women as caregivers, but ideally within their own homes. The agency viewed themselves as guides who could teach working-class women and girls supposedly "proper" forms of domesticity.[70] They advocated for the idea of a protected childhood that, in their view, sometimes meant advocating for placing children in state-run institutions rather than allowing them to be exploited by private employers.[71] Their reforms also emphasized and promoted a gendered division of caring labor in Puerto Rican communities.

The Children's Bureau study dealt with the social transformations happening in urban areas during the 1920s and proposed a liberal reform plan to regulate the effects of capitalist development on the region. The reformers wrestled with how to address the social instability and poverty that had plagued working-class communities for over thirty years due to US colonialism and capitalist expansion. During this period, massive labor strikes and worker organizing challenged US corporations' exploitation of the working class.[72] Additionally, there was a significant migration of rural working-class people to urban areas like Puerta de Tierra in search of work and homes. The changes in the 1920s also deeply affected women, with more of them entering the workforce, including in tobacco and needlework companies and the service industry.[73] Many working-class mothers struggled to balance factory work with the reproductive work they were expected to perform at home due to limited childcare options. In response to political and economic changes, the Children's Bureau study proposed social welfare programs aimed at supporting mothers and children, programs that were meant to address the problem of social reproduction that emerged under capitalism.

As the Children's Bureau study envisioned a new liberal reform plan that would be supervised by social feminists from both Puerto Rico and the United States, it largely overlooked the earlier history of Puerto Rican liberal reformers who had regulated care workers. Previously, under the Spanish colonial government, Puerto Rican liberal elite reformers had worked to regulate the lives of working-class women and children of African descent.[74] Their primary goal was to funnel these women and children into positions as servants, providing caring labor to wealthy families. However, the working-class women from these communities had long resisted the imposition of these regulations and forms of control.[75] The Children's Bureau study failed to take this history into account. Instead, it criticized contemporary practices of child servitude, condemned the Puerto Rican elite for employing childcare workers, and argued that these employers should be educated to discontinue these labor practices.

Perhaps the most glaring oversight of the study was that it failed to acknowledge the historical and contemporary labor activism of working-class women care workers. Scholars have shown how working-class domestic workers had long resisted authorities seeking control of their lives and labor under Spanish and US authority.[76] They have also shown how women who were accused of being sex workers had also resisted the reform projects that had targeted their communities.[77] Additionally, working-class women, many of them care workers, were increasingly participating in labor organizing, agitating for better labor conditions, labor protections, and broader rights in Puerto Rican society.[78] By not considering the role of these women in labor activism, the study further excluded them from mainstream narratives about labor organizing in Puerto Rico. These silences around women's reproductive labor would have a lasting effect on future labor studies in the following years.

The projects initiated by the Children's Bureau highlighted the significance of women's work in society. They focused on instructing professional and working-class women and girls in "mother work."[79] Beatriz Lassalle led multiple initiatives that trained volunteers in professional casework, advocating that charity was a science and should be the state's responsibility. Her first project was establishing a "fresh air camp" that brought hundreds of children from Puerta de Tierra to the rural town of Barranquitas (figure 1.3).[80] The children received medical consultations with doctors and dentists and were taught proper "hygiene" practices. Her second project was working with Red Cross officials to expand "Home Services" under its Family Welfare Bureau, which provided direct-relief funds to some families. She also collaborated with Red Cross officials to construct maternal health, child health, and hygiene clinics in Puerta de Tierra. At these clinics, Lassalle trained volunteer visiting nurses to use casework methods to follow up with patients who visited the clinics, mainly through "home visits." These volunteers provided education in infant care, showed Children's Bureau films from the United States, distributed educational pamphlets, and began a course for "little mothers" for girls between the ages of twelve and fifteen. The programs developed during this period focused primarily on training in gender-specific forms of labor, including reproductive labor in the household.

As part of their work on the Children's Year, the directors carried out three social scientific surveys to examine groups targeted by reformers who could become clients of social welfare programs. The Puerto Rican version of the survey aimed to cover the same topics as previous studies conducted by the Children's Bureau in US communities. The first survey was a census of working-class women defined as "abandoned mothers" by the agency.[81] In the Children's Bureau report, Bary discusses six "typical cases"

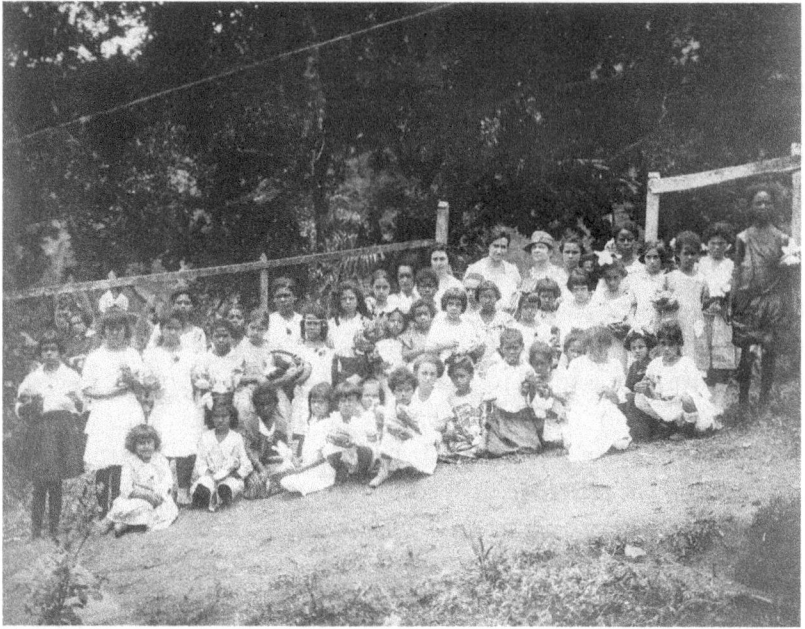

FIGURE 1.3. First Fresh Air Camp in Puerto Rico, 1921. Helen Bary is standing directly to the left of the woman in the back wearing a hat. Courtesy of the American National Red Cross photograph collection, Library of Congress, Washington, DC.

meant to "help visualize the situations" described in the report. These descriptions reveal some of the main concerns of the reformers who collected the data. They listed the women's first names and ages, their marital status, the number and ages of their children, and the location of the children's father, if known. They also focused on how the women supported themselves and their families and whether they received assistance from anyone. The women ranged in age from twenty-two to thirty and had between one and four children. Three out of six women worked outside the home: one in the tobacco industry, another as a laundress, and the last as a seamstress. The reformers also emphasized cases where the male partners or husbands of the women had been engaged in infidelity or gambling, casting a particularly negative light on fathers who were seen as not adequately providing for their families.

The Children's Bureau's census of "abandoned mothers" was conducted by Woman's Christian Temperance Union members. In Puerto Rico, this organization had a long history of regulating working-class women's lives through its campaigns against prostitution and the creation of anti-vice neighborhood police forces.[82] The collaboration between this organization and the Children's Bureau illustrates how older forms of social regulation came under the umbrella of the state, providing the data used to initiate new forms of regulation and surveillance by social welfare officials and public health clinics. Newer social welfare programs were often grafted onto older reform projects, continuing older forms of intervention under new organizations. Through their work on the census, the focus of these reformers turned from "prostitutes" to "abandoned mothers" as a leading cause of concern in Puerto Rican society. This transition reflected a transformation in the language social reformers used to discuss working-class women and their sexuality.

In her final report, Bary argued that the problem of "abandoned mothers" in Puerto Rico was a result of the archipelago's history of slavery, economic inequality, and racial hierarchies. She began by arguing that Puerto Ricans are racially different from white US Americans and that most Puerto Ricans are of African descent. She argued that "while some families have prided themselves upon preserving their blood unmixed, the population, in general, is a product of the mixture of races."[83] She then explained how Puerto Rico's history of "slavery or dependence" had shaped familial and marital relations, leading to "attendant irresponsibility for self-support" and "tendencies towards irregular unions."[84] Furthermore, Bary ties her interpretation of Puerto Rico's racial politics to high rates of paternal abandonment, suggesting that Puerto Rican men's supposed failure to support their families is the reason for poverty in local communities. However, she noted that the "prevailing opinion of the women who made this survey" was that the "basic trouble was economic conditions." According to Bary and her collaborators, men's lack of steady work prevented them from being proper breadwinners and led them to abandon their families.[85]

Bary also argued that "abandonment" was closely tied to labor migrations, which had resulted in workers moving to Puerto Rican cities and to the United States. After US colonization, these migrations increased dramatically and led to the displacement of workers.[86] She underscored the stories of women whose male partners migrated to New York City in search of work but did not provide support for their families. For instance, she described the case of "Dolores," a mother of three young children whose husband had "deserted her two years ago." Dolores and her mother "made blouses" and "with difficulty supported the family."[87] She later received help from the Red Cross and used their networks to contact her husband in New York. However, he still "sent little help" and said he "went north to get better opportunities but had not earned enough to bring the family north."[88] In this case, the Red Cross stepped into a new role and used its connections to US social agencies to track migrants to the United States. In some cases, they arranged for money and resources to be sent back as remittances to family members on the archipelago. The roots of what would become a lasting practice linking Puerto Rico and the United States through social service agencies can be seen in the work conducted with these early cases. As labor migrations increased in the following years, these cases occurred even more often.

While the reformers of the Children's Bureau study emphasized the regulation and control of working-class women, they also clearly defined the work of motherhood as something that should deserve support from society and the state. This was a significant departure from previous commonplace political discourse that often ignored the needs of working-class women. During the period, there were ways that the reformers' proposals overlapped with the demands of working-class women. This was the case of working-class women's organizing for better wages, working conditions, and labor protections.[89] During this period, both working-class women and professional social workers were members of the Socialist Party and witnessed numerous proposals that addressed women workers' concerns about labor standards. The social workers recognized that there was a major social transition underway as capitalism resulted in more working-class women entering the labor force. They also saw how women workers often worked long hours for low wages that were not enough to support their families.

One of the main issues that reformers encountered was the growing number of working-class women who entered waged work outside the home and desperately needed childcare. Working-class women who were a part of the Socialist Party tried to make this a central concern of the party, with limited results.[90] Socialist women emphasized how women working in factories and the service industry needed childcare or day care options to allow them to work while ensuring their children's safety. In addition, some social workers who were members of the Socialist Party helped create day care programs for women workers as a part of the reforms that they developed.[91] In the second part of its survey, the Children's Bureau focused on the needs of working-class children who were living in unstable economic conditions. These children often had mothers who were unable to care for them because they were working outside the home and did not have access to childcare.

The Children's Bureau conducted two additional surveys on what they called "homeless" children, the first on boys and the second on girls.[92] The

Children's Bureau directed this census in three major cities: San Juan, Ponce, and Mayagüez. Lassalle was chosen to direct these studies and met with representatives of the insular police force, who gave her lists of children who had been reported as homeless. The children were later interviewed by caseworkers individually. The final report on children focused on how the group labeled "homeless" was actually composed of child laborers who worked mainly as servants in local homes. According to the final report, written by Bary, "the great mass of homeless children work as servants in private families. Such servants are found in almost every household, and it is only by such work that many of these children escape starvation."[93]

The study focused on how these children were circulated throughout the city and how the large majority had been informally adopted to care for other children and do domestic work in urban households. It emphasized that the circulation of child domestic workers in Puerto Rican society was commonplace.[94] The report argued that the circulation of child servants was "partly the outgrowth of slavery" and that "in large numbers of cases the former slaves continued to live as previously and their children grew up loosely attached to the family of the former owner."[95] The study framed child servitude as the result of racial politics in Puerto Rico and the continued racism faced by people of African descent. It documented how many children circulated through the city, living in private homes of their employers, under the auspices of a broad understanding of "informal adoption" that was really about the continuation of coerced forms of labor.

In the study, Bary also interprets how racial relations in Puerto Rico after slavery have created a persistent form of racialized servitude. This argument provides an interesting and more nuanced analysis of power and exclusion in Puerto Rican society than most other colonial reports of the period. She notes that there are much higher rates of people of "modest means" having three or four servants, something that "people in the states, in similar conditions, would not expect."[96] She attributes this practice to "the race problem," which she argues "has had much to do with a careless attitude toward the education of these child servants, almost all of whom are of mixed blood." She concludes that elite Puerto Ricans have "considered it not unsuitable that the colored people should remain servants and therefore have thought it unnecessary for them to receive an education."[97] The most significant point of her analysis is that cultures of servitude and child circulation in Puerto Rico have maintained racial divisions and hierarchies of inequality.

A closer look at the studies Lassalle conducted reveals how child servants were imagined within the data collection for the two reports on girls and boys, respectively. These studies outlined a gendered division between the types of jobs that were given to homeless youth. In the report on homeless boys, 161 boys were "interviewed and investigated."[98] Many boys did not know where their parents were, but some had working mothers, of whom "6 were washerwomen, 2 were seamstresses, and 2 were cooks." Among the boys, "38 were servants, 104 were engaged in street trades, of whom 24 were bootblacks, 18 newsboys, 7 street vendors, and 55 odd-jobbers; 6 were farm workers; and 13 were engaged in miscellaneous work."[99] Most had never attended school and were living in a variety of conditions not considered proper "homes" by Lassalle and the researchers, such as staying at the houses of employers, with friends, or in rented rooms or boardinghouses. Thirty-seven said they slept "anywhere."

The report includes "outlines of some interesting cases of homeless boys" interviewed for the study. There are eight boys profiled in the study. All were given racial classification directly following their first names; four are listed as "white" while the other four are listed as "colored." In the case of one of the "white" children, Angel, who was eight years old, the case record documents how he migrated to the city with his mother after his father passed away. When they arrived, his mother "found work at a hotel, but the boys were not allowed to stay with her." In Angel's case, he was separated from his mother because her job, likely as a domestic worker at a hotel, did not allow her to keep him with her while she worked. Afterward, Angel went "from house to house asking to work for his board and room." Eventually, he "was taken in by a family to run errands and entertain children"; however, he later was "found to be too naughty and was discharged."[100] Like many other children in the city, Angel sought work as a servant in San Juan by going door to door looking for jobs. The case file also documents a commonplace practice whereby child servants were placed in charge of taking care of other children in the employer's household. Angel was employed with the understanding that he would be a caretaker for the younger children in the employer's house.

Another one of the case records reported on the story of a fourteen-year-old boy named Mario, who was labeled as "colored" in the report and living in a car at the time of the study. The report documented how Mario's mother had passed away and noted that "his father was living [in] another town with another woman." It notes that "after his mother's death Mario had left home, and his sister had been placed out in a free foster home." According to the report, "He slept in an automobile which he was hired to look after" and was "dirty and in rags."[101] In this case, the language of the reformers condemns the father for not caring for Mario and his sister. It also suggests that there were gendered differences in the ways that girls and boys were able to find foster homes or jobs as child servants. The story suggests that placing his sister into a foster care arrangement was easier, which is a noticeable pattern in the records. The report highlighted how boys without parents might find it more difficult to find steady employment in private households.

In a second survey Lassalle conducted of homeless girls, the gendered logic of child servitude and care work continued to take center stage. According to the report, "When a baby is born it is not unusual for the family to take a child of from 7 to 12 years of age who becomes the personal servant of the infant."[102] These children were young girls who were taken into homes to be private servants and often grew up without access to education. According to the report, "There has been no social conscience against this practice," and "in many cases the child's services are not really needed and she is taken into the house more in charity than for any selfish motive."[103]

The discussion of homeless girls in the report does not include case file information, although the process of collecting data about them is described. The collaboration between the reformers and insular police officials is highlighted here, as "questionnaires were sent to all district chiefs of police asking them to list girls who had come under their observation as being in need of such care."[104] Out of the 119 forms that were filled out, there were investigations into conditions and interviews. According to the study, "65 were classed as "homeless," "vagabonds," or "delinquent" and 54 as "servants.""[105] The report mentions reformers' concern with many of the girls living in "conditions of extreme moral hazard" and that some had notations of "prostitute" or "often found on the streets at very late hours" in their files. This concern with "moral delinquents" reflects how the girls' experiences were often viewed differently than that of the boys and were bound up in concerns over sexuality and morality that grew out of the earlier work of reformers and police to regulate working-class women through restrictions on prostitution. The sexual politics of women's work is also interesting in this study; the roles of servant and prostitute are depicted as overlapping in the descriptions and conditions described in the report.

The Children's Bureau argued that to eliminate "homelessness," one of the goals of social reforms should be to encourage compulsory education and to educate "public opinion" against practices of child servitude, particularly within elite women's organizations.[106] The study suggests that cultural practices in Puerto Rico are to blame for child circulation, along with the inability of working women to take care of their children. The report also stresses tensions over whether children, regardless of race or class, should have a right to protected childhood. These arguments may have come as a shock or challenge to the well-off society women who supported the Children's Year project, who were likely some of the employers of these children. However, it is also just as likely that these elite women continued to believe themselves to be enlightened employers who could instruct other families in the proper way of keeping child servants. Either way, tensions over the role and rights of Puerto Rican servants reflected a change in how popular understandings of childhood turned toward the idea that specific regulations and institutions should protect it.

The Children's Bureau report emphasized the difficulties surrounding care work and child servitude in Puerto Rican communities. The study aimed to create programs targeting working-class women and their children for gendered reforms intervening in their intimate lives. While the reformers believed that pushing women toward caregiving roles could positively change Puerto Rican society, they failed to examine the legacy of liberal reformers in the same communities where they worked. These earlier reformers had used child welfare systems to place children in positions as child servants. The Children's Bureau overlooked this history and argued that a new group of social workers, including Lassalle, should be placed in charge of a new wave of reforms and institution building to end child labor in Puerto Rico.

Institutionalizing Social Welfare and Building Social Welfare Programs

Before the Children's Bureau study was published, Helen Bary returned to the archipelago on a follow-up trip and investigated the results of the Children's Year activities. Her report describes how many initiatives Lassalle created were being institutionalized and made permanent by the insular government. These changes had begun in 1923, directly after the Children's Year, when the insular government decided to allocate $60,000 for prenatal and baby clinics. That year, a Social Welfare Bureau was created in the Department of Health to oversee work in the clinics. Lassalle was also enlisted to create a course in social work for students in the Normal School program at the University of Puerto Rico. The first cohort of sixty students participated in a two-week class in basic preparation for social work and attended numerous lectures given by public health professionals. Lassalle later recounted stories about driving around San Juan in the mornings before the course to pick up the program's key lecturers.[107] According to Bary, "The first half of the course was required and the second was elective, but no falling off in attendance occurred after the required period was completed."[108] As a result, social work methods were already widely institutionalized only three years after Lassalle had returned from her studies at the New York School of Social Work.

In addition to providing visiting nurse services, these social workers also entered new roles as field researchers, collecting data through casework that the government used for further studies of poverty. They also developed large-scale social investigations of child welfare conditions, drawing on methods developed by the Children's Bureau, to gather data and write reports. These reports were used as tools to argue for creating new social legislation and building social welfare institutions in the upcoming years. In 1924, these efforts resulted in reorganizing the social welfare activities in a new Social Service Bureau augmented by a board a year later. The Child Welfare Board was comprised of the Departments of Justice, Agriculture, and Education, and Lassalle and Angela Negrón, a representative of the Asociación Feminista (Feminist Association) and secretary of the Bureau of Social Medicine and Puericulture. Their presence and that of suffrage leaders Isabel Andreu de Aguilar and Grace Lugo Viñas on the board signaled a continued interconnection between women's rights organizations and state-sponsored social service administration.

By 1924, the Social Service Bureau within the Department of Health had a staff of eight, including four social workers in the field. According to one of the organization's earliest reports, there had been some tensions during the start of the organization as "many believed it was primarily for the dispensing of charity while others believed that the social workers had supernatural abilities to remedy all the evils that surround those masses of the less fortunate which are to be found in every country."[109] The meaning of social work and the casework practices developed were negotiated within Puerto Rican agencies during these early years. Throughout this time, an emphasis on a scientific application of social services was central to the administration of the program, which also created a database of information about clients. According to the Department of Health, the Social Service Bureau developed a "complete record system" that "was immediately adopted and by this means it has been possible to have an exact understanding of each case, as to antecedents, heredity, family history, previous residence and conditions, social status, past and present, and the actual economic situation."[110] This work, which saw the Puerto Rican state collecting increasing amounts of data about poor families, represented a major shift in the lives of Puerto Ricans. Social workers supervised a rapid expansion of the state's collection and bureaucratic management of case file information.

Casework practices were used throughout the new government agencies, spreading across the archipelago. The number of clinics expanded rapidly during the first years of the Social Service Bureau. According to reports from 1925, there were already dispensaries with social workers in San Juan, Santurce, Puerta de Tierra, Barrio Obrero, Ponce, Mayagüez, Aguadilla, Caguas, Guayama, Juncos, Carolina, Comerío, and Villalba. The clinics treated between seventy-one and 320 patients each, and the work reported included house visits, care, instructions and demonstrations, visits of investigation, and prenatal and baby clinics. In Santurce alone, Department of Health agents reported 806 house visits; other areas listed similarly high numbers. The social workers continued to push the boundaries of public health work into the homes of Puerto Ricans throughout the 1920s.

Some of the cases social workers dealt with in these dispensaries reflected earlier reformers' concerns over the regulation of the intimate relationships of Puerto Rican families. One of the agency's main goals was "to bring about better social relationships and ideas of responsibility, as the number of unmarried and separated couples as well as the number of unmarried mothers is high among the poorer classes."[111] Social workers intervened in particular familial cases and encouraged couples to get married. In one case, when social workers discovered that a man and woman who came to the clinic were not legally married, they spoke with them about the "advisability of establishing legitimate relationships"; later, they reported being invited to the couple's wedding. The concern with marriage is reflected over and over, with reports stating that "many marriages have been affected through the influence of the social welfare agents over the families with which they come in contact, and much stress has been brought to bear also upon the parents as to school attendance."[112] The social workers targeted families who came to their clinics, often for medical reasons, for interventions in familial practices.

In addition, casework conducted by the Social Service Bureau reflected the impact of migration to the United States. In one case, three "orphaned" children cared for by a grandmother were brought to a local baby clinic. These clinics were run as a part of the maternal health programs created by the social workers in the Department of Health. Here, the agents discovered she was in financial difficulty and "could not pay her rent."[113] The social workers discovered that "the nearest relative was a brother in New York," and he was "located through the Charity Organization Society of Brooklyn and was requested to help support the children."[114] In response, the young man sent money back to the family to help care for the children, and other extended family members were found in Puerto Rico. Ultimately, "an aunt offered her home to the oldest boy, the second child's godmother took her and the smallest boy went to live with his godfather."[115] After all the children were placed in new homes, and the grandmother "was given a home in the Asylum for the Aged," the social workers reported on the case as a great success.

This case hints at new patterns of intervention and institutionalization that were becoming increasingly popular because of social work interventions. Common family cases, like grandmothers caring for young children, were becoming subjects of regulation by caseworkers advocating for institutionalized care. Here, the result was profound, as a family's life was drastically altered when social workers' interventions separated them, likely against their will. This case reveals how social workers from the agency often took on cases that were initially brought for medical reasons. It also illustrates how social workers continued to use connections they had with US agencies to contact migrants in the United States for assistance with cases in Puerto Rico. This case hints at how the influence of social welfare officials continued to broaden during the 1920s.

By 1927, agents of the Department of Health went so far as to say, "We have introduced the *visiting nurse* and *social worker* as important factors in the social development of the community and have impressed the public with the importance of their work and the desirability of extending their fields of activity."[116] The role of these professional women in Puerto Rican society was widespread and continued growing when the agency arranged for new groups of women to be sent to the United States for professional training. These women were explicitly sent with the idea that when they returned, they could rework some of the other institutions on the archipelago, including local orphanages and prisons, a school for the blind, and a sanatorium for patients with tuberculosis. It took a while for them to receive their professional degrees and return to the archipelago, leading to a gap between when the government invested in the field and the beginning of most programs. The increasing number of professional social workers eventually led to the field's professionalization in 1929, when the Porto Rico Association of Trained Social Workers was founded. The organization, one of the first professional organizations of its kind, reflected the critical role that participation in social work had come to play in Puerto Rican society.

* * *

DURING THE 1920S, the creation of new social welfare reform projects opened a unique opportunity for Puerto Rican women to advance their political agendas. As women like Lassalle entered new roles as professional social workers for state agencies, they became professional care workers whose identities as elite women were seen as having prepared them for reform work. The politics of maternalism shaped these early social welfare projects, as did their investment in the prevailing notion of the possibilities of US colonial institutions in bringing "modernity." The main target of the projects they would develop were working-class women and children whose lives and labor became the subject of their studies and interventions. As the chapter highlights, many working-class people who were the subject of colonial reforms were care workers, caregivers, and servants. Puerto Rican social welfare reformers emphasized ending child servitude within the newly created social welfare projects of this period. Still, they failed to grapple with reformers' roles in shaping these practices of racialized and gendered servitude or supporting the colonial and capitalist institutions creating this overarching labor system. As the profession began to expand, this earlier generation of social worker activists would find their maternalist ideas increasingly challenged by new practitioners, some of whom were socialists who would emphasize the need for broader forms of social change to address the poverty, inequality, and lack of support of reproductive labor by the state under capitalism in Puerto Rico.

At the time, the government hearings over the extension of social welfare policies in Puerto Rico became important arenas for debates over US citizenship. Creating the Children's Bureau was a decisive moment in developing social welfare policies in the United States, and questions emerged over how US colonies and territories would be covered under these reforms. The Children's Bureau study resulted from the close collaboration between Puerto Rico and the US government, who both advocated for full coverage of Puerto Rico under federal social welfare policy. When there were Puerto Rican hearings over the extension of the Sheppard-Towner Act, Puerto Rican and US officials used the Children's Bureau report as evidence that Puerto Rico needed relief funding and that the United States should invest more broadly in the welfare of Puerto Ricans. Including this report in the hearings showed how Puerto Rican and US women were active in trying to shape the social aspects of Puerto Rican citizenship during a formative moment. Both groups were advocating that Puerto Ricans were deserving of federal social support precisely because Puerto Rico was a colony of the United States.

As an economic crisis loomed with the Great Depression on the horizon, the field of social work was also poised to become a central part of a new period of social reform. The social workers who had become leaders in the 1920s and had already cut their teeth working with US government agencies like the Children's Bureau would be called on to oversee new relief efforts and social welfare agencies. After the late 1920s, the profession grew even more quickly when New Deal agencies recruited many working-class women to be trained as professional social workers or social welfare aides. These women would bring their agendas to the profession as they brought the concerns of working-class women, socialists, and supporters of the growing independence movement with them into their professional careers. However, even as the profession changed, it would still be marked by tensions and conflicts with working-class communities who were the targets of these reforms. As Puerto Rican communities confronted a new crisis, Puerto Rican women activists of various backgrounds would continue to be central figures in debates over social welfare policy and reform, care labor, and the politics of reproduction.

Labor, Welfare, and Gendered Citizenship in New Deal Puerto Rico

On June 1, 1936, the *New York Times* ran an article, "Women Ask Relief for Puerto Ricans," covering five female delegates to the National Conference of Social Workers in Atlantic City, New Jersey, and their efforts to extend Social Security to Puerto Rico. María Pintado, Celestina Zalduondo, Mercedes Vélez, Carmen Rivera de Alvarado, and Geraldine Froscher were all staff members of the Puerto Rico Emergency Relief Administration (PRERA), a program that was originally created as a branch of the Federal Emergency Relief Administration of the United States.[1] The article worried that "almost lost in the millions of words uttered here last week . . . on behalf of the 'forgotten man' were the Spanish accents of five young women, arguing the cause of a whole island of forgotten people."[2] Created only a year before, the Social Security Act of 1935 brought a sweeping set of reforms that established a new federal social welfare system in the United States. However, as a territory of the United States, Puerto Rico had been excluded from coverage.

The social workers' demands for inclusion under the Social Security Act shed light on how women employed on New Deal projects in Puerto Rico were active in political organizing. Among the five women mentioned in this newspaper article were feminists, former suffragettes, ardent socialist labor reformers, and future leaders of the Puerto Rican movement for independence. In the 1930s, these women participated in a historical moment that sparked a powder keg of political mobilization in which Puerto Ricans challenged the emerging US colonial status quo.[3] As government agents working for PRERA, these social workers played an essential role in the struggles that ensued in these projects over reform, development, and decolonization.[4] They were particularly involved in debates over the extension of New Deal social policies to Puerto Rico, as the legislation was being extended in partial and differential ways.[5] When these programs expanded, they became central figures in administering them and played vital roles in shaping the transformation between state and society that resulted from these social policies.

This chapter explores how Puerto Rican women contributed to struggles for Puerto Rican rights and citizenship through their involvement in shaping social reforms and social policy. In the 1930s, the entry of numerous middle-class and working-class women transformed the social work profession. The Puerto Rican government recruited and trained these women to work on state projects, including New Deal agencies and vocational education programs.[6] The new social workers held diverse political beliefs that impacted how they performed their work in local communities. This included socialist women who believed social workers should collaborate with working-class people to achieve social change. It also included women invested in various forms of nationalism, some of whom believed in fighting for the archipelago to become independent from the United States.[7] As social workers became more and more politically engaged, tensions would arise between women with different political visions. At the same time, conservative political forces in Puerto Rico also began to target the field of social work as one that was pushing for unwelcome societal change. Despite these challenges, Puerto Rican social workers would become political leaders in various social movements in the following years.

As social workers developed social welfare programs focused on gendered reforms in working-class communities, their work was increasingly shaped by working-class women's demands for work and better labor conditions. When social workers began working in rural communities, they were charged with creating gender-segregated educational programs that would funnel women into roles as housewives, household workers, and needleworkers. They also encountered working-class women deeply involved in labor organizing who demanded steadier incomes, better jobs, and labor standards.[8] For these women, especially those who were needleworkers, the space of the home and workplace had been blurred as they worked for wages while still providing reproductive labor in their communities.[9] When the same social workers became the administrators of New Deal programs, they developed work-relief and direct-relief programs that aided working-class women.[10] Some of the monetary funds they distributed were explicitly meant to support the social reproduction of the working class through funds directed at mothers and children. However, working-class women would be disappointed that New Deal programs had resulted in the expansion of "relief" programs and not the secure and well-paying jobs they had demanded.[11] In the end, social workers' efforts to regulate gender and labor in Puerto Rican society would lay the groundwork for a rapid expansion of the state into working-class people's lives.

During the 1930s, there was a struggle between Puerto Ricans of different classes and backgrounds and between Puerto Rican and US government officials regarding the creation and administration of New Deal social welfare programs.[12] This chapter focuses on the political organizing of Puerto Rican women within social welfare programs and the debates over social welfare policy. It examines how the creation of gendered labor policies and the administration of New Deal relief programs that targeted women workers affected both Puerto Rican professionals and working-class women. The chapter also considers how Puerto Rican social workers, including those from working-class backgrounds, organized politically, formed professional organizations, and became deeply involved in struggles over the rights of Puerto Ricans to social welfare benefits. These struggles were focused on the archipelago and the growing diasporic population in the United States that had resulted from labor migration. Throughout the decade, Puerto Rican women fought for social change in a tumultuous period marked by rapid economic transformation and political instability.

The chapter concludes by emphasizing the significance of Puerto Rican political activism around applying the US Social Security Act to Puerto Rico. It highlights how the professionalization of social work and the increasing mobility of social workers who traveled to the United States for training gave rise to new forms of social worker organizing and activism on behalf of Puerto Ricans, both on the archipelago and in the United States. Social workers became critical figures in advocating for the extension of the Social Security Act to Puerto Rico and joined broader dialogues about the archipelago's political relationship with the United States and the rights of Puerto Ricans. In 1939, they participated in a series of US congressional hearings about Puerto Rico's potential coverage under the Social Security Act that resulted in the United States finally extending parts of the maternal and child welfare and public health titles. However, the partial administration of this legislation meant that by enacting partial coverage, the US Congress was deciding to create differential territorial social citizenship rights for Puerto Ricans. This moment would usher in a lasting pattern of partial social welfare coverage for Puerto Ricans that social workers and working-class communities denounced. However, the mobilizations around social welfare policy in the 1930s would lay the foundation for continued Puerto Rican coalitions advancing reforms to social policies in the post–World War II period.

Social Workers, Political Organizing, and Rural Reform after 1928

In 1930, a new generation of Puerto Rican social workers, including many from middle-class and working-class backgrounds, began work on rural reform projects where they developed community-oriented forms of social work. The practice of social work they innovated, which they understood as community oriented, was deeply informed by their participation in nationalist and feminist social movements. Among the social workers of this generation were women who supported various political parties, including a group of activists who would become leaders in the movement for Puerto Rican independence. The social reform projects they developed targeted working-class families and regulated working-class women and girls' labor, care work, and reproduction. As social workers created these labor, education, and public health reform projects, they gradually stretched the work of the state into the intimate lives of working-class families. They also articulated their political vision of how Puerto Rican society could be transformed through the practice of social work. This vision was connected to their nationalist belief that strong families would build a stronger nation. They also recognized that women's labor, within and outside the home, would be essential to producing the social changes they envisioned.

The social welfare programs developed by social workers in rural reform projects of the period were part of broader gendered reforms advanced by the state. Scholars have shown how, in the 1920s and 1930s, the Puerto Rican government and US institutions created various social and economic campaigns that targeted working-class communities for change.[13] In part, this was a reaction to the realization that over twenty years of US colonialism had not produced the social transformations, modernization, or benefits to working-class communities that some had hoped. The new reform campaigns that were developed grappled with the reality that US colonialism and capitalist development had left most Puerto Ricans deeply impoverished. The programs targeted the rural peasant, or *jíbaro*, who was described in state discourses as "backward," "primitive," and in need of the guiding hand of the more educated and privileged classes.[14] While earlier interventions by colonial officials had mustered similar concepts, the Puerto Rican elite of this period reworked discourses, casting themselves as able to carry out social and economic transformations where US officials had failed. In addition, many of these reforms specifically targeted gendered reforms because of the widespread entry of working-class women into the waged labor force.

In 1930, twenty-eight young women who had recently graduated from the University of Puerto Rico's Normal School applied for a new training program in social work developed by the Department of Education.[15] The cohort was chosen to be placed in a new type of rural educational initiative called the Segundas Unidades Rurales (SUR), or Second Unit Rural Schools.[16] The schools were meant to provide secondary education in rural areas that represented a new turn toward vocational education with an emphasis on community development. These programs aimed to provide "practical" education, shaping new workers and citizens, rather than centering the curriculum on academic training.[17] They were part of a larger state project, begun in the late 1920s, that sought to "modernize" Puerto Rico through intervention in the lives of the rural poor. Before the social workers departed for their new positions the women took summer courses at the University of Puerto Rico in social work, including casework methods and public health. In a photograph of the social workers from this period, they are shown gathered together, attending a conference at a public health clinic in Caguas (figure 2.1). They were expected to travel to rural areas and begin conducting casework and initiating community development projects in the communities surrounding the schools.

Among the social work students of this generation were women like Carmen Rivera de Alvarado, who had strong connections to socialist, feminist, and independence-oriented activism.[18] Rivera de Alvarado was raised in a socialist household, and her practice as a social worker was deeply impacted by her youth witnessing socialist and anarchist women in roles as political leaders.[19] She applied for the social work program because it was an opportunity to help support her family during the Depression and to participate in major social transformations. According to Rivera de Alvarado,

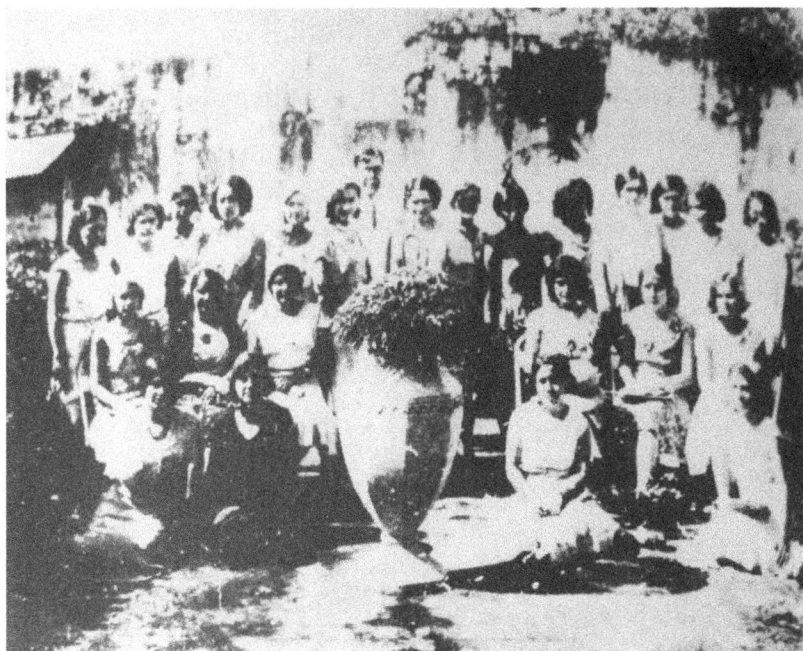

FIGURE 2.1. Social workers at a public health clinic in Caguas, 1931. Source: Carmen Rivera de Alvarado, *Lucha y visión de Puerto Rico libre* (Río Piedras: T. Rivera de Ríos, 1986), 128.

the interview process was difficult, and she wasn't initially accepted into the program because she didn't have the right family connections. However, after she protested her rejection, she and several other women who were not from elite families and who were socialists were admitted.[20] The entry of these women into the profession would change it from one primarily identified with elite women in the previous decade, opening new possibilities for working-class and middle-class women to join its ranks. The social workers would receive training in social work at the University of Puerto Rico taught by US and Puerto Rican reformers, including women of an earlier generation, like seasoned social worker Beatriz Lassalle del Valle.[21]

The social workers in the SUR were trained in rural social work and community-oriented social work, which emphasized rural development and "modernization." In part, this resulted from the type of rural social work they learned from Dorothy Bourne, a social worker from the United States who was the director of the training program (figure 2.2).[22] Bourne and her husband, James Bourne, were friends of President Franklin D. Roosevelt and

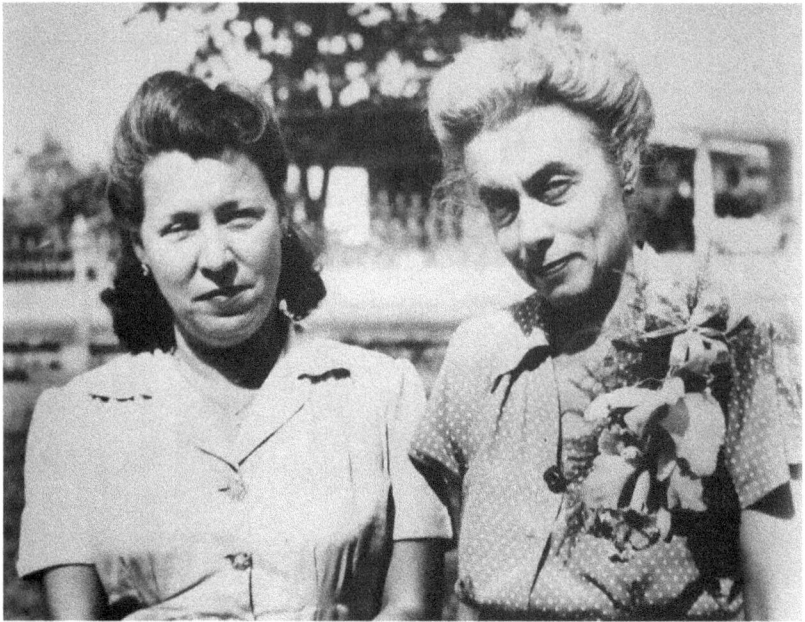

FIGURE 2.2. Dorothy Bourne (*right*) and Carmen Rivera de Alvarado, as seen in a framed photograph displayed at the Department of Social Work at the University of Puerto Rico, Río Piedras, 2012. Photograph by the author.

his wife, Eleanor Roosevelt, who became leaders of New Deal programs on the archipelago.[23] The goal of social work in the SUR was to promote vocational education. Social workers were first called "visiting teachers" and tasked with making the schools operate like community centers. The director of the SUR, Francisco Vizcarrondo, wrote of social workers that "her principle duty is to visit families, study their needs and help them solve their social, economic and sanitary problems."[24] The entire first group of social workers placed were all women, and the role was defined as one that emphasized visiting the homes of working-class families, often speaking with women about their homes and children.

Within the SUR, social workers developed programs that promoted gendered divisions of labor and female domesticity, which also underscored the value of social reproductive labor to national development. The rural social work project aimed to promote vocational education that would train rural inhabitants to be workers on small independent farms or waged workers in industries like needlework, construction, or canneries. The vocational education program was deeply gendered, with farm work imagined as seg-regated between the male breadwinner and housewife and industrial work being segregated along gendered lines, with women increasingly working in the needle trades.[25] The importance of gendered occupational segregation in the programs can be seen in the social workers' role in managing "model homes" at the schools. The model homes were places where working-class children were instructed in gender-segregated vocational education, play-ing out the role of farmer/male breadwinner and housewife.[26] Girls were instructed in home economics programs, which mainly envisioned women's work as care work and work mainly done within the home as housewives, or sometimes done outside of it caring for wages. The home economics pro-gram was described as preparing the "country girl" to "be a useful woman in society, contributing in great measure to the happiness of the rural home."[27] Programs like the model homes promoted women's work and the labor of social reproduction within the patriarchal home as dignified and valuable work that supported both the family unit and national development.

In rural communities, reformers working in the SUR witnessed increasing numbers of rural working-class women entering waged work, and they were drawn into debates over how to regulate this labor and improve working con-ditions. The SUR taught some women skills that would prepare them for waged work outside the home, particularly in the growing needlework trades. For girls, the courses of study included hand embroidery, machine embroidery, lace making with machinery, lace making by hand, *mundillo* lace making, cooking, and "social welfare."[28] For many working-class women, their par-ticipation in the home needlework industry had made their homes the site of waged labor, which they did in addition to reproductive labor. At the time, growing numbers of working-class women also organized labor unions and advocated for and debated proposed labor protections.[29]

Social workers in the SUR sometimes found their work dovetailing with that of social workers employed by the Puerto Rican Department of Labor, including those spearheading reform efforts under the Women's Bureau of the Department of Labor.[30] They were called on by other government agen-cies to share information about new labor standards and regulations that impacted women and children, mainly through regulating child labor. Dur-ing this period, the seasoned social worker Felicia Boria, a socialist feminist labor organizer, was the head of the Negociado de la Mujer y el Niño en la In-dustria (Bureau of the Woman and Child in Industry), which was a part of the Department of Labor.[31] Boria had been born in Puerta de Tierra to an Afro-Puerto Rican father who was a dockworker, and she grew up surrounded by labor organizing.[32] She was an active member of the Federación Libre de Trabajadores (Free Federation of Workers) and had been the secretary of socialist leader Prudencio Rivera Martínez.[33] At the time she helped oversee the application of new labor standards to Puerto Rico and also later became a leader in the social work field.

The work of SUR social workers regulating and managing labor in rural areas included investigating whether children were employed by industries, which they sometimes determined through home visits, and which placed them in positions like that of truant officers, enforcing children's school attendance.[34] In their roles promoting and regulating women's waged labor in gender-segregated occupations, social workers increasingly embraced the idea that women's waged labor represented a growing reality for Puerto Rican families and communities.[35] Some social workers' connections with labor organizers and reformers made them increasingly supportive of labor protections for women wage earners.

Social workers' involvement in social reform was also closely connected to their work supporting public health projects that addressed maternal health and distributed birth control. Scholars have documented how maternal health programs in Puerto Rico were sites of significant interventions into the lives of working-class women's reproductive lives.[36] Within maternal health clinics, Puerto Rican and US government officials and pharmaceutical companies tested new forms of birth control and sometimes promoted sterilization. Historian Laura Briggs has shown how through their work in maternal health programs, social workers like Carmen Rivera de Alvarado embraced ideas of "progressive eugenics," in which ideas about eugenics were melded with progressive programs aimed at providing health and material assistance to poor people.[37] Briggs further notes that the forms of eugenics advocated by these reformers were often a part of liberal and leftist social projects in which women reformers played a key role. After working at the SUR, Rivera de Alvarado would specifically oversee the development of birth control clinics throughout the island. Rivera de Alvarado understood her promotion of birth control as something that was empowering to working-class women who did not have access to the same tools to regulate their reproduction as elite women.[38] However, the programs she helped create would soon become the subject of major controversy and debate on the archipelago as the programs directly conflicted with various political actors and the Catholic Church.[39] In addition, the programs, and the vision of eugenics she espoused, would later be decried by feminist activists who viewed them as having disempowering and violent legacies in working-class communities.[40]

As the social work program at the University of Puerto Rico expanded and growing numbers of Puerto Rican women entered professional roles working on gendered reform projects, they also found employment on social scientific studies. Through their roles on social science projects, social workers became a part of a growing number of women collecting data for health and social science research on the archipelago. Scholars and government agencies used this data in numerous texts and reports about rural communities. For example, information about the social work conducted in the SUR became the subject of a larger social science research project that drew on the case file information collected by social workers. The project was published as a study in *Rural Life in Puerto Rico* by Dorothy Bourne and Luz Ramos, the director of home economics at the University of Puerto Rico.[41] The Bourne and Ramos study explored the living conditions of rural workers and attempted to measure and document how modernization and development could effect change in their lives.

Among the social workers trained at the University of Puerto Rico in these years, one group became leaders of the nationalist and independence movements on the archipelago in the following decades. In the 1930s, the University of Puerto Rico campus was a hotbed of political activism, and some social work students quickly joined organizations dedicated to the archipelago's independence. Among them was Blanca Canales, a young woman who attended meetings at the home of nationalist leader Pedro Albizu Campos while training to be a social worker.[42] Canales brought other social work students with her to the meetings, including Isabel Rosado Morales, after which both women became leaders in the independence movement.[43] The group also included Carmen Rivera de Alvarado, who later wrote about the life-changing impact that her years as a student had on her political formation as a socialist and advocate of independence.[44] These social workers linked their work in rural social work with their nationalist activism, envisioning the social work they had developed as something radical, something different than mainstream social work, something that Canales called "social work of the people."[45]

The participation of social workers in creating new reform projects in the SUR opened a new space for them to be educated and join larger political projects. As these social workers created gendered reform projects that targeted working-class women, they also became involved in debates and discussions over women's labor and rights in Puerto Rican society. Some of these reformers would also link their social work in local communities with their feminist, socialist, and nationalist activism in other concurrent social movements. Within only a few years of the creation of the first social welfare training program at the University of Puerto Rico, there was a cohort of young women ready to move forward with political activism entwined with their vision of social work.

Women, Work, and Struggles over "Relief" in New Deal Puerto Rico

On August 19, 1933, President Franklin D. Roosevelt named James Bourne, the husband of Dorothy Bourne, to be director of the newly founded PRERA, which managed new social service and relief programs in Puerto Rico, initially modeled on existing US programs.[46] In collaboration with Puerto Rican officials, US officials spearheaded the administration of this reformist colonial project, which marked the beginning of the New Deal in Puerto Rico. Bourne noted in PRERA's first annual report that the Great Depression and two major hurricanes had left Puerto Rico "perhaps at the lowest point in its history," with a growing population and widespread poverty. However, despite these hardships, "given the opportunity Puerto Rico can become a self-sustaining and creditable part of the American nation."[47] Bourne and many other US and Puerto Rican officials believed PRERA provided "the opportunity to prove this." In this vision, the New Deal might even result in the full integration of Puerto Rico into the United States. His reflections also highlight how, from its creation, PRERA was viewed as distinct from US programs of relief because it was also imagined as an agency that would develop and modernize Puerto Rico.[48] Bourne was charged with transforming the archipelago via an ambitious development project to rework the decades-long imperial project already underway in Puerto Rico. The underlying imperialist notion, however, predicated on racist assumptions that Puerto Rico needed the guiding hand of US civilization, remained largely unchallenged during the New Deal.[49]

Although the US-based New Deal project rested largely on providing relief to male breadwinners supporting their families, these concepts were far from the real and lived experience of Puerto Ricans. Women's activism in Puerto Rico during the period pushed the state to recognize that women were workers who depended on wage labor to support their families and communities. Demanding work, not relief, these women questioned the gendered discrimination that they faced within New Deal organizations. The early PRERA programs embraced the idea of Puerto Rican women as breadwinners via work-relief programs and expanding vocational education programs for women and girls, creating relief and training programs for women across economic classes. Bourne's wife, the social worker Dorothy Bourne, had already developed the social work training program for the Puerto Rican government and trained Puerto Rican women for placement in rural schools, whose curricula specifically targeted women, work, and reproduction.[50]

In implementing these New Deal reforms, the Puerto Rican government was actively categorizing people along gender, race, and class lines that had immediate consequences in their daily lives. PRERA's assistant director, Rafaela Espino, noted that the Social Service Division was especially important—the "parent Bureau of the whole Administration"—because the entire PRERA project, and arguably the New Deal as a whole in Puerto Rico, rested on separating out those whom state officials had determined deserved relief.[51] Social workers developed casework methods and means of testing to determine eligibility for relief, while also creating a bureaucracy to manage this new knowledge about the population. They built both direct-relief programs that distributed food and monetary payments and work-relief programs that offered paid employment on state-run projects.[52] The gendered segregation of social work had continued under the New Deal, and the vast majority of social workers were women.[53] In their new administrative roles in PRERA, they became the representatives of the New Deal in Puerto Rico and played a central role in administering PRERA relief and labor programs.[54] In so doing, they also reinforced separations in Puerto Rican society along both class and gender lines. The creation of work-relief programs specifically for women who had high school and college degrees also enabled applicants for relief to become PRERA administrators and social workers.

A "white-collar" work program placed workers considered skilled or educated into administrative positions in the agency itself. Because there were not enough trained social workers to staff the PRERA programs, its directors decided to hire untrained social work aides, managed by the trained social workers who became the agency's directors.[55] According to Espino, "In the beginning, investigators were taken from relief rolls on the basis of their own need for relief rather than preparation for the service."[56] While the agency tried to hire only district directors and bureau heads with professional social work training, the demand for social workers was too high, and aides were also placed in executive positions. Thus, growing numbers of applicants for relief entered administrative roles in PRERA, expanding the professional ranks. In its placement of aides, the New Deal opened up new spaces for social mobility: Not all government agents came from elite or middle-class backgrounds.[57]

While some women qualified for professional jobs like those in PRERA, the majority of applicants were sent to a separate Women's Work Division. This agency was created to give "relief to a comparatively large group and class of people" who "are not well enough prepared to be able to take advantage of the White Collar Relief."[58] The majority were employed in a state-sponsored home needlework program and were given cloth pieces they made into garments in exchange for relief tokens. The program had a "secondary relief aspect, because the majority of items were distributed to other relief applicants through the Social Service Division." In this way, relief applicants were put to work creating goods that could be used by other poor Puerto Ricans. The creation of a government-sponsored needlework program shored up the already existing home needlework economy that, despite declines during the Depression, remained the largest employer of women on the archipelago.[59] Through their work in this industry, Puerto Rican women already had become active members of the labor force and were providing crucial financial support to their families. And the centrality of labor programs for women within PRERA illustrates the growing concern among policymakers about providing work for women, unlike the US-based New Deal project focused on male breadwinners.

One way women in the needlework industry organized in the period was by creating unions of the "unemployed" that led massive strikes around the archipelago.[60] Women's demands for work challenged assumptions that Puerto Ricans were content with receiving state relief.[61] Women faced greater job insecurity, because regulations of the needlework industry had led many companies to abandon Puerto Rico to find cheaper labor elsewhere. Moreover, women often felt alienated from labor unions. Their main concern involved their right to employment, and they were sometimes willing to accept lower wages in order to support their families.[62] This in turn caused friction between them and labor organizations and reformers.[63] Felicia Boria, a social worker who became the director of Puerto Rico's Bureau of Women and Children in Industry, spoke openly about the negative impact that protective legislation had on many working women. Administrators believed that the need for training women in needlework would "remain after relief work [had] ended."[64]

PRERA social workers created twenty-five new "industrial schools," similar to the ongoing vocational programs in home economics that were already taught in the public schools. PRERA estimated that 13,216 people (including students and their families) were financially benefiting from these work-relief salaries. The quantification of this number suggests that New Deal reformers were acutely aware of the centrality of women's and girls' work in supporting families and communities. Women and girls were "given courses in cooking, sewing, administration of the home, hygiene and care of the sick, and servant training." The program also provided immediate work relief, in that students were paid one dollar a week for their participation. This was in addition to the larger goal of the program, according to its directors: to "prepare girls to earn a living."

Social workers also managed a larger network of other programs that targeted women and children, including distribution centers where direct relief in the form of food and financial support were provided to some workers and their families. In addition to work relief, social workers helped develop an expansive health service network that provided free medical care, milk stations to distribute milk to mothers of small children, and school lunch programs in public schools, run in collaboration with parent and teacher associations.[65] PRERA also developed nursery schools for poor families, which social workers claimed "lay the foundation for a 'sound mind in a sound body' and thus prevent these tots from becoming social problems when they are adults." Social workers also created maternal health programs, some of which disseminated birth control, which became a topic of great controversy.[66] The maternal and child welfare programs that were created by social workers during this period would remain central parts of New Deal reform programs initiated on the archipelago in the years that followed (figure 2.3).

Throughout their public health work, social workers and public health nurses lectured working-class people about proper nutrition and parenting. In doing so, they drew on popular ideas of progressive eugenics that promoted the idea that a healthy nation would result from interventions in the health, hygiene, and moral lives of poor citizens.[67] Such discourse and attendant policy often targeted the bodies and lives of working-class women for reform and created a host of racist policies that were deployed by the US and Puerto Rican governments. New Deal reforms and relief were also instrumental in shaping racial politics in Puerto Rico. Scholarship on such social reforms as public health projects, slum clearance programs, and the creation of public housing projects has drawn attention to how these programs served as places of exclusion where Puerto Ricans of African descent faced

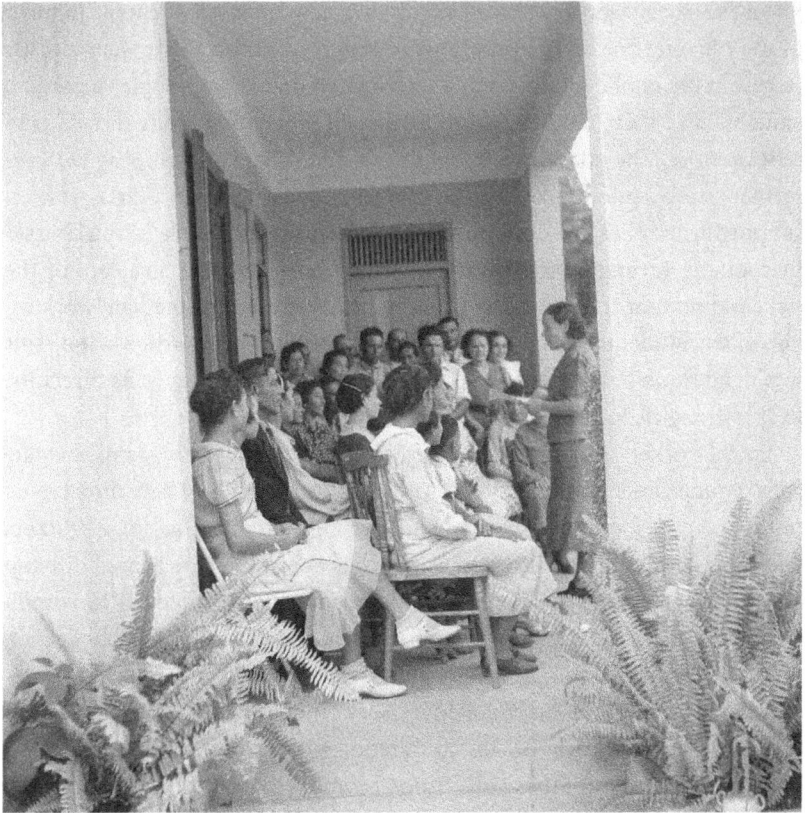

FIGURE 2.3. Class in maternal and child welfare directed by the Puerto Rico Recon-struction Administration in January 1938. Photograph by Edwin Rosskam. Courtesy of the Farm Security Administration, Office of War Information Photograph Collection, Library of Congress, Washington, DC.

discrimination and marginalization.[68] In any case, it is clear that through their work for PRERA, social workers had become state experts whose work specifically targeted interventions in the lives of working-class women and the creation of relief programs for women.

Social Workers, Liberal Reform, and Political Mobilization in the 1930s

As social workers developed and implemented PRERA's activities, they be-came increasingly important political actors in Puerto Rico. Their work in the organization also provided them with a platform from which they claimed a new professional status and advocated for the archipelago to be covered by the federal social welfare provisions that emerged out of New Deal reform. At the same time as social workers gained increasing political power in Puerto Rico, New Deal agencies, their representatives, and the social workers staffing them also came under harsh criticism from opponents. Social workers fought among themselves about professionalization, and tensions emerged between them and both New Deal reformers, who had different visions of what the goals of these reforms should be, and opponents of the growing power of the New Deal liberal political coalition that began to dominate Puerto Rican politics. The arguments sparked by these tensions would eventually lead to the dismantling of PRERA and its relief programs in favor of a new economic development program, which would shift the emphasis of New Deal programs on the archipelago while continuing to employ large numbers of social workers. By the late 1930s, professional social workers and the vision of broad social welfare coverage they promoted would become an increasingly important force in Puerto Rican politics. Moreover, these social workers would also become central figures in the movement for broader coverage for Puerto Rico under federal social welfare provisions.

The challenges faced by social workers during the 1930s resulted from PRERA's being linked to the rise of a new liberal and reformist political coalition led by Luis Muñoz Marín, a politician's son who emerged as one of the architects of this new vision of colonial reform. The most transformative of these reforms was the drafting of the Chardón Plan, a new development and land redistribution program that Luis Muñoz Marín had played a central role in creating.[69] The Chardón Plan outlined a project of agricultural rehabilitation that would break US sugar estates into small farms and distribute them to farmers. The US and Puerto Rican reformers who produced this vision argued that a planning approach, led by liberal social scientists and Puerto Rican technocrats, could gradually transform Puerto Rico into a modern and industrialized society. The first step in this direction was the creation of a new relief agency called the Puerto Rico Reconstruction Administration (PRRA) in 1935. The new agency was placed under the directorship of Ernest Gruening, a liberal journalist, future territorial governor of Alaska, and later Democratic senator from Alaska. In 1933, Gruening was named director of the Division of Territories and Possessions of the Department of the Interior. Within this new organization, social workers would continue to be charged with ushering in societal transformations; however, the focus of the programs would shift.

The main role of the PRRA was to expand development-oriented work-relief programs. Gruening and his supporters believed this new approach would create lasting change in Puerto Rico, rather than providing immediate relief and direct assistance as PRERA had done. Puerto Rico began liquidating the older agency shortly after the new agency was created, despite the protests of many former administrators. Those who had worked for PRERA were critical of the new agency, which they believed ended programs that were working well and that should be continued. In particular, they drew attention to the fact that the new organization reflected the state's reorientation toward creating new labor camps for men that targeted them as male breadwinners. In short, it was a move away from work-relief programs for women. This move also alienated many of the New Dealers who had first worked on the archipelago, such as the Bournes. However, the new agency's creation did not mean a total end to relief programs, and many social workers found work in the new organization (figure 2.4). Among them was Rafaela Espino, whom the Puerto Rican government hired to oversee the transition from the PRERA to PRRA. In 1935, Espino helped develop a new Unidad de Servicio Social (Unified Social Service) in the PRRA.[70] She noted that after 1936, this program was broadened into the Section of Social Service, which focused on working with rural families. She also noted that in each of the twenty labor camps created, there was a *visitante social* (visiting social worker) and that, out of these, twelve were trained social workers while the others held bachelor of arts degrees. Through their work for PRRA, social workers like Espino continued to play central roles in shaping the New Deal project in Puerto Rico. However, tensions over resource allocation and the roles of New Deal officials and social workers in the government would continue to plague the agency moving forward.

At the same time that social workers organized professionally on the archipelago, they faced growing challenges to their authority and their work from those opposed to the New Dealers' role in the growing liberal political coalition. As New Deal employees, the social workers saw their activities linked to the reforms put forward by US and Puerto Rican agents in the liberal coalition. Those who viewed the emerging New Deal liberal political coalition as a threat to a more conservative political vision, as well as supporters of the growing independence movement on the archipelago, critiqued social workers. Social workers faced some of the harshest reprisals and attacks on New Deal agencies because of the work they did as New Deal agents. Opponents of the New Deal group and Muñoz Marín saw New Deal organizations like PRERA as part of a politically biased patronage program,

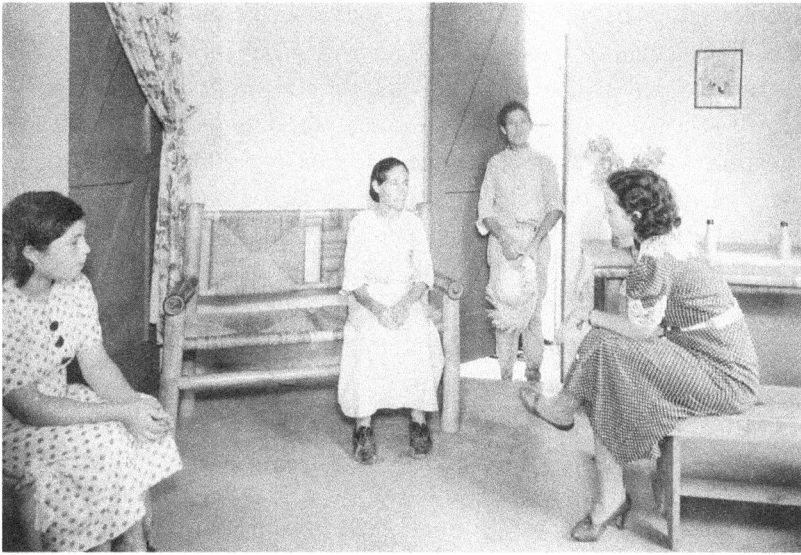

FIGURE 2.4. Social worker (*right*) employed by the Puerto Rico Reconstruction Administration meeting with a family. Courtesy of La Colección de Fotografías de la Puerto Rico Reconstruction Administration, Colección Puertorriqueña, University of Puerto Rico, Río Piedras.

and they questioned social workers about the objectivity of the agency and its distribution of resources.[71]

Social workers responded to the shifting political terrain they faced within New Deal agencies and the growing influence they held in New Deal reform programs by beginning to organize professionally. They hoped to claim a new status both within local communities and in their relationship to the US administration on the archipelago. Professional organization revealed tensions among social workers around class, status, race, and education, even as new alliances developed that would have lasting impact on the political mobilization of women in Puerto Rico. Tensions among social workers mirrored the ongoing and overlapping class and racial hierarchies that had plagued the Puerto Rican suffrage movement during the period.[72] Elite women pushed for the exclusion of women they considered lower in status because of their class and racial backgrounds.[73] Professionalization generally also provided the social workers with a new platform for organizing around the inclusion of Puerto Ricans under federal social policies and for an expansion of the benefits of territorial citizenship.

Some of the first discussions about professionalization surfaced shortly after the creation of PRERA, when a number of social work aides were hired to staff the agency. Some social workers, objecting to the aides being considered social workers, proposed that the profession be regulated.[74] The members of the Porto Rico Association of Trained Social Workers—a group educated in US schools, including many older social workers who had been involved with earlier charitable and public health organizations before the New Deal—led this call for professionalization. They argued that social work should be licensed and that both aides and social workers who had been trained at the University of Puerto Rico should have to apply to be licensed.[75] The social worker Georgina Pastor, who had been educated at the University of Puerto Rico, noted that "the word 'trained' in the title of this Association came to be a type of insult" aimed at social workers who didn't have US educations.[76] Pastor also stated that its members "obviously were trying to create a classist organization, representing the so called 'niñas bien' [rich girls] of the middle and upper classes." According to another social worker, Blanca Canales, most of the group "began to look down on social workers" and "said that we didn't have the necessary education to call ourselves social workers."[77] The struggle among social workers continued as their numbers increased dramatically because of the demand for their services in the New Deal projects.

New Deal administrators responded in varied ways to the campaign to license social workers. Some, believing the need for practitioners of social work outweighed these concerns, were against regulation. Some explicitly believed regulation was a way of policing the upward social mobility of working-class women—in other words, that it was a way to restrict the expansion of a field that created more professional jobs for women. Despite these protests, in 1934, social work was regulated with the passage of a new public welfare law, later considered the first law of its kind in the Americas.[78] Shortly afterward, a *junta examinadora* (review board) was created by the insular government, which issued permanent and provisional licenses to social workers. The first junta, appointed by the Puerto Rican government, was comprised of social workers representing what were considered the main groups within the field. Then a new professional organization that included all licensed social workers, called the Sociedad Insular de Trabajadores Sociales (Island Society of Social Workers; SITS), was created in April 1935. The organization elected as its first president, the socialist social work leader Carmen Rivera de Alvarado.[79] Professional organizations provided new platforms for social workers to organize around their own labor and to debate and discuss the politics of labor in the greater community.

Attacks on PRERA sought to undermine social workers' authority in a variety of ways. Critics argued that social workers were promoting immoral living among their clients. The Catholic Church joined the charge against New Deal programs by specifically targeting the creation of maternal health programs that provided birth control. Catholic priests in Puerto Rico, including Father Raymond McGowan, also argued that social workers lacked proper professional training and were running a disorganized agency. As evidence, McGowan pointed to articles published in PRERA's journal *La Rehabilitación* that, he claimed, promoted free love and birth control and advocated against marriage, the family, and the home. Dorothy Bourne countered that while there were flaws in the social work program, the program had done much good.[80] Bourne sidestepped many of the questions about birth control, saying that such questions were in the hands of doctors and nurses rather than social workers. However, the attack was successful in restricting the social work programs that were under way and also in putting pressure on political figures to end the maternal health programs that they had already created.

As disagreements between New Deal agencies and their opponents fermented, new tensions within the liberal coalition intensified, and social workers were caught in the crossfire. Some of the most damaging political challenges to New Deal agencies like PRERA would come from within their own ranks, out of tensions between US and Puerto Rican agents and their differing visions about the archipelago's needs and future. After the Ponce Massacre on March 21, 1937, the political tensions within the New Deal agencies came to a head. Nineteen people were killed and two hundred wounded when police attacked a march protesting the arrest of nationalist leader Pedro Albizu Campos. US officials in Puerto Rico responded in different ways to the uprisings. For her part, Dorothy Bourne published an article on the state of social welfare in Puerto Rico that addressed the Ponce Massacre and argued that the colonial situation in Puerto Rico could not be ignored or avoided. A primary issue that faced any project on the archipelago, particularly that of social workers, she contended, was a "colonial psychology" that impacted all of their work and hindered what they were trying to accomplish.[81] Bourne's sympathies were with the social workers: She became increasingly disheartened by the limitations of the colonial project that she had played a central role in constructing as she worked alongside and became close friends with nationalist women like Rivera de Alvarado.[82]

On the other hand, Gruening grew reverently anti-independence and more broadly antinationalist, a stance that would lead to a political break with Muñoz Marín and other Puerto Rican liberals.[83] He had arrived there with a liberal vision of Puerto Rican politics and optimistic about the role of the United States in transforming the archipelago, and he was shocked to witness the growing support for the independence movement in Puerto Rico. Shortly after the Ponce Massacre, Gruening began a purge of state officials he deemed sympathetic to supporters of independence, attacking, among others, the leaders of PRERA, including the Bournes.[84] Despite Gruening's attacks, James Bourne was kept on the staff of PRRA and given the directorship of the relief aspects of the agency. However, he abandoned the position afterward because of the political tensions that continued to plague the agency's work.[85] Nevertheless, the political shake-up within government organizations resulted in the dismissal and blacklisting of a number of social workers seen as ardent nationalists or potential supporters of the independence movement. Finding a job as a social worker with nationalist politics became increasingly difficult, as government agencies became politically charged terrain. However, many survived the political purge of workers during the period and continued to play central roles in state agencies.

As social workers continued to face political challenges on the archipelago, they became increasingly involved in professional organizations. They also found that the social welfare organizations they created provided a new and expanded platform for engaging in US politics and discussions about the extension of federal policy to the archipelago. Working for New Deal organizations, they had seen firsthand the impact of US welfare policy in Puerto Rico, and they began to seek ways to influence the implementation of those relief programs in Puerto Rico. The professional organizational meetings they held became spaces where social workers discussed how to influence and lobby the US government and Congress for increased funding and coverage under social welfare provisions. The first assembly of the professional social work organization SITS, in Río Piedras, was a formative moment in the development of the field because it created a new platform for political organization and debate among social workers. Its members used these meetings to lobby the insular and federal governments for the expansion of social welfare services.

Social workers also organized for more local agencies and for federal coverage under the Social Security Act of 1935. The first task the social workers' professional organization addressed was developing strategies to advocate for the creation of a Department of Public Welfare in the Puerto

Rican government, a task that would require changes to the Organic Act of the archipelago. One of the organizers, Carmen Rivera de Alvarado, noted that "cent by cent they raised the funds to send a delegation to Washington in April 1936 to solicit the Resident Commissioner, socialist Don Santiago Iglesias," to present a law authorizing the creation of this department.[86] They also discussed the recent passage of the Social Security Act and began to articulate demands that its policies cover Puerto Rico. The organization raised more money to send delegations to US social work meetings and exerted pressure on US reformers to change the law. Social workers also wrote emphatic letters to the US Congress arguing that the archipelago should be included under the Social Security Act.

The social workers sent leaders in the field to present their work in front of the House of Representatives. The group included Beatriz Lassalle, Celestina Zalduondo, and María Pintado de Rahn.[87] This group exemplified how social work in Puerto Rico had rapidly become a platform for women's political activism. Lassalle had been collaborating closely with social welfare officials in Washington, DC, since she had been enlisted to work with the US Children's Bureau in 1920. Zalduondo also had already established herself in the field working for the Department of Public Health in Puerto Rico as a psychiatric social worker before becoming director of Social Services under PRERA and then working closely with US reformers in Puerto Rico under the New Deal.[88] Pintado de Rahn was another social worker with extensive connections to US social workers. She had studied at Smith College and the School of Social Work in New York (1930–1931) before enrolling at the School of Social Services at the University of Chicago, where she studied with social reformer Grace Abbott and obtained her master's degree in 1936.[89] Abbott discussed the extension of social policy to Puerto Rico with Pintado de Rahn and supported her work in Washington by having "introduction letters" to politicians sent by herself, her sister Edith Abbott, and Sophonsiba Breckinridge.[90] These letters helped the Puerto Rican social workers advance their cause as they continued lobbying.

While at first these petitions were unsuccessful, they signaled new types of organizing by professional social workers that would continue over the ensuing years. Social workers maintained pressure on professional organizations, unions, social welfare leaders, and US Congress members to expand social welfare provisions to Puerto Rico. They framed these arguments around the United States' responsibilities toward all its citizens, challenging the United States to more expansively include Puerto Rico under social policy. Thus, the social work organization that had been created to regulate professional status was now taking on a new role, providing the social workers with a platform to intervene as experts and lobbyists. Social workers' reach and influence would only grow as the labor migrations of Puerto Ricans put the legacy of US empire, New Deal relief programs, and Puerto Rico under a US spotlight in the years to come.

Labor Migrants, Social Welfare, and the Shifting Terrain of Puerto Rican Political Organizing

The migration of Puerto Ricans to the United States in the 1930s changed the discussion about Puerto Rican inclusion in New Deal programs. Although social workers in Puerto Rico were overwhelmed by the local demand for relief, they were also drawn into efforts to help New York City deal with a small but substantial Puerto Rican population. In 1910, fewer than two thousand Puerto Ricans lived in the continental United States, but this number grew to an estimated 52,774 in 1930 and to nearly seventy thousand by 1940.[91] Migrants, while legally entitled to full citizenship in the United States, faced the same types of racist discrimination other "nonwhite" people encountered in the United States. Trying to claim social services and find housing in US cities was one of the first areas where Puerto Ricans encountered racism in the United States.[92]

In the 1930s, in an attempt to address the needs of the growing migrant worker population in the United States, the Puerto Rican Department of Labor created an office called the Bureau of Employment and Identification.[93] Because migrants were often thought to be foreign and were frequently denied jobs and services, the agency provided identification cards that Puerto Ricans could use to prove their US citizenship.[94] During the same period, the Puerto Rican government gave grants to sponsor numerous Puerto Rican social workers to study and work in the United States. Some of these social workers specifically became involved in the Puerto Rican government's efforts to address the racism and xenophobia that Puerto Rican labor migrants faced. Through their work advocating on behalf of migrants, social workers became increasingly involved in Puerto Rican demands for access to the benefits of US citizenship in the continental United States.

When migrants applied for social services, their rights to the benefits of US citizenship came under close scrutiny.[95] While the number of Puerto Rican applicants for relief was actually quite small, the New York City press, fueled by imperialist and racialized visions of Puerto Ricans, printed numerous articles about the "Puerto Rican Problem" of migration and relief dependency. At the same time, many New York social service agencies actively discriminated against applicants, using stricter residency requirements as a justification. Some welfare agencies in New York even created "resettlement" programs for Puerto Rican applicants, which returned migrants to the archipelago.[96] While the number of these cases might have been small, their creation initiated a new relationship between social welfare agencies in New York and Puerto Rico.

United States social service agencies corresponded with emerging Puerto Rican social welfare agencies about migrants through a new Interagency Services Bureau. Puerto Rican social workers examined the cases the United States sent them and sometimes conducted follow-up casework with migrants' family members on the archipelago. In cases where social workers decided that return migration was advisable, information was sent back to New York, and in some cases, the New York agency would fund the client's transportation back to Puerto Rico. Beatriz Lassalle managed the Puerto Rican side of this program.[97] Lassalle hired Frances Adkins Hall, a social worker from the United States who had worked for the Children's Bureau of the US Department of Labor, to establish new ways of handling the cases.[98] Hall's first project in Puerto Rico was to conduct a study, for the National Association of Social Workers branch in Puerto Rico, of social service agencies on the archipelago. She stayed on to reorganize the work of the Interagency Services Bureau in the aftermath of PRERA.

Hall began her work by overseeing a study of the "transportation cases" US agencies referred to Puerto Rican social welfare officials. The first part, "The Problem of the Migration of Indigent Puerto Ricans to and from New York City," was published in the bulletin of Puerto Rico's Department of Health.[99] Students studying social work at the University of Puerto Rico assisted Hall in the work. The research compared casework conducted during the height of PRERA with that done while it was being dismantled; the idea was to trace how the organization's end affected social services, clients, and migration. According to her report, PRERA had provided funding to help with migrant cases and had overseen "resettlement cases," which ended with the liquidation of the agency. In particular, the report noted, changes in New York's residency requirements after 1937 placed Puerto Rican migrant applicants for assistance at a disadvantage. As a result of this research, Lassalle asked Hall to oversee the revamping of the Interagency Services Bureau's casework processes, which the bureau hoped would reduce the amount of staff labor needed. Hall created form letters and new systems to track the "transportation cases." In doing so, she was contributing to ongoing bureaucratic production aimed at managing information about migrants. The work that Lassalle and Hall conducted points to migration as a growing concern of social service workers.

At the same time that Puerto Rican officials began managing migrant casework, they also sought to shape US policy by appealing to US elected officials with Puerto Rican constituents—most importantly, to Vito Marcantonio, an Italian American congressman in New York City who became a central advocate for Puerto Rican migrants in the United States.[100] A socialist who supported labor organizations, Marcantonio built a relationship with the Puerto Rican community and employed Spanish-speaking assistants specifically to help Puerto Ricans. Marcantonio increasingly operated in a colonial field of politics, and Puerto Rican government agencies corresponded with him about numerous concerns.[101] On both the local and state levels, Puerto Ricans sought political representation through Marcantonio because they had no other channels of support. In 1936, Geraldine Froscher, the director of interagency services for PRERA, wrote to Marcantonio about the liquidation of the department's agencies. Froscher, a feminist who had lived and worked in Puerto Rico for many years and participated in the suffrage movement, warned Marcantonio that the end of PRERA programs and social services would result in increased migration and demand for social services in the United States, particularly in New York City.[102]

The social workers suggested that unless social citizenship rights were extended to the archipelago, further disequilibrium would ensue, and Puerto Ricans would be drawn to the United States, where their citizenship was worth more and where they could access relief benefits that were increasingly unavailable on the archipelago. Froscher's letter also points to how the connections New Deal agencies in Puerto Rico had developed between social welfare offices via interagency services allowed them to track migrants and, to a certain extent, regulate migration. She stated emphatically that "unless some provision is made to continue the present set-up of relief in Puerto Rico, or a Dept. of Public Welfare is established in Puerto Rico, we will be unable to continue the assistance that we have been able to give . . . in having Puerto Ricans, who are without legal residence in New York, returned to Puerto Rico."[103] Among the agencies that PRERA helped, Froscher listed the New York State Department of Social Welfare, the New York City Department of Welfare, the New York City Department of Hospitals, the Emergency Relief Bureau, and the Bureau of Unattached and Transients. By highlighting the collaborative work of Puerto Rican New Deal agencies and

US social welfare agencies, Froscher revealed how new conduits of people and information had been created.

New Deal welfareism had bound Puerto Rico and the United States ever more tightly together in a territorial and colonial relationship deepened further by the growing labor migration of Puerto Ricans. The connections between Puerto Rican citizens and the United States could not be undone without invoking consequences that Froscher and others believed would result in more displacement and migration. Initially, New Deal social workers' petitions to Congress for inclusion under the Social Security Act had been unsuccessful, but the migration of Puerto Rican workers and the questions that arose about their rights to benefits provided a new context in which Puerto Rican citizenship was debated and scrutinized. In 1939, when a set of congressional hearings raised the possibility of Puerto Rican coverage under the act, Marcantonio would become one of its most ardent supporters.[104] He would later claim that his work alongside Puerto Rican activists for the partial inclusion of Puerto Rico under the Social Security Act was one of his greatest congressional victories.[105] The demands of Puerto Rican workers and migrants, the organization of Puerto Rican activists, and the professional coalitions of social workers and reformers would all contribute to meaningful change in Puerto Rican social citizenship under US empire.

Legislating Inequality through the Partial Inclusion of Puerto Rico under the Social Security Act

In the end, a new political mood both in Washington, DC, and on the archipelago, as well as years of Puerto Rican social workers' and reformers' lobbying and organizing for access to federal social welfare provisions, helped bring about change, and a broad set of amendments to the Social Security Act in 1939 opened portions of the Social Security Act to Puerto Ricans. While historians have investigated the impact of these amendments on the continental United States, the resultant partial coverage for Puerto Rico has received little attention. But congressional hearings about these amendments did offer a platform for Puerto Rican representatives and their allies to present their case for inclusion under federal social welfare provisions.

The 1939 amendments to the Social Security Act extended the occupational insurance benefits to widows and children of those already covered, dramatically changing its coverage.[106] However, the amendments also reinforced divisions between entitlements for mainly male white workers and "needs-based" programs for single women and their families, which further restricted access to social provisions along racialized and gendered lines. This division would become known in popular discourse as a rift between "Social Security" benefits (meant mostly for white male workers and their families) and the stigmatized and means-tested "welfare" programs (meant for single women and children). The 1939 amendments resulted in part from the political mobilization of social welfare experts in the Children's Bureau of the US Department of Labor, who oversaw the application of certain titles of the act.[107] The Children's Bureau already had a long history of working with Puerto Rican social workers and conducting studies in Puerto Rico, and it was amenable from the start to Puerto Rico's receiving more federal support.[108]

At the same time, Puerto Rico's shifting relationship with the United States and the emergence of a new political party on the archipelago effectively reframed the discussion around Puerto Rican status and inclusion under federal programs. In 1938, Muñoz Marín broke with the Liberal Party and founded the Partido Popular Democrático (PPD), a populist party that sought "bread, land, and liberty" for its people through a program of social reform, social justice, and a "peaceful revolution."[109] Central to the party's goals was the administration of reforms that would help working-class people, in particular the rural working-class *jíbaro*, who became the symbol of PPD leadership and was depicted on the party's flag. The PPD also built on the political networks between the United States and Puerto Rico that were created under the New Deal, and it sought to use social science to guide the development of the archipelago. These changes culminated with the redefinition of Puerto Rico as an Estado Libre Asociado (Free Associated State) or commonwealth. While it would take more than a decade for this change to occur, the new political platform the PPD developed in 1938 had immediate transformative consequences for Puerto Rican citizens. One of the changes was a renewed discussion about Puerto Rican access to federal provisions under the Social Security Act being pushed forward by coalitions of reformers, including Puerto Rican social workers and their allies.

The congressional hearings leading up to the 1939 Social Security amendments provided the perfect venue for Puerto Ricans to present their case. Santiago Iglesias, the nonvoting resident commissioner in Congress, spoke on behalf of Puerto Rico during these hearings, testifying that these amendments provided a crucial opportunity to cover both Puerto Rico and the Virgin Islands under the Social Security Act.[110] "Since the Social Security

Act was first considered by Congress 4 years ago," he noted, "Puerto Rico has been desirous that this law be extended to the archipelago for the benefit of the people there." Iglesias lamented that Puerto Ricans had no say in how they were covered, and he emphasized the US Congress's power and responsibility to make these changes on their behalf. Invoking the symbolic rhetoric of Puerto Rican citizenship, Iglesias drew attention to the "1,800,000 loyal American citizens" whose exclusion from the benefits of the act was "unfair."[111]

The limitations on territorial citizenship and their lasting economic consequences also became the subject of congressional testimony. Harold Ickes, the US secretary of the interior under President Roosevelt, submitted a written statement to the hearings, claiming that the "need for aid of this sort in those possessions is at least as great as the States and Territories." He further noted that "Puerto Rico has suffered particularly from legislation designed to benefit American people" but whose "benefits . . . were not applicable to its citizens." Moreover, Ickes saw "no just reason for discriminating against these possessions" by continuing to exclude them from coverage under the Social Security Act. Emphasizing Puerto Ricans' lack of congressional representation, he suggested members of Congress should endeavor to ensure that Puerto Ricans "not suffer economically through their lesser political status." In underscoring how territorial citizens experienced US citizenship, he illuminated the specific economic ramifications of their lack of representation—an issue that would have lasting consequences for Puerto Ricans but that was often elided in political discourse.[112]

Perhaps the most important testimony given at the hearings was Katharine Lenroot's. In her testimony, the director of the Children's Bureau—which oversaw the administration of the maternal and child welfare provisions of the Social Security Act under Title V—highlighted that she had always supported Puerto Rican inclusion under the bill. She also identified the increasingly important role of Puerto Rico as an outpost of US empire, another key issue surrounding Puerto Rican incorporation, stating that Puerto Rico was a "natural link" between the United States and Latin America. Stressing her long-standing relationship with US-trained Puerto Rican social workers and public health administrators, Lenroot asserted that the archipelago was prepared to run the programs if coverage were extended. The Children's Bureau's interest in expanding the reach of its offices into Puerto Rico was, in part, the result of US cultural imperialism and an implicit understanding that US-based reformers could produce transformative colonial policies on the archipelago.[113] The agency already had a long history of involvement in Puerto Rico, and it saw extending social policy to the archipelago as a natural extension of work already under way.

During the congressional hearings on Social Security, Lenroot was questioned about Puerto Rico. This line of inquiry revealed some of the ways US imperialism shaped social legislation. For example, congressman Thomas Jenkins (R, OH) suggested that "of course we recognize the population of Puerto Rico is very dense" and that "they are in a warm climate"; thus, "racially they are very different from the American people, generally speaking." There were numerous such reflections on Puerto Ricans as an inferior people, one distinct from the continental US population. Moreover, Jenkins concluded that because of this racial difference, "their requirements and needs" were "not quite the same" as those of people in the United States. Because Puerto Ricans were "poorer" than those living in the continental United States, uplifting the archipelago would entail "taking on a much bigger load toward them than we are toward our own people."[114] Imperialism and the racialized understandings of Puerto Rican people that it engendered were crucial components of deciding how Puerto Rico should be treated under social policy.

The ways Puerto Rico was understood racially also shaped its partial inclusion under the Social Security Act. In the end, only Title V, popularly known as the "maternal and child welfare provisions," and Title VI, or the "public health" sections, of the Social Security Act were extended to Puerto Rico. The extension of the public health portion of the act mainly proved uncontroversial because US officials supported the construction and maintenance of public health clinics, which had long been a mainstay of the US government on the archipelago. In the congressional hearings, commonplace generalizations about the "overpopulation" of Puerto Rico were specifically cited as evidence of the need for increased public health funding for the archipelago. Of course, the very notion of overpopulation was predicated on US imperialist policy, which was framed by popular understandings of the Puerto Rican people as racially inferior.[115] Moreover, these ideas intersected with US eugenics discourses that emphasized the population control of poor and nonwhite communities, described in terms of "public hygiene," in order to improve the health of the national body.[116] The two titles of the Social Security Act extended to Puerto Rico in 1939 provided very specific types of access to the provisions that were framed by US understandings of Puerto Rican difference.

The titles that were extended thus covered dependents rather than workers, who still could not apply for benefits under the social insurance titles of the act. The division of these types of benefits into separate public assistance acts (meant for dependents) versus social insurance provisions (for male breadwinners in industrial occupations) divided citizens into gendered categories with long-lasting effects. Most applicants for assistance were working mothers, who were imagined as state dependents needing charity but not entitled to the same benefits as male workers.[117] These programs marked a major shift away from creating New Deal programs in Puerto Rico under PRERA, which had recognized women as workers and created work-relief programs to benefit their families. That the broader social insurance titles covering some industrial workers were not extended to Puerto Rico, while the public health measures were, in a sense figured the entire population of the archipelago as dependent.

The Puerto Rican social workers who had advocated for the extension of the Social Security Act would be in charge both of managing the maternal and child welfare programs and of providing assistance to the public health programs. Despite this victory, the social workers had fallen short of their goal of achieving full coverage under the act. They would continue to fight for inclusion by sending lobbying delegations to the United States. Their efforts were renewed with the populist reforms spearheaded under the ascendant PPD. The PPD government ran on a platform of "social justice," arguing for the expansion of social welfare programs and benefits for Puerto Ricans.[118] In 1943, the toil of social workers and their allies bore fruit with the creation of the Department of Public Welfare. From the beginning, the Department of Public Welfare in Puerto Rico was developed with the understanding that it provided an infrastructure onto which the Social Security Act could be grafted. The 1943 legislation became known as the "Law of $7.50," because it established a maximum payment of that amount per month to families or individuals who were defined as "in need." The department's creation resulted in the expansion of social welfare offices throughout the archipelago, and social workers took over the social programs initially created under the New Deal.

DURING THE 1930S, the creation and expansion of New Deal social welfare programs were deeply connected to gendered reforms in Puerto Rican society. When working-class communities grappled with the economic disaster caused by the Great Depression, they called on newly created New Deal government agencies to help support their struggles to navigate the crisis. For many working-class women, these demands were centered on insisting on ample and better-paying jobs that would allow them to support themselves and their families. Many working-class women had already entered the waged labor force in the preceding decades, and more sought employment to help them confront the economic challenges of the time. While early relief projects did provide some women with employment at state-run needlework cooperatives and as assistants on New Deal projects, the broader call for more jobs for working women was not emphasized as the programs developed. Instead, the work of these agencies centered on reform projects that regulated the reproduction and labor of women. This included the creation of gendered vocational education programs that prepared women for gender-segregated occupations that pushed them toward caring labor in their own homes and the homes of others. The state focused on gendered reforms, often led by newly professionalized women reformers, that provided education and relief but failed to give working-class women the work and security they sought.

The New Deal also ushered in the rise of a new group of social work leaders and activists from more diverse backgrounds than the previous generation of reformers. As agencies sought more trained women social workers to staff expanding social reform projects, they opened the field to some middle-class and working-class women who were not from the same elite backgrounds as the maternalist society women of the first cohort. In the early 1920s, in a newly created social work program at the University of Puerto Rico, young women received training that would later prepare them to direct New Deal reforms. These women continued their work in social movements and brought their politics into the profession, advocating for socialism, feminism, nationalism, and independence. Additionally, many working-class women became social work "aides" and worked on New Deal projects without the same training as university-educated social workers. This led to debates between social workers over who was taking up the mantle of professional identity. While these tensions resulted in some regulations around the social work profession, they also marked the expansion of the field and the recognition of the increasing numbers of women of working-class backgrounds in the profession. Subsequently, social workers became essential leaders in each of the political parties in Puerto Rico, including those who advocated for statehood, independence, and liberalism, which would bring the PPD to power.

The partial extension of the US Social Security Act to Puerto Rico in 1939 would also become an essential benchmark in future discussions about the social aspects of Puerto Rican citizenship. While coverage under the act was restricted, including Puerto Rico under some of these policies was a starting point for activists who would continue to push for broader access to federal social programs. As was the case in 1939, these debates would often involve struggles between US and Puerto Rican policymakers and advocacy by social workers who used their social welfare expertise to support these benefit programs. Discussions about social welfare policies continued to include concerns about the Puerto Rican migrant community and debates over their rights to social welfare benefits and migration policy. For social workers, these dialogues were crucial in their political organizing around Puerto Rican citizenship. Moreover, when the titles were extended, social workers played a significant role in shaping new social welfare programs during the 1940s and 1950s as part of the broader reform project of the PPD. As they moved into administrative roles managing these programs, they would participate in a renewed debate about working-class women's deservingness of benefits brewing on the horizon.

3

Working-Class Women, Claims for Benefits, and the Politics of Deservingness under the Puerto Rican Populist State

In 1950, in the urban barrio of La Perla in San Juan, Camila Pérez struggled with social workers over the means-testing practices they had developed in her neighborhood. Pérez became a client of the Department of Social Welfare in Puerto Rico when she applied for benefits at a public health clinic where she was receiving treatment for chronic tuberculosis.[1] She sought assistance to support her children because her illness made it difficult for her to work, and her husband had migrated to the United States. However, Pérez faced conflict with social workers over how she reported the financial support she was receiving from her husband. The social welfare benefits she was allocated were reduced after she signed a document stating that she had lied about his income on an application. Later, Pérez forcefully argued that social workers had pressured her into signing this document and that she had never lied. Over the months that followed, she protested the reduction in benefits that resulted and fought with social workers over how her income was recorded. She insisted that she deserved more funds because of the caregiving labor she provided for her family.

The heated exchanges between Pérez and social workers over her income and labor were recorded in the case file that social workers created when she applied for benefits. This case file provides a detailed record of Pérez's work history, which centers mainly on her experience as a care worker and caregiver. Social workers documented how Pérez had spent her childhood sewing and taking in laundry alongside the women in her family. She later spent part of her youth as a child servant who worked in the households of others in exchange for room and board. As an adult, she continued to weave her way between waged and unwaged work, later finding jobs as a waitress and a laundress.[2] She sought assistance when she could not continue working as a care worker for wages, although she was still actively a caregiver for her children. She hoped the archipelago's new social welfare programs would help support her family, but the path to receiving benefits soon became rocky. The case file documents fifteen years of her struggles with social workers over her application for assistance.

Pérez's intimate battle over means-testing was not unique. Instead, her story is echoed by those of other working-class women care workers and caregivers who applied for social welfare benefits from the Department of Social Welfare in Puerto Rico during this period. This agency was created in 1943, shortly after the Partido Popular Democrático (PPD) came to power, ushering in a sweeping set of populist reforms that included expanding social welfare programs as a part of its liberal political platform.[3] For the PPD, creating more expansive social welfare programs for working-class families was seen as a central part of its program of social change.[4] Shortly after its social welfare programs expanded, thousands of women applied for assistance, making claims on the state. Many of these women believed they were entitled to assistance as workers and citizens after they witnessed and participated in the widespread labor and political activism on the archipelago that resulted in demands for change that brought the PPD to power.[5] However, when working-class women became "clients" of these new social welfare programs, they encountered new means-testing practices and narrow criteria of deservingness that contradicted their broader understandings of entitlement.

Historians of gender and race in Puerto Rico have shown how this period was marked by profound changes in the relationship between working-class women and the state as Puerto Rican and US government agencies developed regulatory measures that deeply impacted women's lives and labor. This chapter builds on scholarship like that of historians Laura Briggs, Eileen Findlay, and José Flores Ramos that has emphasized how state-sponsored programs focused on public health became arenas where women's reproduction and sexuality were targeted and regulated.[6] In particular, it examines how working-class women experienced becoming clients of social welfare programs, which has often not been the focus of previous studies. The chapter also builds on Puerto Rican women's labor history that has demonstrated how women navigated complex terrains of labor participation in the home and outside of it, moving between waged and unwaged work.[7] Previous studies have considered reproductive labor, but most scholarship has focused on needlework and factory work. This chapter documents and analyzes the labor histories of welfare recipients, and it is, therefore, a labor history of people who are not often considered workers. It argues that the labor histories of welfare recipients can shed new light on the history of reproductive labor, care work, and caregiving in Puerto Rican communities.

This chapter examines the struggle over social welfare benefits that emerged after the creation of social welfare programs by the PPD. It considers how working-class women care workers became clients of the welfare state and how the creation of new public welfare offices and clinics impacted their lives. As historian Solsiree del Moral has demonstrated, the regulation of the intimate lives of people of African descent and Black Puerto Ricans was particularly acute under the social welfare projects that emerged after the rise of the PPD.[8] In this chapter I emphasize how, as working-class women became clients, they struggled with social workers in welfare offices over how women's labor was valued or recorded. These struggles intensified as social workers developed forms of means-testing that were increasingly regulatory and that sometimes obscured or minimized working-class women's reproductive labor. In response, working-class women continued to push back against how social workers recorded information about their labor and invasive social work practices. However, despite their efforts, these social work practices would contribute to broader social understandings of working-class women welfare recipients as dependents and nonworkers.

The chapter also shows how the same social workers developing means-testing practices during this period became central figures in producing US social scientific studies of poverty that would have lasting impacts on Puerto Rican communities. These studies of poverty depicted Puerto Rican communities as pathological and often portrayed working-class women as social deviants who were prone to welfare dependency.[9] This chapter argues that the ways that researchers understood working-class women's reproductive labor shaped the outcome of two major studies by US social scientists. On the one hand, Oscar Lewis produced a study of Puerto Rican communities in the mid-1960s that emphasized the dependency of Puerto Rican women, overlooked their labor, and shored up his theory about the "culture of poverty." On the other hand, Helen Safa, writing in the mid-1970s, emphasized women's labor, leading her to conclude that women were productive members of society who played essential roles in sustaining the community in the face of rapid industrialization.[10] However, in the end, Lewis's vision would become the most influential, as his ideas about working-class women as undeserving members of society would be taken up by Puerto Rican and US policymakers to justify the increased regulation of working-class communities.

The stories of women care workers and caregivers at the heart of this chapter shed light on how working-class women navigated the social transformations taking place in Puerto Rico in the mid-twentieth century. They also show how, as many Puerto Rican workers migrated in search of work, both within Puerto Rico and outside of it, they faced an increased fraying of the social bonds that had previously sustained their communities. While social welfare agencies' records are full of stories of how people experienced the breakdown of former traditional social networks, they also demonstrate how working-class people reconstructed new forms of communal support and interrelation far beyond their households. These stories also show how Puerto Rican women consistently pushed back against the devaluing of their reproductive labor in society and asserted their deservingness of state support and social rights, despite the persistence of negative descriptions and tropes that were deployed against them in society.

Working-Class Women, Care Work, and the Creation of Social Welfare Programs under the Partido Popular Democrático

In the 1940s, the San Juan region bustled with urban growth as migrants across Puerto Rico traveled to the city searching for work. The metropolitan area grew steadily during this decade as neighborhoods where workers lived expanded. Working-class women moved through a rapidly changing city and provided much of the labor that sustained its growth. They served freshly cooked meals of *arroz con pollo* in small cafes, cleaned the homes of well-to-do families in wealthy neighborhoods like El Condado, and did seemingly endless loads of laundry in local fountains and rivers. Women who had recently arrived from the countryside were schooled by seasoned urban dwellers on which market stands had the best prices and which movie houses had the most exciting films. They also passed along information about how to find a day's work taking care of children for a local mother or a more long-term live-in position as a domestic worker. In images from the period, women are shown moving through the city and claiming the quickly expanding working-class neighborhood as their own (see figure 3.1, for example). As working-class women navigated the shifting terrain of urban San Juan, they followed in the footsteps of earlier generations while encountering new challenges.

During this period, working-class women also began visiting public health clinics and social welfare offices recently created by the Puerto Rican government to seek health care and monetary assistance. At public welfare clinics, women waited for their appointments in the shade and wrangled unruly toddlers as they made small talk to pass the time. Among these groups might have been pregnant women seeking help because of early contractions or those who feared their nightly chest pains might mean a diagnosis of tuberculosis. When they arrived, some may have already known about the new programs offering funding for maternal child welfare, old age assistance, and disability.[11] Together, they waited until they gradually wound their way to the front of the building and met the nurses and social workers who greeted them and began to collect information about their lives in a case file. The social workers held bundles of documents in their arms, pulled out an intake form or a blank sheet of paper, and quickly scribbled down notes in their documents. This process resulted in many working-class women becoming clients of social welfare programs for the first time.

The creation of these new social welfare offices was the direct result of the expansion of the state after the ascendent populist party, the PPD, came to power. These changes began in earnest with the PPD's victories and deepened when the party oversaw the creation of a new "Commonwealth" government, the Estado Libre Asociado (Free Associated State).[12] During this period, working-class women became the targets of new social reform programs developed under the new government.[13] This chapter explores the stories of working-class women care workers and caregivers who became clients of social welfare programs. The social welfare programs created by the PPD emphasized creating divisions between working-class women based on whether they were seen as "deserving" or "undeserving" of public assistance funds and support. The divisions around who was perceived as deserving were shaped by the political agenda of government officials as well as a broader understanding of gender, sexuality, and race in Puerto Rican society.

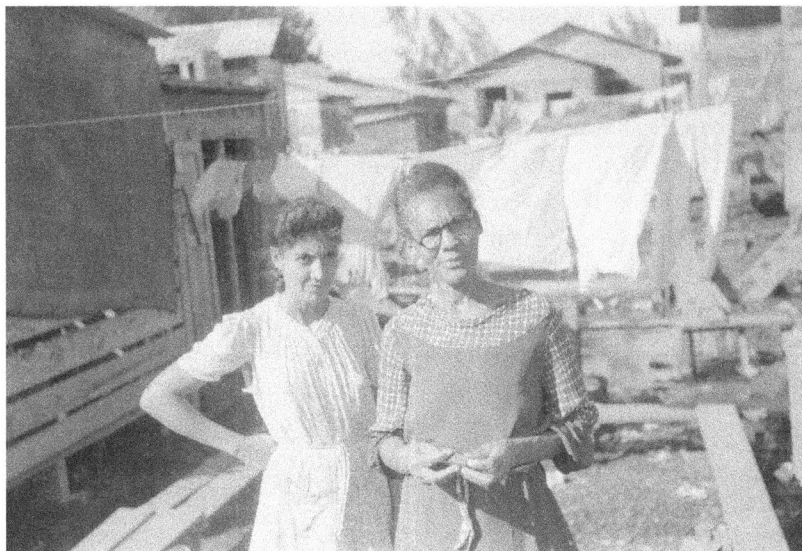

FIGURE 3.1. Two women residents of the neighborhood called El Fanguito, San Juan, Puerto Rico, January 1942. Photograph by Jack Delano. Courtesy of the Farm Security Administration, Office of War Information Photograph Collection, Library of Congress, Washington, DC.

Scholars have shown that, after the PPD came to power, the social reforms ushered in were intimately linked to the production and regulation of ideas about gender in Puerto Rican society.[14] The PPD promised working-class Puerto Rican communities that they would provide reforms that would restrain the ravages of industrial capitalism and US colonialism. The party targeted working-class communities in its populist campaigns by using the symbol of the *jíbaro*, a rural male worker.[15] As historian Eileen Findlay has shown, the PPD often aimed to shore up traditional ideas about gender and masculinity, as the party promised working-class men jobs and good wages that would allow them to be both breadwinners and heads of households.[16] The PPD's focus on male workers as heads of household and strengthening the patriarchal family also deeply impacted working-class women, as their societal role as workers and breadwinners in their families was increasingly overlooked.

The creation of social reforms that targeted working-class women was shaped by officials' ideas about sexuality and race. As Laura Briggs has shown, the Puerto Rican government continued to develop various "social campaigns" during this period that were focused on regulating the reproduction of working-class women.[17] The outcomes of these social reform campaigns were also shaped by the racist beliefs of reformers who often defined women of African descent as deviant.[18] These social programs often focused on creating social divisions between "good" and "bad" women. Women who were "decent" were the targets of expanding home economics programs and professionalization opportunities in fields like social work. Those who were seen as "bad," especially those who were understood to be prostitutes, became the targets of social reform campaigns that built on earlier waves of regulation. Among the most invasive were eugenics campaigns, which emphasized reducing the population of Puerto Rico by promoting birth control and sterilization.[19] As this chapter shows, the administration of social welfare programs also became a place where divisions between women were made.

In 1943, the Puerto Rican government created the Department of Public Welfare (DPW), which became the primary agency overseeing various new social welfare programs on the archipelago.[20] The creation of this department resulted from the passage of the Ley de Bienestar Público (Public Welfare Law) of 1943, which stated, "The provision of social services and economic assistance to individuals or families prevented from providing for themselves the essential means of decent life is a basic responsibility of the government."[21] The DPW was managed and run by an expansive network of social workers who oversaw its social programs, social welfare clinics, and residential institutions. The creation of this agency was made possible by the expansion of social welfare infrastructure in rural and urban areas in previous decades. The new agency oversaw programs that included assistance to needy families, old age assistance, assistance for people with disabilities, foster care services, and other programs for children, as well as running residential social welfare institutions. The agency soon began administering relief programs and distributing direct aid to thousands of working-class individuals and families throughout the island. Within ten years of the creation of the DPW, social workers were managing the agency's main central office, five district offices, and seventy-six Unidades de Bienestar Público (Public Welfare Units) across the archipelago.[22] Through these offices the workers managed a budget of nearly $4.5 million, $3 million of which was distributed through direct-relief programs. However, they would forcefully argue and demonstrate that this budget was severely limited and did not come near meeting the demand and need for social services they encountered.

For social workers, the DPW heralded a moment of victory in their long fight to create state-sponsored social welfare programs on the archipelago.

Social workers and feminist reformers in Puerto Rico had been advocating for such a social welfare agency for decades, and they believed that its creation represented a broader societal and state recognition of the needs of women and children. Social workers described the DPW's initial creation in heady ways as they saw the moment as a hopeful one that promised positive social transformations. It also heralded an even more expansive role of social workers and professional women within state institutions and their involvement in governance. In addition, the demand for social workers to staff the expanding agencies of the DPW outpaced the number of trained social workers who had experience in the field, and there were efforts to broaden training programs. Throughout the 1940s and 1950s the Puerto Rican government also advertised in local newspapers that there were social work positions available. In one such advertisement in a 1953 edition of the newspaper *El Imparcial*, the Puerto Rican government noted that there were twenty open positions for child welfare social workers in twenty different towns across the archipelago.[23] Applicants for these positions had to hold a bachelor's degree already and would be eligible for scholarships to receive graduate training at the School of Social Work at the University of Puerto Rico. However, despite these promotional efforts, there were still not enough social workers to fully staff the social welfare agencies that were created.[24]

The newly created social welfare programs were mainly focused on providing monetary assistance to working-class women and their families through a system that focused on the "family wage," a gendered approach that would shape the outcomes of its programs.[25] This approach sought to offer support when a male breadwinner was absent while reinforcing the patriarchal family structure. Historians of social welfare have demonstrated that this structure of distributing assistance had lasting consequences on society, as it produced and regulated ideas about family, gender, and sexuality.[26] This was particularly evident in the maternal assistance programs that were established. Social workers were tasked with ensuring that households had a heteronormative family structure with a male breadwinner whenever possible. When no such breadwinner existed, social workers saw their role as providing the financial resources that were missing due to the absence.

In the Puerto Rican context, social workers' and policymakers' investment in reproducing the "family wage" through social welfare programs were coupled with recognition that working-class women were already working outside the home for wages. Therefore, their approach toward working-class women differed from that of other contexts, such as in the United States, which social welfare scholars have discussed. Social workers acknowledged women as waged workers, as there was already a significant movement of working-class women into waged labor on the archipelago. Additionally, social workers accepted that many women were unmarried, had relationships outside of marriage, or had children when they were not married. This was because, despite efforts by US and Puerto Rican policymakers to promote marriage, many Puerto Rican women remained unmarried. Social workers also recognized many single mothers working outside the home for wages and invested in assisting this group.

Social workers also decried the limited funding available to DPW social welfare agencies and increasingly oversaw means-testing practices to determine clients' eligibility for benefits. The main form of monetary aid distribution from 1943 to 1950 occurred through a program known as the "Law of $7.50" because it offered a maximum payment of $7.50 per month to clients.[27] According to the director of the Division of Social Welfare, Celestina Zalduondo, in the first year of the program there were 76,762 applications that received assistance from this program, which included 30,733 new applications at local social welfare clinics, 21,606 applications that were grandfathered into the program from earlier social welfare programs, and 24,423 cases that were reinvestigated to see if they were deserving of benefits.[28] In 1946, social worker Luisa Igesias de Jesús noted that the Puerto Rican government only provided direct assistance through the $7.50 program to thirty-three thousand out of eighty thousand families who sought to "claim the right to receive public assistance."[29] To manage the distribution of this assistance, social workers developed a broad system of means-testing that relied on casework with clients initiated in public health agencies and social welfare offices. The underfunding of social welfare programs also meant that not all the eligible applicants received assistance.[30] There were also numerous cases where individuals were eligible for more than seven dollars and fifty cents, but the cap was still applied. As the social welfare programs expanded and more people applied for the limited available funds, this justified more strident means-testing practices. After 1950 there was a gradual expansion of these funds because of the extension to Puerto Rico of more titles of the Social Security Act; however, assistance remained low.[31]

In addition to working with clients in Puerto Rico, the growing migration of Puerto Ricans to the United States also led to numerous social workers being tasked with dealing with cases related to migration. The DPW oversaw an expanding Interagency Services Bureau, created specifically to manage the circulation of information between Puerto Rican and US social welfare agencies about migrants.[32] The unit referred cases from

US social welfare agencies, courts, religious organizations, hospitals, and other organizations. At the same time, social workers from the DPW also sent requests for information to US social service agencies, including departments of social welfare in the United States as well as the National Desertion Bureau to inquire about cases of clients that came to their offices. During the fiscal year of 1947–1948, this unit received 6,043 new cases and responded to over 17,936 letters about these migrant cases. In the years following the creation of the DPW and its expansion throughout the archipelago, questions about migration and migrant rights were often central concerns of both clients and social workers.

The rise of the PPD in the 1940s resulted in the immediate extension and growth of social welfare programs in Puerto Rico. Many of these programs were initially made available to working-class women and their families who were in need of assistance. The creation of these programs marked a new form of state intervention in Puerto Rican communities, as well as a time where the social workers, as agents of the state, were charged with determining eligibility for these benefits. Programs like the direct assistance that was provided through the Law of $7.50 quickly extended the role of social workers into Puerto Rican communities. As increasing numbers of working-class people applied for benefits, it also put pressure on the state to hire more social workers, create new social welfare clinics, and have a more robust system to distribute aid. There was also growing frustration among working-class people over the limited funding available in these programs, the means-testing practices developed by social workers, and the social regulation of their lives that resulted from the programs' expansion.

Working-Class Women's Struggles to Claim Benefits and Negotiate Means-Testing

The Department of Public Welfare case files, which were created after the PPD came to power, provide a detailed record of the interactions between working-class women clients and government officials in public health clinics and social welfare offices across the archipelago. These files show how working-class women claimed benefits and negotiated their applications for assistance. The records also document how the state managed and administered these programs and determined eligibility.[33] They reveal how a struggle between clients and social workers ensued within the clinics over how working-class women's labor would be defined and valued. These struggles often centered on means-testing practices that working-class women who applied for benefits were forced to undergo. These practices were developed to separate supposedly "deserving" from "undeserving" applicants.

Many of the new welfare recipients of the social welfare programs created during this period were care workers and caregivers. The social work case files offer a window into the history of women's labor in Puerto Rico that shows how the space of home and work were intertwined and the categories of "productive" and "reproductive" labor were often blurred. These files are full of the stories of women who provided the social reproductive labor that sustained their families and communities. They did this work under vastly different conditions—some forced, some for wages, some without wages.[34] They also sometimes paired their domestic work with work in factories and other industries. The records also show that one of the main aspects of means-testing practices was that social workers were trying to "make sense" of women's labor, including their care work and caregiving, by developing processes that would allow them to quantify and label it.

During this moment, one of the particularities of women's labor force participation was that the shift to industrial occupations did not mean an end to their work in domestic and service positions. Instead, most working-class women continued to be domestic and service workers, and many navigated their way in and out of waged and unwaged work, toiling in their homes and newly built factories.[35] In the case of domestic work, there was also a persistence of racial occupational segregation, rooted in the legacy of slavery, that resulted in many women of African descent working as domestics. Scholars have shown how domestic and care workers in Puerto Rico, particularly women of color, were paid meager wages and often faced the most precarious working conditions.[36] Therefore, as industrialization occurred in Puerto Rico, it did not displace the need for service and caring labor, often done by the most marginalized workers (figure 3.2). Care work and caregiving labor in Puerto Rican society was shaped by social hierarchies of race, gender, and class that generally left working-class women, especially those of African descent, with the least resources. During this period, racialized labor segregation persisted, and many Afro-Puerto Rican women continued to be employed as care workers.

While the case file records document the gender, race, and class divisions in Puerto Rican society that were enacted through divisions of caring labor, the information that social workers provided on forms was often incomplete. Some social work forms had spaces where racial descriptions of clients could be listed. However, this information is often absent or partially recorded. Instead, social workers included more detailed descriptions

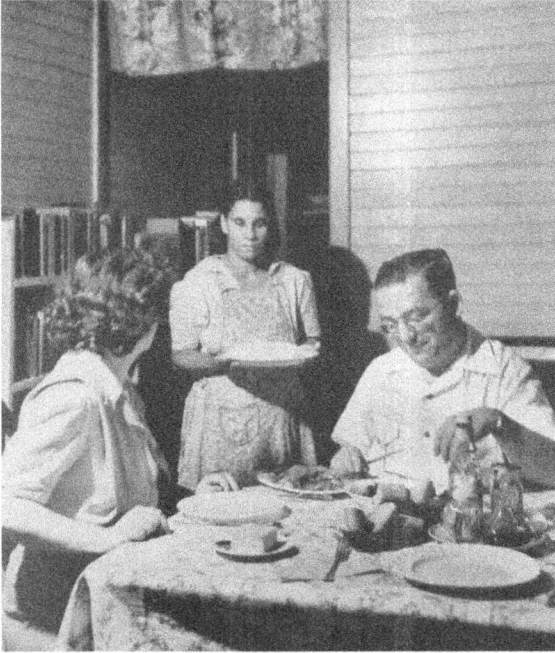

FIGURE 3.2. Domestic worker serving food at the home of her employers. Photograph by Charles E. Rotkin. Source: Lewis Cutter Richardson, *Puerto Rico, Caribbean Crossroads* (New York: US Camera Publishing and the University of Puerto Rico, 1947), 69.

of how they perceived their clients' race within the narrative portions of the life histories and background sections they authored. Solsiree del Moral has shown how social workers described clients' skin color and race, often with detailed descriptions of characteristics that were meant to emphasize their African descendance.[37] In the case files of care workers, social workers described clients' skin color, hair color and texture, and phenotype in various ways. For example, in a description of two teenage sisters who were clients, there was a listing of the first sister as white on a form and then physically described in the narrative case file as "trigueña blanca," a term in Puerto Rico that signified that her skin was "wheat-colored" or not completely white, and her sister was described as "color blanco . . . pelo grifo," which meant that she was white but had densely curly, or "kinky," hair"[38] The case file notes different qualifiers for the "whiteness" of the sisters, and in this way the social workers marked each of them as being partially of African descent. These files also show that while social workers were concerned with demarcating racial divisions in society on their forms, they did not always do so uniformly. Instead, they often had longer descriptions of race that nonetheless served the purpose of making visible racial divisions and hierarchies in Puerto Rican society.

When social workers conducted interviews with clients, they often produced long background studies about their clients' lives that focused on the labor history of applicants. These narratives focused on documenting how women had worked in the past and what types of work they had done. They included caregiving in the home that was not waged, as well as waged employment of various sorts. In some instances, social workers would also describe how and why women could no longer work, providing details about why they couldn't care for their children or work for wages. The information they collected was used to determine whether a client would be eligible for state support that compensated certain cases, such as funding for maternal and child welfare, disability, or old age assistance. As social workers collected information about Puerto Rican women's labor and their income for means-testing, they produced a detailed record of Puerto Rican women's labor histories. The case files also emphasized women's caregiving and care work, which was not often documented in other labor records.

Within the case files, social workers used various descriptions of care workers' and caregivers' labor. Sometimes, care work and caregiving were collapsed into broad categories. For example, the occupation of women was often described as "oficios domesticos," which was a catch-all term for various forms of labor performed at home. On some occasions, a woman's occupation was listed as simply "domestic," which was a category that could refer either to a stay-at-home mother or to a domestic worker who worked outside the home for wages.[39] When women worked as domestic workers outside the home, more specific language was sometimes used to define their waged labor. For instance, the file of Edna Colón noted that she "dedicated herself to domestic work in the homes of other families" and that she "did all the housework."[40] It was also typical for the occupation in the files to broadly describe a woman as "cooking, washing, and ironing" or for specific domestic or service work types to be listed, such as when women were listed only as cooks or washerwomen.

Many of the files deal specifically with young women, teenagers, and girls who were domestic workers and servants. There were many examples of children living in the families of their employers and doing household tasks, either in exchange for room and board or for wages. For example, in the case of one of the sisters mentioned previously, the social worker noted that the young woman had "never attended school and in actuality, she was rented out to help the family economically."[41] The case file says of her that "the work that she does is taking care of the little boy of a neighbor." There were also cases where the employers paid child servants' wages directly to their parents or guardians. These children, who were often forced into positions as care workers, usually had little control over the terms of their labor, and their living conditions could be strictly controlled by their employers.

Social workers developed new forms of documentation to record women's labor in the informal economy while conducting means-testing. One such case involved Soledad Campos, a grandmother who applied for assistance to support her grandchildren under her care.[42] The complexities around recording the labor of women who were both care workers and caregivers can be seen in her file. The social workers noted that the children's mother had left for New York City while the father had gone to work on a sugar plantation. Campos, who did not make enough money to support her grandchildren as a part-time cook, applied for social welfare benefits. The social workers asked her to sign a document stating how much she earned monthly. Campos signed a form stating that she earned ten dollars a month selling food she cooked. This is just one of many similar documents that record how social workers kept track of information about women's labor in the case files. These documents were a form of receipt that created a new state record of various forms of domestic and service work women performed for wages.

The case file of another client, Gabriela López, documents how a woman of African descent navigated her application for social assistance while trying to advocate for her right to benefits.[43] During a social work interview, López recounted how she had been born into slavery on a plantation in Puerto Rico. To establish eligibility for the social welfare programs, she had to provide her personal history, including when and where she was born, and other details. She had spent most of her life living in the city of Guayama before she migrated to the San Juan area later in life.[44] López had worked her entire life, first as a child when she was enslaved alongside her family, later as a seamstress during much of her working life, and finally as a domestic worker in the city. She went to the public health clinic because she was experiencing health issues and needed health care. At the office, she was offered monetary assistance from the Department of Public Welfare's new programs aiding elderly people. Her story provides a window into how working-class women care workers experienced applying for social welfare benefits.

In the years that followed this initial application, López struggled with social workers over numerous aspects of their means-testing protocols. She had numerous heated exchanges with social workers over how they recorded her labor, documented the assistance and mutual-aid support that she received from friends, and calculated the amount of financial assistance she should receive. While at first she was given seven dollars and fifty cents monthly, the maximum funding under the program, the amount was later reduced by social workers who said she was receiving monetary assistance from a friend.[45] These social workers had López sign a document saying that she was receiving one dollar a month for doing seamstress work for a friend. However, she later protested that this had been an occasional job and that she had not received any money from her friend for over a year.

López's case file shows how caregiving and support networks among Puerto Ricans were important to working-class communities and how social workers understood and recorded information about these networks. Means-testing practices produced data and documents about labor that were used to determine benefit payments. These documents also sometimes quantified resources that friends and others gave to a client's personal and community network. This confrontation also points to how "facts" that were recorded by social workers were sometimes contested by clients. The production of knowledge in social work case files resulted from the negotiation of complicated power dynamics and struggles between these individuals. The arguments that ensued sometimes made their way into the narratives recorded by social workers, as they did in López's case, but it is likely they largely went unrecorded.

Social work case files often documented the caregiving networks within working-class communities. For example, the case file of the previously mentioned domestic worker Edna Colón noted that she "lives off the charity of a friend, who gives her food once a day."[46] However, this assistance was not a secure stream of financial support for the social welfare applicant, as the friend had plans to move to New York to "reunite with her mother who lives there." In this instance, the case file further noted that the food given to the applicant cannot be considered a "secure resource."[47] This case highlights how migration reshaped Puerto Rican communities as more people moved to the United States. It also illustrates how social workers sometimes perceived the support clients received from friends as one of their primary resources.

The case files often contain stories of caregiving networks that highlight the forms of interdependence and mutual support common in working-class communities. These networks extended beyond traditional nuclear or biological families and included individuals who were considered kin, friends, and acquaintances. Social workers recorded these networks in their narratives and wrote information about how resources were circulated within these broader networks. Thus, the case files document how new relationships were being formed in displaced communities. They also indicate that wider caregiving networks between working-class people were crucial in sustaining them as they encountered rapid social, economic, and political changes. Furthermore, the records demonstrate how these broader social networks became increasingly essential to working-class communities as migration to the United States increased.

The social welfare case files contain numerous examples of working-class women struggling with social workers over the content of the files they produced. These files reveal conflicts between clients and social workers regarding how their labor and income were documented in the paperwork. This included receipts that recorded women's work in the informal labor economy or resources they received from their family, friends, or members of the broader community. The cases of Soldedad Campos and Gabriela López provide examples of such struggles. Both women protested how social workers recorded their resources and income and argued that the resources they had access to were unreliable. They argued that their low incomes should make them eligible for more extensive benefits under the social welfare programs they had applied for. They argued that their low income should qualify them for comprehensive social welfare benefits.

During this period, the Puerto Rican Department of Welfare began administering a state-sponsored caregiving program known as the housekeeper, or *ama de llaves*, program; it placed paid caregivers in clients' homes.[48] In the 1947–1948 fiscal year, there were over one thousand children in Puerto Rico who were receiving this service, and social workers argued that there were many more that were eligible for it, if the program was further expanded.[49] This program was an extension of a similar service that provided temporary assistance to social welfare clients in the United States. Historians Eileen Boris and Jennifer Klein have documented how programs like the housekeeper service program were responsible for funneling US working-class women, many of whom were women of color, into low-wage positions as care workers.[50] They have also demonstrated how the program was part of a broader shift toward privatizing health care in the United States. The state recognized this caring labor was necessary and chose to employ working-class women to care for others rather than invest in more robust state institutions.

In Puerto Rico, the *ama de llaves* program mainly provided temporary care for children. Social workers referred families to the program when they thought that temporary caregiving would allow a family to stay together rather than having children placed in an institution or into foster care.[51] The housekeeper was responsible for providing childcare as well as cleaning and cooking. The women employed by the program were working-class women who often lived in the same neighborhoods as the families where they were placed. The program was seen as providing employment opportunities for women who could potentially be welfare recipients themselves. Social workers interviewed the housekeepers before placing them in positions, and they also met regularly with them to ensure that the clients' needs were being met. The housekeepers also served as a source of information about their clients, reporting to social workers about the conditions in their homes.

In an article titled "Visitando un ama de llaves" (Visiting a housekeeper) in the social work journal *Bienestar Público*, social worker Carmen Villarini described the work of Modesta Pinto López, a housekeeper who was a part of the Department of Public Welfare's housekeeper program.[52] Pinto López had been placed in the home of a widowed father whose wife had passed away a year before. The father had four children in the home, and the article suggests that he was provided assistance through the housekeeper program because his children were not attending school after their mother's death. Villarini describes how the children were doing much better with Pinto López in the house, and the article includes photographs of the housekeeper that depict her taking care of the children. In one of the images, Pinto López is shown styling the hair of the youngest girl, and both housekeeper and child are smiling (figure 3.3). Villarini also describes how Pinto López attended official meetings with other workers in the program at the local offices of the Department of Public Welfare, and how these workers were required to attain regular health certificates administered by the Department of Public Health. When Villarini was leaving the home, she spoke with the children's father and inquired about his plans after the four-month temporary housekeeper service ended. He told her that he was about to start making more money, and that he was going to ask if Pinto López would continue working for him for a wage but noted that what he could offer would be less than what she was being paid by the housekeeper program.[53] The social worker approved of this plan and also agreed to continue following up on the case after the formal participation in the housekeeper program ended. The story is one in which a woman hired in the housekeeper program, which was paid by social welfare funds, was also being encouraged to take a role later as a private household worker.

Numerous case files from the period show how working-class women clients and their families were assigned housekeeper services. For example, Emilia Gomez, a janitor at a local school, applied for the program because she needed assistance caring for her baby and two nephews while in the hospital for treatment.[54] The housekeeper services were seen as a stopgap that

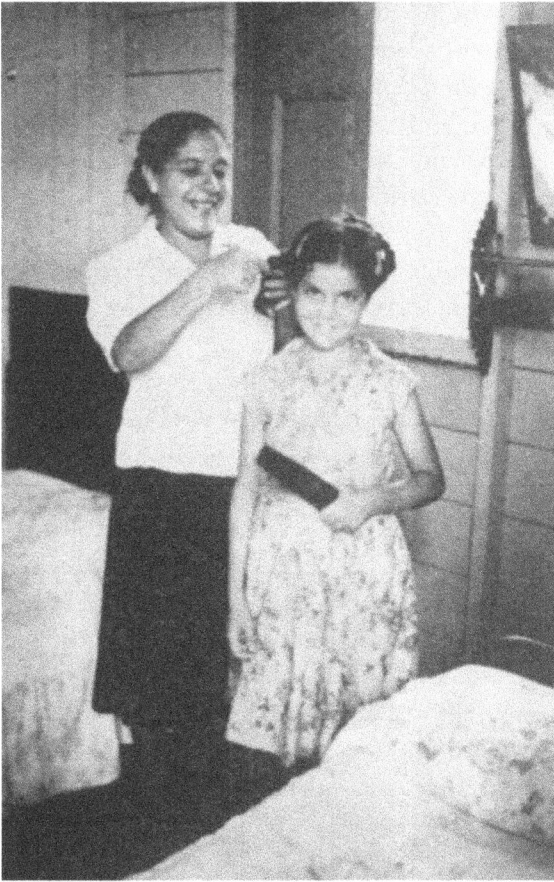

FIGURE 3.3. Housekeeper, or *ama de llaves*, Modesta Pinto López with one of the children in her care. Source: Carmen Villarini, "Visitando un ama de llaves," *Bienestar Público*, June 1948, 24.

enabled the children to be cared for at home until she recovered and returned home. Therefore, the social workers recommended that she be provided housekeeper service for one month. The social worker who met with her wrote that she "explained how the housekeeper program works" and argued that the boys might behave better if someone watched them while she was at work. She also noted that the housekeeper would "leave them a prepared lunch" and "perform all the work she did not have time to do."

In Gomez's case, the social workers identified and hired housekeepers from her neighborhood. After the first housekeeper didn't work out, they hired Daniela Meléndez, who also left the position after working for a short while.[55] The case file notes that Meléndez, "*ama de llaves* of the children, came to our office today to give notice that she was leaving her job that day because her mother was leaving [for the United States] and taking her as well. She came to get the money owed to her so she could take it with her." The case file describes that she was being paid twenty dollars a month for her work as an *ama de llaves*. This is one example of how social workers were constantly discussing migration in the case files and specifically how migration was impacting caretaking networks, including the attempts of the state to provide support through the housekeeper program.

The broader migration of children's caretakers and caregivers to the United States is a central theme of social work case files from the time. For example, in the case of Camila Pérez, recounted at the beginning of this chapter, a woman wrestled with social workers over her application for assistance while navigating her husband's migration to the United States.[56] Pérez was unable to continue working as a care worker because she was very sick with tuberculosis, and she was receiving intermittent financial support from her husband in the United States. After social workers confronted her about supposedly lying on a form about how much money she had received from her husband, the social welfare agency spent considerable effort following up on the case details. The social workers had her sign a handwritten note, creating a receipt that recorded the fifteen dollars that she had received from her husband that month. She would later argue she had been forced to sign this document and it was untrue. The case file also recorded the escalating tensions between Pérez and the social workers.

As social workers further developed means-testing practices, they increasingly relied on regulatory methods that invaded clients' privacy. In the story of Pérez, we see how, in addition to the information in her file undergoing increased scrutiny over time, there is also increased animosity throughout the casework process.[57] The social workers visited her home numerous times to try to meet with her about the case. In addition, they interviewed other people who knew her, like friends and neighbors, to get more information about her and the income to which she supposedly had access. Pérez's story is just one of many in which social workers conducted means-testing that included unannounced home visits, and had confrontations with clients who were suspected of lying.

The intensification of means-testing significantly impacted not only the applicants but also their families and communities. The case of Carolina Romero is an example of the struggles between clients and social workers over how money from partners was recorded in the case files.[58] After Romero applied for assistance to help support her children, she recounted her labor history, saying that she was not making enough money to support them. She told social workers that she had previously worked as a laundress for three dollars a month before she found a part-time job at a shirt factory where she was paid five dollars a month. Her husband also had unsteady employment and health problems, and together they were struggling to put food on the table. Subsequently, the social worker began a means-testing process that would last years.

In Romero's case, the social workers were unhappy with not being able to have a clear monetary value listed for her husband's income. Both Romero and her husband explained that his employment as a manual laborer was irregular, and he had been facing health issues that prevented him from working regularly. To prove this, his employer submitted a document stating that it was difficult to calculate how much he would earn monthly as they could not predict when they would get jobs or how much they would pay. Nevertheless, the social workers were displeased with this response. They mentioned in her file that she was "hostile" toward them, and her husband was deemed "non-cooperative" because he did not attend meetings at their offices.

Throughout Romero's case, when social workers did not receive the information they requested, they escalated their efforts by visiting the client's home and neighbors. Initially, the social workers made several unannounced visits to Romero's home, threatening to revoke her assistance benefits if she did not provide the information.[59] Later, they began to broaden their fact-checking methods to determine eligibility for benefits. This involved visiting neighbors and others in the community to gather information about Romero. After organizing this information, the social workers returned to Romero's home. They confronted her about the apparent contradictions between the information she provided and what they had gathered from other sources. Consequently, her case was suspended, with social workers claiming that her husband refused to provide transparent information regarding his income and contributions to the household. The social workers accused Romero of lying and subjected her to increased investigations and intimidation and revealed information about her private life and income to neighbors.

The case files show that clients had to subject themselves to intense means-testing to receive small amounts of money from the state. They often struggled with social workers over recording small amounts of money they, or others in their family or network, made. They were also required to document income and resources that were often very unstable or might change regularly. Receiving social welfare benefits came with many strings attached. In addition, they had to open their private life to intense scrutiny, which included the possibility of home visits where social workers would collect information about their case. The files also show how social workers often commented on clients' demeanor within the files. There was an expectation that clients should be pleasant and grateful for the benefits they received. When social workers felt that clients were being difficult or not acting in the way that they expected, negative information about them as "troublesome" would be recorded in the case files. In other words, to have the best chance of receiving benefits and the support of case workers, clients must have felt that they had to perform as if they were grateful and not complain about the invasive forms that means-testing was taking during this period.

The case files also demonstrate how even when working-class women were working outside the home, they were often unable to support their families because of the low wages they received. In the case of Romero, we see one such example of a social welfare client moving back and forth between waged occupations in care work and employment in factory labor.[60] These factories paid meager wages that were often insufficient to support their families or pay for childcare. In some instances, working-class women were trying to pair low-wage employment in factories with receiving social welfare benefits that would help subsidize this income.[61] The invasive practices that social workers developed were trying to make it difficult for women to work in these jobs and receive social welfare benefits. The reality for working-class families was that, even if they were able to receive a combination of low-paying waged work and small social welfare payments, it was not enough to provide financial stability.

Working women also struggled constantly with how to find childcare or day care services when they worked outside the home. As women moved into the workforce, they could often not provide the same social reproductive labor they had previously for children and others in their households and communities. In addition, the wages they received were too paltry to provide adequate resources for families or for them to provision for the care labor they needed, which resulted in many families not having enough money or support for social reproductive labor. Social workers themselves documented the scarcity of childcare resources available to working women in their writings from the period, noting that there were limited attempts to create day care services in urban areas, such as the Centro de Cuidado Diurno de Escuela José Gautier Benítez in Santurce, but that these types of services were far too restricted. One study of the period noted that the mothers of children in this program included needleworkers, domestic workers, teachers, and washerwomen.[62] It also noted that professional women, including nurses and social workers, were struggling to find care. The failure of private or public institutions to provide childcare plagued working-class and professional women, and social workers argued that it created strains on families that would only be solved if broader day care services were available to all women.

After the first decade of the expansion of social welfare programs under the PPD, many working-class women navigated applications for social assistance and encountered social workers for the first time. At first much of the work done by social workers emphasized the value of women's caring labor, which was viewed as essential to sustaining communities deserving of state compensation. However, over time, means-testing practices that sought to quantify and regulate women's labor often ended up minimizing and erasing its value, helping to produce the idea that women were nonproductive and not deserving. As social workers deployed their shifting understanding of labor and deservingness, working-class women pushed back against how social workers made sense of their lives, labor, and entitlement. These working women insisted on the value of their labor and emphasized that social reproductive labor counted as an important form of labor. The story of welfare recipients' struggles around the terms of their labor demonstrates how these women were politicizing caring and social reproduction in their everyday lives. These stories also provide an important counterpoint to the commonplace narratives that swirled around them about how Puerto Rican working-class women were pathological and welfare dependent.

The Contested Production of Poverty Knowledge and Understanding of Working-Class Women's Deservingness

During the 1950s and 1960s, Puerto Rican social workers played an essential role in social scientific studies of poverty that the PPD encouraged. Many of these research studies were led by US scholars, and Puerto Rican social workers served as their research assistants.[63] These studies were profoundly shaped by how researchers and scholars viewed and valued working-class women's reproductive and caring labor to society. For example, a comparative analysis of two crucial studies of Puerto Rican poverty demonstrates how differences in the perception of women's labor shaped their outcomes. The first, Oscar Lewis's *La Vida: A Puerto Rican Family in the Culture of Poverty* (1966), described working-class women as nonworkers whose deviant lifestyles were supported by social welfare benefits.[64] The second, Helen Safa's *The Urban Poor of Puerto Rico: A Study in Development and Inequality*

(1974), emphasized the outsized labor of working-class women in Puerto Rican society, centering on how their reproductive labor was fundamental in sustaining families and communities in the face of rapid social change.[65] Anthropologist Jorge Duany has argued that Safa's work would "debunk the myth of the culture of poverty on empirical and conceptual grounds."[66] Examining the production of these two studies reveals that they were plagued by heated debates over how the individuals working on them interpreted women's labor and poverty.

The narratives produced during this time would have significant consequences in Puerto Rican and US society, as Lewis's ideas about Puerto Rican women's pathology and dependency became influential in popular discourse and shaped social policy. As historian Laura Briggs has argued, social scientific studies about Puerto Ricans emphasized that Puerto Rican women were "demon mothers" who passed along their deviance to their children.[67] In addition, as Briggs has demonstrated, the idea of the "welfare queen" was, in part, "born in Puerto Rico and the Lower East Side" because US officials took up studies like Lewis's La Vida as evidence that "poor" female heads of household reproduced immorality and deviance.[68] In the United States, the welfare queen was a racist stereotype based on the idea that "poor" Black and Latina women were responsible for their impoverishment because of their immorality, avoidance of work, and proclivity toward dependency on social assistance.[69] The welfare queen trope was deployed by politicians after the 1970s to justify cuts to social services, and it was commonplace for Puerto Rican women to be depicted in this way.[70] An analysis of social scientific studies from the period when these narratives were forged also shows that they were sites of struggle.

The PPD encouraged studies of Puerto Rican poverty as a part of its liberal agenda, emphasizing a "planning" approach to help instigate the archipelago's development. Scholars have shown how Puerto Rico became a social laboratory in which the impact of US-backed capitalist development could be studied.[71] Additionally, the Puerto Rican government specifically encouraged social scientists from the United States to develop research studies on the archipelago. The type of research on poverty that was done at this time was part of the broader US production of scholarship that Alice O'Conner has called "poverty knowledge" and that Aloysha Goldstein has noted was shaped by local and imperial discourses about state power, community organizing, and social movements.[72] As Goldstein shows, Puerto Rico would become a part of discussions about poverty in the United States, and Puerto Rican reformers would seek to impact the outcome of studies they hoped would lead to social change.[73] The Puerto Rican government hoped these studies would confirm that the forms of industrialization and capitalist development they were pushing forward were positively impacting society. The researchers sometimes focused on exploring the social, economic, and political changes in Puerto Rico that had been initiated since the New Deal period or, more narrowly, under the reforms of the PPD. The researchers who participated in these studies often portrayed them as demonstrating the results of a "peaceful revolution" brought on by US influence, modernization, and capitalist expansion. Within a Cold War political framework, this vision of social change was seen as a direct challenge to socialist revolutionary mobilization, like that in Cuba, and an alternative path.

From the start, social workers were deeply involved in social scientific investigations under the PPD, building on their work on such studies in previous decades. Some of these studies bridged the forms of knowledge social workers produced in the 1930s with the social changes underway in the 1950s and 1960s. For example, Dorothy Bourne and James Bourne, who had been New Deal officials in Puerto Rico, returned to Puerto Rico under the PPD government to conduct a follow-up study to their earlier investigations of poverty.[74] Dorothy Bourne, who had developed the first social work program on the island, collaborated with many social workers she had known in the 1930s and recruited a new cohort of social workers to work with her. The Bournes published a book, *Thirty Years of Change in Puerto Rico*, to show the social changes that had resulted in the years since they had been involved in New Deal programs.[75] The study reflected positively on these changes, highlighting the advances in public health. However, the authors also noted that rapid industrialization and migration to urban areas had caused destabilization in communities that were not yet totally understood.

During the same period, the anthropologist Oscar Lewis traveled to Puerto Rico to begin a research project on poverty, partly at the urging of social workers from the University of Puerto Rico. Lewis was a leftist scholar from the United States who had already written extensively on the history of Latin America and was interested in the social transformations taking place in Puerto Rico during the PPD years and the formation of migrant communities in the United States.[76] The research for his Puerto Rican study would include analysis of survey data alongside interviews with Puerto Ricans in urban areas on the archipelago and in New York City. Lewis's inclusion of Puerto Rican migrants living in the United States made his work an early example of transnational research about migration. It also meant that the study results would be more broadly of interest in both Puerto Rico and the United States.

From the start, Lewis's research was encouraged by the Puerto Rican social work leader Rosa Celeste Marín. Marín was the head of the School of Social Work at the University of Puerto Rico, and she actively recruited Lewis to come to Puerto Rico.[77] At the university, Marín was at the helm of a major study of what she called "multiproblem" social welfare cases.[78] She was particularly interested in exploring the history of families living in extreme poverty and theorizing how their conditions could be changed. After Lewis agreed to begin working in Puerto Rico, Marín put him in contact with various social workers and social work students who might be able to assist him in conducting research on the archipelago.[79] In addition, she spoke with him about different promising research areas and her hope that his expertise could contribute to the ongoing efforts of social workers and the Puerto Rican government to eradicate poverty.[80] While Lewis was grateful for the invitation and the connections he received, he didn't want his study to be too closely linked to the field of social work, as he perceived the interview information that social workers collected as being too prescriptive and dry. He ended up creating a research team comprised of Puerto Rican researchers of diverse educational backgrounds and enlisting outsiders he had worked with on his earlier studies.

Among the Puerto Rican researchers Lewis hired was Francisca Muriente, a Puerto Rican woman who had grown up in a working-class family in a rural area before moving to San Juan to study social work at the University of Puerto Rico.[81] After Muriente was selected to work with Lewis, she interviewed working-class people in the neighborhood of La Perla and soon became the most prolific researcher working on the study. Her ability to connect with those she was interviewing and get them to talk about the most personal aspects of their lives was unparalleled among the other researchers. Ultimately, she was responsible for producing half the interviews collected for the multiyear project, even though more than fifty researchers worked on the study.[82] In *La Vida*, Muriente's name was changed to "Rosa González," and the La Perla neighborhood was called "La Esmeralda." The entire narrative structure of *La Vida* relies on following Rosa as she enters the working-class neighborhood of La Esmeralda and describes it as an outside observer who is also a native of Puerto Rico.[83] Lewis uses Rosa as an avatar who descends into the city streets of the neighborhood, enters the homes of poor people in the community, and develops close and intimate relationships with her research subjects.

Later in life, Muriente became a social worker, and, using the name Rosa González, she published an article in a social work journal that offered recollections about her time working on the project. She described how she came from a "poor rural family" and was interested in learning about how "poor people in the urban area lived."[84] She recounted how at first she entered the La Perla neighborhood with her notebook, but her informants gave "cold," and she believed untrue, responses to her questions. However, over time she began to make connections in the community as she played with children and later was cared for by a kind woman while ill. She began to realize that a way to gain confidence in the neighborhood was to help women with their work and to listen to their stories. She described, in particular, helping a woman tend to her pigs, a task that she had done growing up. As they worked, Muriente told her that she herself "had to work a lot in her life," and the woman began to "tell her life story," first emphasizing her own work history and later more intimate stories about her family.[85] In another moment, in order to make time to conduct interviews with another woman, Muriente traveled with her to her job as a domestic worker and "helped to clean the house" while her informant cooked.[86] Over time she began staying overnight in the neighborhood and building closer relationships with those she was interviewing.

She would note that, as a researcher for the study, she began to build lifelong connections to the community of La Perla. Her relationships with her research subjects facilitated and shaped her work for Oscar Lewis. She developed close relationships with the families that became the center of most of her research interviews while working on the project. When her parents visited her in San Juan, she brought them to meet the families she had interviewed. She also noted that although people in the community at first viewed her as an outsider, she built relationships with them over time because she believed they came to see that she treated them as equals and was in solidarity with them.[87] The way that they saw her may not have been as she imagined, but her relationships facilitated a form of research that went far beyond what Lewis would have been able to do without her. Later she also traveled to New York to follow some of the families who had migrated there, and thus helped make the study a transnational one that emphasized migration to the United States.[88] She stayed in touch with the families over the years that followed and visited them regularly. In addition, after Lewis left Puerto Rico, Muriente continued to work in La Perla, helping establish a community health clinic in the neighborhood that solidified a longer connection to the place.[89] For Muriente, her work on the

Lewis study was just the beginning of a longer experience working in this neighborhood.

While the interview data that Muriente collected for Lewis was wide-ranging and linked to demographic data about the families in the study, the narratives that Lewis produced about them were presented in a sensationalist way. Reviewers would note that the study lacked sufficient political, social, or economic context to make sense of the narratives.[90] Lewis wrote the book for a US audience, and it was graphic and narratively driven, and soon became a bestseller. In the book, he advanced broad generalizations about Puerto Ricans and poverty to advance his theories about the "culture of poverty," which focused on the social transmission of poverty through poor families. His narratives also focused on hypersexual descriptions of Puerto Rican women, who were depicted as bad mothers who contributed little to society. The outcome of these narrative choices resulted in a book that quickly became a lightning rod for controversy once published.

Lewis received pushback about the narratives he produced for the study while he was writing it, including from Muna (Munita) Muñoz Lee, a Puerto Rican sociologist and daughter of PPD leader Luis Muñoz Marín. She argued with Lewis over the way that he presented the narratives about Puerto Ricans without providing adequate context for understanding the political and social worlds in which they lived.[91] In particular, she took issue with the way that these narratives portrayed Puerto Ricans as apolitical and inferred that people in extreme poverty were not involved in political organizing. Muñoz Lee protested the erasure of working-class Puerto Ricans' long-standing political participation in social movements over previous decades. For her, Lewis's production of narratives about a docile Puerto Rican population was particularly troubling. However, Lewis did not fully engage her criticisms or change the book; instead, he moved forward with a version that portrayed La Perla residents as he had originally planned.

La Vida produced images of Puerto Rican "poor" women as social deviants who did not work or make valuable contributions to society. It did not examine working women's labor or address how they supported or cared for their families. Instead, it broadly argued that the forms of care and mothering that they did provide were pathological and that this mothering was transmitting the "culture of poverty" to the next generation. The study emphasized that these individual women's behaviors needed to be reformed, as did the social conditions under colonialism and capitalism that had produced the situations in which they lived. Those who took up Lewis's ideas would go one step further, arguing that the state should not fund or support these women's mother-work or caring labor. In the years that followed, conservative politicians would use the results of the study to suggest that these women were deviants who were undeserving of state-funded social support because of the negative role they played in society.

When *La Vida* was published, it caused a storm of controversy among Puerto Ricans, including the frustrated responses of many of Lewis's Puerto Rican interlocutors. Puerto Ricans perceived the portrayals of themselves as unfavorable and believed that Lewis provided a lurid view of Puerto Rican poverty. Many also believed that the book would have damaging results, and some foresaw the long shadow it would cast as policymakers took it up. Over the following years, selections from *La Vida* were included in training manuals for social workers and other books meant to introduce people from the United States to Puerto Rican communities.[92] For those who republished the materials, they were seen as providing an honest account of poverty in Puerto Rico and valuable analysis. In the years that followed, US policymakers would take up this research and use it in dialogues about Puerto Ricans and social welfare.

During the same period, an alternative story about Puerto Rican poverty and working-class women emerged from the work of anthropologist Helen Safa, who also conducted extensive research on the archipelago. Safa began working for the Puerto Rican government in the 1950s, after participating in an educational trip to Puerto Rico.[93] She later wrote her master's thesis on Puerto Rico, and the Puerto Rican government later helped fund her doctoral studies at Columbia University in New York City. From 1959 to 1960, while conducting her doctoral research, Safa worked with the Puerto Rican government's Urban Renewal and Housing Administration.[94] She planned to write her dissertation about Puerto Rican communities' experiences as they relocated from "shantytown[s]" in Puerto Rico to newly developed housing projects. The first part of the study focused on a neighborhood in San Juan that she called "Los Peloteros," but which was likely El Fanguito. Safa followed how the neighborhood residents were relocated to a new urban public housing development, and how their lives were uprooted and changed dramatically.[95] The study she produced created a historical record of a community that the Puerto Rican government later demolished as a part of urban renewal.

To collect the interview data that she needed for the study, she relied on Puerto Rican research assistants, including social workers working for the Urban Renewal and Housing Administration.[96] She also worked closely with members of the Puerto Rican government, who helped her identify people to interview for the study. This research study would mark her first close collaboration with Puerto Rican interviewers, which would continue over the long years of her career where she worked in Puerto Rico. Safa would end up mentoring several Puerto Rican anthropology students, and some of her research assistants would become important scholars and political figures in Puerto Rico.[97]

During her initial research in Puerto Rico, Safa found that the communities that moved to housing projects faced many challenges as displacement disrupted the close social bonds they had formed in working-class neighborhoods.[98] Moreover, many of those who had been relocated missed the networks of support they had previously relied on. When Safa began to write up the results of her study on the housing development, her conclusions were not in line with the positive spin that the PPD wanted to maintain about their social reform programs. Safa's study was critical of the social programs created and highlighted the difficulties that working-class people faced living in housing developments. Safa conducted research that delved into the role of women in the community. Her findings revealed that many women were employed outside of their homes and were the primary breadwinners in their households. She highlighted the active involvement of Puerto Rican women in both domestic and professional spheres.[99] Her stories showcased working-class women's hard work and perseverance, portraying the strength of Puerto Rican working-class communities in the face of significant social changes.

When Safa presented her research to her collaborators and government officials in Puerto Rico, they were dissatisfied with the findings. Safa later revealed that the Puerto Rican government put intense pressure on her not to publish her research.[100] The PPD government officials felt that their investment in Safa and their support of her education had not produced the desired outcome. Despite the pressure, Safa completed her dissertation as planned. After Safa finished her follow-up research in Puerto Rico several years later, she published the results of her dissertation as the book *The Urban Poor of Puerto Rico*. It was later translated into Spanish. The follow-up research focused on further developments in the working-class communities that had been the subject of Safa's original investigation. She noted, in critique of the PPD, that its members "found it difficult to reconcile their defense of the interests of the poor with their courtship of American capitalism."[101] She critiqued the limitation of welfare state development in Puerto Rico under the PPD and argued that in order to eradicate poverty in Puerto Rico there would have to be more "radical social change." The study, as published, ended up being a well-received and important investigation of Puerto Rican poverty.

The Urban Poor of Puerto Rico included a rich set of images, some of which provide vivid depictions of Puerto Rican care and intimacy. These photographs of Safa's research subjects were taken by photographer James Weber. In some of the images, Weber photographed families in their homes, sharing moments of tenderness and joy.[102] The photographs' depiction of Puerto Ricans caring for each other makes a powerful visual argument about their humanity that stands in contrast to the dehumanizing narratives that were produced in some studies of poverty. Among the images are pictures of mothers, fathers, and grandmothers tenderly holding or watching over small children. In one such image, a Puerto Rican toddler grabs onto her mother's legs as her mother looks down with a smile (figure 3.4). This photograph, and the caption's emphasis that "the mother-child tie is very close," offers a positive portrayal of Puerto Rican motherhood.

In her work, Safa is directly in dialogue with Oscar Lewis in various ways and mentions how her research contradicts his conclusions in *La Vida*. Safa notes in the book that she disagrees with how Lewis has characterized Puerto Rican people as being apolitical; she instead highlights the various ways that working-class communities are broadly involved in political struggle.[103] She states, "We found little of the hopelessness and apathy that Lewis claims characterizes families in the culture of poverty."[104] Later in her life, she would also note several times that Lewis had a negative vision of the Puerto Rican people that was focused on how they were apathetic and docile—and that she saw a completely different thing as she worked in the Puerto Rican community.

In the study Safa particularly works to contradict narratives about Puerto Ricans as prone to welfare dependency. She offers a sharp critique of the limitations of social welfare programs and the difficulties that Puerto Ricans who apply for welfare benefits face. In the study she notes that nearly half of the "households headed by females in Los Peloteros received some public assistance."[105] She argues that many Puerto Ricans now find that "public welfare is demeaning" and that they "resent the constant prying into one's private life that public welfare imposes," which includes "checking to see if one is working (even taking in a few pieces of laundry) or if one's child is legitimate or if one is living with another man."[106] She cites one of the women from her study, "Raquel," as saying, "What they pay is a pittance, . . . they are always waiting to see if someone comes and they say look, she is washing

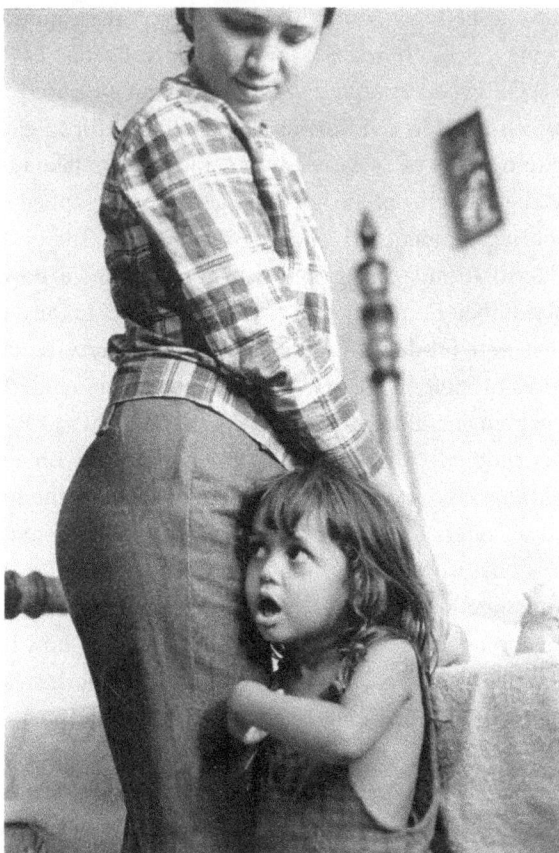

FIGURE 3.4. Puerto Rican mother and child. Photograph by James Weber. Source: Helen Safa, *The Urban Poor of Puerto Rico: A Study in Development and Inequality* (New York: Holt, Rinehart and Winston, 1947), 47.

clothes and earns so much," and then describes how benefits are often cut.[107] Safa also underscores that the payments are so low that it is still impossible for women and families to live off the proceeds.

Safa's work on her first book in Puerto Rico laid the foundation for further scholarship by her on working-class women in Latin America and how these women often supported their families. A later book, *The Myth of the Male Breadwinner* (1995), built on and expanded this research. In this research, she deployed a socialist-feminist analysis, arguing that previous studies of Latin American countries undergoing rapid industrialization and development often overlooked the importance of social reproduction. For Safa, this meant that they had not paid careful enough attention to how the exploitation of women workers, and women workers' "double-day," had facilitated the transition to twentieth-century capitalist economies. Her work was an early example of how some socialist-feminist scholars have emphasized the significance of social reproduction to the history of capitalism. Some of Safa's research assistants, like Carmen Pérez-Herráns, further developed the field of feminist labor studies in Puerto Rico. They pushed for critical interpretations of industrialization under colonial capitalism in Puerto Rico and investigated how these social and economic changes impacted working-class women.[108]

In Puerto Rico, there were tense reactions to the social scientific knowledge about poverty that was produced by the studies of scholars like Lewis and Safa. When the Puerto Rican government invited scholars to Puerto Rico to study the island's development, they hoped that these scholars would produce studies that reflected positively on PPD governance. However, one of the main issues that both Lewis and Safa raised was that capitalist development in Puerto Rico hurt poor communities. Lewis concluded that the adverse outcomes were somehow also being reproduced within Puerto Rican communities through the deviance of working-class women. He argued that the conditions that Puerto Ricans were facing were making them more apathetic and docile. For Safa, there was a different set of conditions at play, and she argued that the capitalist development underway in Puerto Rico had very destabilizing impacts on society that were difficult for working-class communities to face. In particular, she highlighted the alienation that Puerto Rican communities experienced as they were displaced from the communities where they had previously lived. She noted that people in the housing developments were still living in poverty, and they were confronting difficult conditions within them without the networks of social support that they previously had access to.

Lewis's research gained more widespread recognition when politician Daniel Moynihan drew on it to produce his study of Black families in the United States, which became known as the "Moynihan Report."[109] The report argued that Black poverty in the United States was caused by matriarchal familial structures, particularly in households headed by Black single mothers who were said to pass along deviance to their children. Moynihan's work also claimed that female heads of household were prone to "welfare dependency" and portrayed them negatively, even though he supported social welfare funding. However, his ideas were taken up by conservative political figures and used to argue for dismantling public assistance programs.[110] Consequently, policymakers initiated a rollback of social support for working-class communities, which had a profound impact on Puerto Rican women because the archipelago's social welfare programs were a partial colonial variant of those in the United States.[111] As federal funding for public assistance was cut in the United States, the amount extended to the archipelago was also reduced, leaving women in poverty.

While the research and writing of scholars like Helen Safa contradicted the claims made by Oscar Lewis in *La Vida*, commonplace negative narratives about Puerto Rican women as pathological and welfare dependent continued to circulate long after these studies. While the PPD had sought to have social scientists come to Puerto Rico to confirm and support that their development programs had been a great success, the results of these studies were more mixed than they would have liked. And, while social workers may have initially sought to create broad social support systems that would help working-class communities, their research on social scientific studies of the period was sometimes used in ways that had not been foreseen. The data those social workers produced, like the narratives that Francisca Muriente wrote for Oscar Lewis, were sometimes used to create sensationalist and damaging portrayals of working-class women. However, the work of Safa also suggests that there were profoundly different interpretations emerging in social science and society. For the next generation of Puerto Rican feminist scholars that Safa worked with, questions of social reproduction and women's labor under colonial capitalism would emerge as central questions for further investigation and political mobilization.

DURING THE 1940S, the creation of new social welfare programs under the PPD provided access to welfare benefits to a rapidly expanding number of clients. Many of these clients were working-class women struggling to navigate the social, economic, and political instability caused by colonial capitalism and the mass displacement and migration of workers. As they claimed benefits from these programs, they hoped they would receive support to help them take care of themselves and their families. And while these programs did bring much-needed resources to some applicants, they also ushered in an expansive new regimen of means-testing and social regulation of working-class people's lives. The case files of social welfare agencies show how working-class women struggled with social workers over the terms dictating means-testing. In the following years, growing numbers of applicants would undergo these often regulatory practices to receive small benefit payments that were insufficient to provide adequate support. For most working-class women, these means-tested benefits were more limited than the expansive social support they had desired.

The work of means-testing required separating out social welfare applicants who the state believed were deserving from those who were not. This chapter traces how this process resulted in social welfare projects of the period, moving from a broader focus on the state expansively supporting women's reproductive labor to a gradual erasure of this labor from state records. As social workers began quantifying reproductive labor and clients' meager resources, at first, they created a detailed record of women's labor that state agencies often overlooked. Some believed they should provide these women with monetary support that would also help facilitate their broader social reproductive labor and also help their families, communities, and society. However, this data was eventually mainly used to restrict access to benefits, and its collection incentivized applicants to obscure this labor or not have it recorded. Over time, these means-testing practices would erase women's labor from the historical record and emphasize more narrow and restricted ideas of deservingness.

In the decades that followed, the production of new ideas about poverty in mainstream discourses often nefariously cast working-class Puerto Rican women as undeserving of state benefits and as prone to welfare dependency. Within social scientific studies, Puerto Rican and US social workers, social scientists, and government officials debated and discussed why poverty persisted on the archipelago. In the late 1950s and early 1960s, a common and damaging narrative emerged within these debates that Puerto Rican mothers were pathological and that they passed along negative behaviors to their children. Some scholars and activists pushed back against broad portrayals of working-class Puerto Rican women as "welfare queens" who were hypersexual, apolitical, and undeserving of citizenship. However, these negative depictions of Puerto Rican women remained in Puerto Rico and the United States, and they became part of the fodder for discrimination against Puerto Rican migrants.

As the Puerto Rican government became more deeply involved in sponsoring labor migration to the United States, many working-class women would arrive in US cities where these stereotypes would negatively impact them. They would also become embroiled in even more politically charged debates over their reproductive and caring labor in which working-class women and social workers sometimes struggled against one another and other times worked in solidarity. These decades-long political mobilizations over labor and welfare would disprove time and again the narratives about Puerto Rican women's apolitical nature that continued to circulate in public discourse.

Part II

CARE WORK AND
WOMEN'S ACTIVISM
IN THE PUERTO RICAN
DIASPORA

Care Workers, Household Labor Organizing, and Puerto Rican Migration after 1944

On November 28, 1946, a group of Puerto Rican women picketed in front of the Chicago offices of Castle, Barton, and Associates, the private employment agency that had brought them to the city to become domestic workers. Puerto Rican students from the University of Chicago, as well as labor rights organizers, joined the protestors and supported their demand that the agency be accountable for the terrible labor conditions that migrant contract workers faced in the city.[1] The women on the picket line had been recruited from the Puerto Rican cities of San Juan and Ponce, where around six hundred women had signed labor contracts drafted by the private agency and overseen by the Puerto Rican government's Department of Labor. When the women arrived in Chicago, they were met with low wages, long hours, and deductions from their pay for transportation and other costs. They responded by walking away from their jobs, forming alliances with other migrants and the Puerto Rican community in the United States, and seeking alternative forms of employment in the city.

Months earlier, Castle, Barton, and Associates had advertised in Chicago newspapers that Puerto Rican domestic workers were available and had solicited requests from potential employers. Lured by the promise of workers willing to accept half the city's going rate, employers were willing to pay transportation costs up front. They sought to undercut a rising wage scale that resulted from local domestic workers organizing for better wages and legal restrictions on immigrant labor.[2] Working-class Puerto Rican women could travel to the United States because they were colonial US citizens and were willing to sign contracts and move in search of employment. However, when they migrated to the United States and encountered difficult labor conditions and exploitation, they quickly protested.[3] The history of working-class domestic workers' resistance and their alliances with professional social workers and feminist labor reformers reveal Puerto Rican women's ongoing participation in debates about the value of care work and reproductive labor. Their political mobilization around care work put pressure on Puerto Rican and US politicians to reform the labor migration that they were actively promoting and create lasting changes in migration in the years that followed.

The migration of Puerto Ricans to Chicago to become domestic workers has attracted scholarly investigations because it represents a crucial flashpoint in the struggle for Puerto Rican migrants' rights in the United States.[4] As scholars have shown, this domestic worker migration generated broad public conversation and debate over the rights of Puerto Rican workers to move to the continental United States and raised the question of their status—that is, would the legal entitlement of Puerto Ricans to full US citizenship rights and benefits once they moved to the United States, as opposed to the restricted version of territorial US citizenship they received as colonial subjects while living in Puerto Rico, be respected?[5] These questions emerged at a moment when the colonial relationship between Puerto Rico and the United States was being reworked under the leadership of a new Puerto Rican populist government that rose to power during the same period. This government launched a development and industrialization program to promote emigration, sponsoring labor migrations that would place workers in US jobs where they often faced challenging conditions. The problems surfaced in these labor migration programs, like those faced by domestic workers in Chicago, put pressure on the Puerto Rican government to regulate and reform its migration policies.

In the 1940s, the Puerto Rican government and the Partido Popular Democrático (PPD) implemented programs to promote and regulate the labor and reproduction of women. As a part of this program, working-class women were encouraged to migrate to the United States, which would ultimately lead to a reduction in Puerto Rico's population. Many of these initial migrants were also specifically recruited to become domestic workers. Additionally, the government encouraged US industries to establish themselves in Puerto Rico to take advantage of the cheap labor provided by women workers. The government also recognized the growing need for care work in the Puerto Rican diaspora, thus promoting women's migration to fulfill this need. In migrant communities, working-class women were expected to care for their families and work for wages. The government also encouraged the migration of professional women care workers, especially those who would help integrate Puerto Rican migrants into US communities, typically through their work as social workers. The migration of Puerto Rican women to be care workers in the diaspora significantly impacted how they experienced Puerto Rican citizenship and belonging. Furthermore, as growing numbers of Puerto Rican women migrated, struggles over migrant rights also became struggles over care, work, and social reproduction in the diaspora.

The history of these Puerto Rican household workers is also a story about their participation in a broader political mobilization of women around household labor reform in the United States. In US cities, Puerto Rican workers discovered that the labor conditions faced by domestic workers were being hotly contested by workers, labor organizers, activists, and government officials.[6] In addition, as Premilla Nadasen has shown, African American women in the United States had long led the charge in domestic worker organizing and labor protections and connected this political organizing to their participation in other social movements.[7] As Puerto Rican women in the United States began organizing around their labor conditions, they built a coalition with professional Puerto Rican women and progressive US reformers to demand that domestic work be regulated through labor reform.[8] Because they had little political or social support, Puerto Rican women resisted degrading labor conditions through work stoppages and walkouts.

The story of Puerto Rican women migrant workers during this period demonstrates the importance of political mobilization and organizing around care work in the Puerto Rican diaspora. Puerto Rican household workers and social workers soon became a part of a reform alliance that pressured the Puerto Rican and US governments to take responsibility for what had happened to migrant workers in the United States. While domestic work remained outside of US labor protections, Puerto Rican domestic workers were able to make demands on the Puerto Rican state by calling for the regulation of migrant contract work by the insular legislature and the colonial government's sponsorship of household worker training programs. Despite these reforms, the response of the Puerto Rican state to worker organizing and labor reform activism failed to create well-paid, safe, and desirable jobs in household work. Nevertheless, the history of Puerto Rican women's domestic work and the struggle for regulation illuminates a formative moment in Puerto Rican women's organizing and activism for labor rights. As growing numbers of Puerto Ricans migrated to the United States, this migration opened new dialogues about gender, rights, and citizenship in the Puerto Rican diaspora that were shaped by both race and gender.

The Puerto Rican Government, Labor Migration, and Gender Politics

During the 1940s, growing numbers of Puerto Rican women, including those who would become domestic workers and social workers, migrated to the United States in search of work as a part of state-sponsored migration programs (see figure 4.1). The Puerto Rican government's development strategies during this period often centered on gendered reforms and targeted working-class women's social reproduction as a central concern of state projects.[9] During this period, the demand for household workers in US homes opened an opportunity for US companies and the Puerto Rican government to oversee and promote the migration of women care workers to the United States. As problems arose with these programs, Puerto Rican social workers who were professional care workers trained at US institutions and were drawn into efforts to regulate and reform household worker migration. Ultimately, working-class and professional women's care work in the diaspora helped shape migration policy and the formation of Puerto Rican communities in the United States.

This migration of Puerto Rican workers coincided with the rise of a new populist party, the PPD, which sought to transform the colonial relationship between Puerto Rico and the United States. Under the PPD, new social reforms were pushed forward that were closely linked to the liberal US and Puerto Rican New Deal leadership.[10] The PPD proposed transforming Puerto Rico's society and economy through a development and industrialization project known as Operation Bootstrap. This modernization plan sought to bring capital and jobs to Puerto Rico by incentivizing US corporations, including tax breaks and cheap labor.[11] US scholars saw Puerto Rico as a laboratory to study industrialization and development, and it became

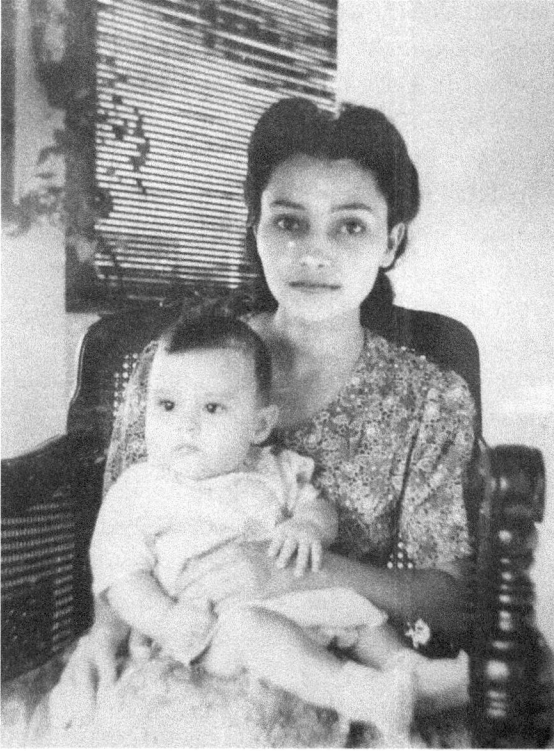

FIGURE 4.1. Formeria Jiménez Amador, the author's grandmother, ca. 1940s, before she migrated from Puerto Rico to the United States to find employment as a domestic worker. Collection of the author.

known as the "showcase of democracy."[12] These policies also continued to bind the Puerto Rican and US economies together and provide the economic and political foundation for the parties' call for creating a new commonwealth status for the archipelago, which was created in 1952.

Many of the PPD's development and reform programs centered on working-class women and questions of social reproduction. These programs partly resulted from the Puerto Rican government's belief that the archipelago was overpopulated and that reducing the population would assist development efforts and reduce poverty. The state worked to reduce the archipelago's population through the promotion of eugenics and the distribution of birth control.[13] It also continued its involvement in training working-class women in gendered vocational education programs that prepared them for care work and employment in waged work that was gender segregated, like needlework. They advertised to US companies that there was a low-wage workforce on the archipelago, including women workers who were paid even less than men.[14] These programs went together with efforts to promote women's labor migration to the United States, which had already occurred for decades but now would be more actively encouraged by the Puerto Rican government. The growing demand for factory and household workers during the war provided another opportunity for the state to become involved in population control through emigration.

In addition to eugenic policies, the Puerto Rican government began exploring opportunities to encourage emigration through labor migration, which had occurred in other historical moments and was now reinvestigated with renewed interest.[15] They formalized the development of this policy by creating an Emigration Advisory Committee in July 1945 that discussed how migration should be encouraged and regulated. One of the ways that officials sought to propel migration was through new contract labor programs administered by the Puerto Rican government and the US War Manpower Commission.[16] The War Manpower Commission was responsible for bringing more than two thousand Puerto Ricans to work in the United States in 1944 alone.[17] Among these workers were many recruited to work in canneries, such as those for the Campbell Soup Company. During the war, more Puerto Rican workers were recruited to the United States to fill agricultural, factory, and domestic jobs.[18]

During the 1940s, the Emigration Advisory Committee also discussed the possibility of transforming the Puerto Rican government's role in the United States through its offices in the United States. The Puerto Rican government had operated the Bureau of Employment and Identification in New York City since 1930. Located in Harlem, this office issued identification cards and helped place workers in jobs in the city, playing a similar role to other private and government-sponsored employment agencies of the period.[19] Like these agencies, it oversaw the placement of workers in jobs throughout the city. In addition, it provided identification cards that proved Puerto Ricans were US citizens and that were meant to help them avoid the discrimination faced by foreign workers. Migrants used these documents when searching for jobs and dealing with employers, landlords, schools, and representatives of social service agencies.[20] The Puerto Rican government viewed the agency as potentially providing a valuable base for addressing issues that had already arisen from Puerto Rican labor migration and integration into New York City.

The Puerto Rican government's efforts to develop the island by promoting the emigration of working-class women were also increasingly reflected in the work of the branches of the state that it created and cultivated in the United States. And in the years that followed, the expanded version of the Puerto Rican Department of Labor's branch in the United States also became involved in promoting and regulating women's work in household employment in the United States. These programs also encouraged the migration of Puerto Rican professional women care workers to work for Puerto Rican and US government agencies as social workers overseeing migration. Over the years, these programs increasingly funneled working-class and professional women into positions as care workers in the Puerto Rican diaspora and in Puerto Rican migrant communities in the United States.

The Puerto Rican Department of Labor's Bureau of Employment and Identification and Domestic Worker Placement

The Puerto Rican government's Bureau of Employment and Identification in New York placed working-class women as domestic workers throughout the city, like many other US private and state-sponsored employment agencies. The placement and training programs it created, which emphasized care work and home economics, pushed Puerto Rican women into positions as domestic workers during the 1930s. According to the agency, domestic workers, trained and untrained, composed the largest number of laborers placed during the period—three times as many as in needlework.[21] While women might not have needed an intermediary to find needlework positions, these numbers suggest that domestic work was an essential source of employment for Puerto Rican women. The Puerto Rican government's role in placing these workers established a pattern that persisted well after the 1930s as it continued to navigate the politics of placing workers in domestic positions that were increasingly racially segregated, were unregulated by labor laws, and left them open to exploitation by employers.

During the 1930s and 1940s, an important aspect of the Bureau of Employment and Identification's work was addressing the xenophobia, racism, and exclusion that Puerto Rican workers faced in the United States. The New York City press and government agencies increasingly portrayed Puerto Ricans as a racial "other" and deployed various racial scripts about communities of color in the United States against them. They often referred to the "Puerto Rican Problem," a catchphrase mirroring that of the "Negro Problem," which suggested islanders were not ethnically or racially a part of mainstream US society.[22] Puerto Ricans were also still seen as colonial subjects who needed Americanization to assimilate properly. When Puerto Ricans were categorized as uniformly "nonwhite," it also sometimes resulted from US officials not recognizing multiple or mixed racial heritages within commonplace US "Black" and "white" binaries. However, while these blanket categories did lead to discrimination, the intensity of racial discrimination was much more severely felt by Puerto Ricans of African descent, who were the targets of racial discrimination both within Puerto Rican and US society.[23]

At the same time, Puerto Rican workers and their advocates had also been active in responding to the social exclusion and racism they faced. These workers protested their poor conditions and demanded that Puerto Rican and US government officials assist migrants in their struggles for economic and civil rights. Puerto Rican activists in New York, including many leftists, also developed harsh critiques of the PPD's policies and its sponsorship of labor migration to New York. These activists highlighted how the liberal agenda of the Puerto Rican government emphasized the interests of development and capitalism at the expense of providing social support and help to working-class Puerto Rican communities on the island or in the diaspora.[24] Some of these activists allied with US congressman Vito Marcantonio, an Italian American socialist politician who supported Puerto Rican labor organizers and independence leaders. Marcantonio's offices frequently provided help to migrants facing discrimination through his Spanish-speaking assistants. Concerned about pro-independence and socialist political organizing among Puerto Ricans in the United States, the PPD developed numerous countermeasures during the period, going as far as sponsoring a campaign against Marcantonio.[25] Despite the pushback that these activists faced, they continued to organize for migrant rights and to be critical of migration policies.

While Puerto Rican government officials of the Bureau of Employment and Identification saw themselves as fighting discrimination in Puerto Rican communities, the work they did placing Puerto Rican migrants into labor markets segregated by gender and race deepened the inequalities workers faced. As historian Lorrin Thomas has documented, Puerto Rican officials in the Bureau of Employment and Identification also struggled over classifying and categorizing Puerto Ricans racially as they conducted their work.[26] Sometimes Puerto Rican officials' understanding of "whiteness" came into conflict with that of US officials, especially as popular understandings of Puerto Ricans as a nonwhite population became commonplace. The agency was often limited to placing workers in occupations that were low waged and unstable, including those in agricultural work and service occupations. For working-class women this sometimes meant placement in needlework and factory jobs, but as these jobs became more difficult to find in later years, it would mean integration into the labor market increasingly in precarious positions doing care work in private homes. As these placements continued, Puerto Ricans were further racialized as nonwhite in the United States through their integration into racially segregated labor markets. In addition, Puerto Ricans of African descent would particularly face limited opportunities and racial segregation as they sought work in US cities.

As the Puerto Rican government sought to find work for Puerto Rican women, including positions in needlework, they encountered a shifting and increasingly segregated economy in which some women's labor was in higher demand than others for specific jobs.[27] Growing numbers of European immigrant women were moving outside the home as wage laborers, leading to increased demand for domestic work at the same time that shifting standards of middle-class domesticity and housekeeping intensified the need for caring labor.[28] Puerto Ricans joined African American women, many of them recent migrants from the South who became domestics when they faced labor discrimination in other fields and were funneled into these jobs by private agencies and government-sponsored employment programs. A study of Puerto Rican migration in the 1930s reported that "it is not unusual, when a woman calls by telephone to inquire about obtaining a Puerto Rican worker and is asked whether she prefers a white or colored Puerto Rican, for the woman to reply that, since she had asked for a Puerto Rican, of course she wants a colored person."[29] Since employers increasingly expected domestic workers to be "colored" and imagined Puerto Ricans as uniformly nonwhite, they judged Puerto Rican women to be suited for domestic work. The employers would actually encounter a racially diverse group of Puerto Rican domestic workers, although patterns of racialized gendered servitude in Puerto Rican communities meant that women of African descent were generally overrepresented in these occupations. By agreeing to place migrant women as domestics in US cities in the 1930s, Puerto Rican government policy served to further mark these workers as nonwhite.

Employer expectations of labor in the middle-class white home further framed the experiences of Puerto Rican women who became domestic workers. But these expectations often diverged from those of the workers themselves. Employers argued that nonwhite women needed training in white, middle-class norms of domesticity in order to properly do their jobs. While these ideas stemmed from a longer history of middle-class reformers instructing immigrant women in how to perform household work, African American women increasingly became the targets of these interventions in urban areas.[30] Puerto Rican domestic workers faced similar scrutiny. Investigators claimed that "whatever merits of Puerto Rican and American methods of household management may be, they are at least very different.

Unless she were employed by a Spanish-speaking family of the lower-income group, the average domestic worker from the archipelago seeking employment in New York, would require training." Casting Puerto Rican women as needing instruction in white middle-class US domesticity was underpinned by popular discourses of Puerto Ricans' racial and colonial difference. One observer, for example, charged that they lacked culinary aptitude: "The average Puerto Rican woman knows very little about the cooking of American food. Some of the vegetables found in Puerto Rico are unknown in New York. The Puerto Rican cook uses too much grease or lard to suit the American taste."[31] In the United States, Puerto Rican women found ideas similar to those taught in Americanization programs on the archipelago, restated and reworked, as they sought employment as domestic workers.[32]

Some labor reformers and domestic workers also supported the idea of training but for a different reason. These activists believed that training could lead to the professionalization of domestic work, which would allow workers to claim the status of skilled laborer, making it possible for them to demand higher wages, better working conditions, the regulation of domestic work by state agencies, and access to social benefits and rights under future labor legislation. Although domestic worker training programs in the United States had long existed, these reformers gained more government funding for education in domestic work throughout the 1930s. The majority of this training targeted African American women. Under the Works Progress Administration in New York City, for example, African American women made up to 93 percent of the workers selected for housekeeping aides training programs.[33] Puerto Rican women also participated in these educational initiatives and were sometimes referred by the offices to private programs in the city. The Casita María settlement house, for example, served the "Spanish-speaking" community with instructional classes for Puerto Rican migrants.[34]

The Puerto Rican Bureau of Employment and Identification was limited in its placements by the reluctance of Puerto Rican women to accept live-in positions. From the beginning, the bureau noted that many prospective employers sought live-in workers. Puerto Rican women were averse to this type of employment, however, preferring to work first in any other type of job or, if in domestic work, then specifically as day laborers. The demand for day labor positions resembles struggles of African American women in the United States, who sought to move away from the exploitation that live-in domestics faced.[35] Generations of African American women distanced themselves from the control of their employers through live-out jobs. African

American women's continued aversion to this type of work may have led some employers to seek out Puerto Rican domestics (some of whom were Afro-Puerto Rican), whose recent migration status and often precarious economic circumstances, employers believed, might have made them more amenable to live-in work. Yet many Puerto Rican women avoided live-in jobs too and pressured the labor agency to explore other options for their placement. However, despite Puerto Rican women's aversions to live-in domestic employment, the expansion of the Puerto Rican Department of Labor's work in the United States in the 1940s resulted in increased attempts to place women in these positions.

The "Chicago Experiment" and Workers' Resistance

In 1946 the "Chicago experiment," which brought hundreds of domestic workers to the city, marked a new moment in the history of Puerto Rican labor migration. During the Second World War, larger waves of Puerto Rican migration occurred as US employers sought cheap sources of labor. US agricultural firms and other businesses recruited some, others were fleeing unemployment and poverty on the archipelago, and after 1942 the new ruling party, the populist PPD, encouraged migration to lower Puerto Rico's population and reduce unemployment.[36] The Puerto Rican state mainly targeted intervention into the lives of working-class women through eugenics policies because their sexuality had long been blamed for social problems on the archipelago, such as overpopulation.[37] The PPD developed new migration policies as a part of Operation Bootstrap, a modernization and development plan that sought to industrialize Puerto Rico by providing incentives to US corporations, such as tax breaks and cheap labor.[38] The Puerto Rican government also developed a contract labor program to encourage and regulate emigration to the United States.[39] These state policies created a colonial migration flow between the archipelago and the United States, resulting in the rapid expansion of Puerto Rican communities in several US cities.

Before the Puerto Rican government developed its own contract labor program, privately owned US agencies conducted most labor recruitment on the archipelago. Domestic workers, for example, were sent to Chicago, Philadelphia, and Atlanta.[40] The largest group consisted of hundreds of women recruited by Castle, Barton, and Associates, which had offices in Ponce and San Juan; they began arriving in 1944. The majority were sent to Chicago, where they established a new Puerto Rican community.[41] The employment agency advertised in Chicago newspapers that Puerto Rican domestic workers were available for hire. Potential employers filled out paperwork requesting domestic workers with particular attributes and skills. Meanwhile, on the archipelago, Puerto Rican women also signed contracts that were overseen by Puerto Rico's Department of Labor. Over half of the women were under twenty years of age; younger teenagers ignored the minimum cut-off age of eighteen and signed up. Numerous recruits thought these jobs would allow them time to study or gain other experiences and opportunities in Chicago.[42]

Racial politics stood at the forefront of incorporating these domestic workers into Chicago. The first advertisements that the agency placed noted that "Puerto Ricans [White]" were available to work, while later reports noted that "colored" Puerto Ricans had been sent to Florida and Atlanta. Unlike the earlier placement of workers in New York, such racial descriptions may have signaled that Puerto Rican migrant workers were like earlier waves of European immigrant workers previously employed in domestic service. Indeed, officials working for the Puerto Rican government also began describing the migration of Puerto Rican women to the United States as being akin to that of European women.[43] The Puerto Rican government benevolently cast the program as providing Puerto Ricans with an opportunity to be integrated into the United States, like European immigrants before them. Racial demarcation explicitly set them apart from African American and Mexican women already working in domestic service in the city. However, despite company efforts to market these women as white, racial and colonial logics and discourses of both employers and US government officials cast the workers as nonwhite.[44] When the workers arrived in Chicago and encountered residential and social segregation, the majority navigated this by entering and befriending Mexican and African American communities, compounding popular and state perceptions of them as nonwhite.

Women responded to the difficult labor conditions, including long hours and low pay, by walking away from jobs as domestics. They did so as soon as they created networks of friends and alliances in the city, which made it possible for them to move out of employers' homes and into temporary housing in hotels provided by the recruiters. When they did so, workers immediately encountered state organizations and agencies that viewed them as subject to the same regulatory regimes as immigrant communities and communities of color in Chicago. Upon realizing they couldn't deport the workers because they were US citizens, social agencies denied them social assistance based on the same Illinois residency requirements often used to discriminate against African American communities and particularly against migrants from the South. They also became the targets of local police, who were conducting an antiprostitution campaign.[45] A number of the women were arrested, likely after socializing at dance and social clubs in the city. Reporters suggested that because of the low wages received in Chicago, the Puerto Rican women had begun working as prostitutes. Concern over Puerto Rican women's integration into African American and Mexican neighborhoods and their socializing with men from these communities framed these accusations.[46]

The domestic workers found cross-class and cross-race allies. The Young Women's Christian Association (YWCA) invited them to social events and teas where they shared their experiences. Gathering with other domestic workers provided a forum for the Puerto Rican women to make friends. They began traveling together to other gatherings, sometimes meeting up with Puerto Rican men in the city as contract workers.[47] The YWCA long had served as a site for discussions on the conditions of household labor, its regulation, and its professionalization through training.[48] At the YWCA, Puerto Rican women compared their work experiences and wages with other domestics; they realized that they were making half the average rate for household work in the city, while working longer hours and getting less time off. The Puerto Rican workers also learned that the agency was trying to undercut the wages of local household workers by bringing Puerto Rican women to the city.[49]

At the YWCA, Puerto Rican workers also found out about the ongoing struggle of household workers, particularly African American women, to attain better working conditions. They met women who were already organizing to create labor standards for domestic work. Among them was the Household Employees League, a group representing domestic workers that met at the YWCA. Its members joined in seeking better working conditions for Puerto Rican women and later joined the picket lines when the workers organized a strike. Puerto Rican women quickly learned that, despite numerous attempts by domestic workers to organize for inclusion under protective labor legislation, state and federal standards excluded this job category. In coming to the United States to work as domestics, they had entered a contentious political field that was in the process of extensive political mobilization and the subject of much debate.

These workers developed allies among Puerto Rican graduate students at the University of Chicago who had connections to Puerto Rican political leaders on the archipelago; notably, Elena Padilla, a young anthropologist, and her roommate Muna Muñoz Lee, the daughter of the leader of Puerto

Rico's senate.[50] The students used their personal connections to raise awareness about the labor conditions the workers faced through an already existing network of Puerto Ricans in the United States. They argued that the terms of the contracts were exploitative and that the contracts themselves could not legally be enforced. There were no US laws specifically regulating domestic work, and when workers attempted to contact the Puerto Rican government about contract violations, there was little response. Together the students and more than fifty domestic workers organized labor strikes, picketed the offices of a private employment agency, and documented the women's experiences.[51] The students also reached out to established social activists and labor leader Jesús Colón in New York City, who arranged for some of the Chicago domestic workers to travel to the New York Puerto Rican community to discuss their conditions.[52] The student allies both brought public attention to what had happened and demanded that the Puerto Rican government investigate the case and intervene. They insisted that the colonial state was obligated to address the conditions that domestic workers had experienced and ensure that similar cases didn't occur in the future. Puerto Rican officials responded by coming to Chicago to investigate, a result of the students' networks on the archipelago and their ability to reach officials.

One of the first Puerto Rican representatives involved in the case was Carmen Isales, a social worker trained at the University of Chicago who helped build social welfare programs on the archipelago.[53] Isales had previously studied at the University of Puerto Rico, and her sister Josephina Isales was also a social worker, so she had deep connections with the social work profession. Later in life, Isales married Fred Wale, a US educator, and became a central figure in organizing community development projects on the archipelago under the Division of Community Education developed by the PPD.[54] As a student in Chicago she had worked with local social agencies that served Puerto Rican workers. Although she worked for the Puerto Rican government as a social worker on the archipelago and, therefore, was a state agent, her interest in the case initially was personal. Isales first learned about the domestic work program when she saw the advertisements seeking workers in Puerto Rico. She was skeptical of the offers she saw in the papers, which suggested that workers would receive thirty-five dollars a week, much more than the ten- or twelve-dollar-a-month average a domestic worker could make on the archipelago.[55] However, Isales knew that in the United States, most domestic workers received closer to fifty dollars a month because while she was a student, she had tried to hire help and was told by friends it was too expensive. Curious about the intentions of the employment agency, Isales decided to investigate the situation when she traveled to Chicago on a vacation, which doubled as an opportunity to check in with administrators at the Chicago School of Social Work about the possibility of finishing her degree.

When she arrived in Chicago, Isales discovered that the Puerto Rican domestic workers were living in "horrible" conditions. She judged their situation to be a "system" of "indentured servitude" that had been formally supported by the Puerto Rican colonial government itself. Isales noted that the Department of Labor agents had a relationship with the private agency and that their primary loyalty was not with the workers.[56] She noted that when the commissioner of labor traveled to Chicago, he was picked up in a company car hired by Castle, Barton, and Associates. When she began her investigation of the workers' conditions, the company immediately accused her of being a communist, something that she recalled was then "the quickest way to stop social justice." Despite the denunciations she received from the company, she found support from the YWCA, which she noted "had always been a pioneer in these cases" and which offered her an office. She then gained the secretarial support of a friend, Juanita Aldea, who helped her investigate the cases and begin corresponding with US and Puerto Rican government agencies. She also met up with the Puerto Rican students already working to organize the domestic workers and joined them in organizing the workers and pressuring the Puerto Rican government to respond to their needs.[57]

Employers frustrated by absconding workers organized to try to recuperate the loss in transportation costs they had paid to the private agencies for the domestic workers to come to the United States. They had planned to gradually deduct these costs from salaries, and when they could not, they demanded that Castle, Barton, and Associates, or the women themselves, repay them. Some employers threatened workers with deportation or arrest by the police if they did not pay for transportation costs. As tensions escalated and the private agency argued it was not responsible, the employers began to sue the workers for breach of contract and for expenses. Isales went to court with the women to help them get the charges dropped.

Isales began her investigation into the case by interviewing thirty domestic workers who had participated in the program.[58] In her report to the Puerto Rican government, she specifically described how employers sought to exploit Puerto Rican women by paying them less than US workers, undercutting even the relatively low wages that they had offered African American women for these same jobs.[59] Isales also drew attention to the lack of coverage of domestic work by US labor legislation, suggesting that women's participation in this type of work made them vulnerable because there were no labor standards. After receiving Isales's report, Fernando Sierra Berdecia, the commissioner of labor of Puerto Rico, arrived in the United States to further investigate the domestic work program.[60] Meanwhile, workers and their allies continued to call attention to the state's complicity in placing Puerto Ricans in unregulated, low-paid, and dangerous occupations. Isales played a central role in relating information about the problems with the contract labor program to the Puerto Rican government and presenting them with information about the broader discussion. What had begun as a vacation turned into a full inquiry and resulted in presenting a persuasive argument to the Puerto Rican government that changes in migration policy needed to be addressed.

While in Chicago, Isales also collaborated with field agents from the Women's Bureau of the US Department of Labor. The Women's Bureau representatives noted that situations like those created by the Chicago program could be averted if the US government regulated domestic work and if state agencies managed migrant labor.[61] On October 8, 1946, a "committee representing public and private agencies," explained bureau director Frieda S. Miller, contacted the agency for "both facts on the rights and responsibilities of employers, workers, and community agencies involved, and help in dealing with the human problems of the workers." This group included welfare agencies, civic and religious groups, individual employers, and later the Puerto Rican workers themselves, who "complained of their conditions of work, deductions from their pay which they did not understand, and of other misrepresentation."[62] One of the main issues that the Puerto Rican workers faced was that most of the workers in social and government agencies did not understand or respect that Puerto Ricans were US citizens and were afforded the same legal protections as other workers.

The Women's Bureau agents worked alongside Isales and the Puerto Rican students to intervene on behalf of the Puerto Rican workers. As Frieda S. Miller noted, "Consideration of all these questions had to be in terms of the undeniable right of Puerto Ricans, as American citizens, to take up residence and employment with exactly the same freedom as any other American citizen. And I may say that that was not very well understood by the community in which they found themselves." But US citizenship did not mean that Puerto Rican women would have labor protections as domestic workers because, as Isales and the other reformers had learned, such labor fell out of the purview of labor standards. Because "there are no laws of any State—with one possible exception, in the State of Washington—which limit the hours of women employed in domestic service," as Miller explained: "In the case of this particular group of migrants, what was done to improve their conditions had to be by way of the acceptance of voluntary standards and the understanding of the importance of those if there was to be a good working relationship." In Miller's vision, the most the Women's Bureau and the other reformers could do was try to negotiate the best possible conditions for workers outside of formal legal protections.

Despite the inability of women reformers to regulate Puerto Rican contract labor or help the workers gain better working conditions, the scandal generated major changes. The workers' strike, the organizing of domestic workers with professional women, and calls for reform by various US officials all pressured the Puerto Rican government to intervene. In response, the Puerto Rican colonial political apparatus mobilized, propelled in its own right by the populist government's desire to continue using emigration as a means of depopulation. It worked to stave off another scandal. The Chicago field agent from the Women's Bureau was invited to Puerto Rico to discuss the case, and Miller happily reported that in the future the Women's Bureau agents would take up central roles as intermediaries between US employers and migrant laborers, like the Puerto Rican domestic workers. The Puerto Rican government enlisted these representatives to join it in creating an insular program that would regulate contract labor using the laws of the colonial state to intervene into the lives of migrant workers while the United States remained disengaged. The organizing and resistance of the domestic workers, local students, and seasoned reformers like Isales and Women's Bureau agents led to this change. The women reformers involved in the Chicago case were quickly enlisted to create a new state-sponsored household worker training program that emerged within a year of the workers organizing and striking.

Regulating and Reforming Labor Migration

In response to calls for an investigation into the experience of domestic workers and other Puerto Rican laborers in the United States, the Puerto Rican government instituted a new set of policies to regulate contract work. They formed a Migration Division of the Puerto Rican Department of Labor in New York City to expand the earlier Bureau of Employment and Identification activities and create other branches in the United States. Demands made by workers, unions, and labor reformers in Puerto Rico and the United States resulted in the expansion of the Puerto Rican colonial government's role in the US administrative apparatus regulating labor. The colonial government responded to demands for supervision of labor recruitment while it broadened the ongoing activities of its New York agency. Thus, the agency expanded, owing to government plans to promote out-migration, labor organizing, and mobilizations recently institutionalized in the Puerto Rican Department of Labor and to workers' and citizens' protests that labor agencies be regulated.[63]

Isales was directly involved in this process as an intermediary. She traveled to Washington, DC, to meet with Luis Muñoz Marín to discuss the labor situation after her investigation. While she was in Washington, she spoke with him and his wife about the conditions that Puerto Rican workers faced. One of the main issues that arose in their conversation was the fact that Puerto Rican workers didn't know what their rights were as US citizens. One of the plans of these administrators was to educate Puerto Rican workers about their rights. She noted that Muñoz Marín was already thinking about a broader public education program along these lines on the archipelago.[64] Besides working on the Chicago study, Isales produced other documents about migration for the Puerto Rican government. She wrote a study of social welfare systems that was reproduced in social scientist Clarence Senior's first study of Puerto Rican migration.[65]

The Chicago case became one of the justifications for creating a more robust labor regulation and migration system. In response to this issue and others created by problems with Puerto Rican labor migration to the United States, the already-established Emigration Advisory Committee also formalized new labor policies. Toward this end they oversaw the passing in the Puerto Rican legislature of a new law in May 1947 that made it necessary for employment agencies to register their programs with the insular Department of Labor.[66] The resulting changes in contract labor migration thus were closely tied to the labor resistance of domestic workers and the calls for reform made by Puerto Rican women professionals. The reforms would also go hand in hand with creating other forms of reform, including household worker training programs. The Puerto Rican Department of Education would soon oversee the creation of household training programs that trained women how to be migrant household workers in the United States (see figure 4.2).

Seeking to prevent another scandal like the one in Chicago, the Puerto Rican government hired Frances Phillips, an experienced domestic worker and labor organizer from the United States, to help develop a new state-sponsored household worker program to regulate contract labor. Phillips, an African American woman, was chosen for the post because of her experience

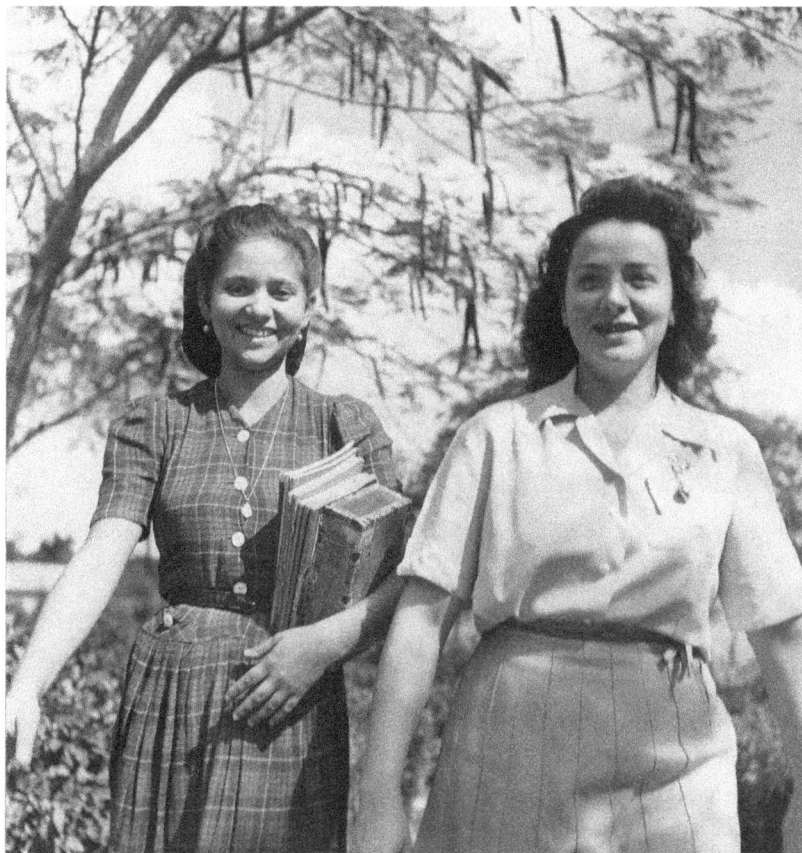

FIGURE 4.2. Student and teacher in the Household Workers Program of the Puerto Rican Department of Education, February 1948. Photograph by Charles E. Rotkin. Courtesy of the Collection of the Office of Information of the Puerto Rican Government, Archivo Fotografico, Archivo General de Puerto Rico, Puerta de Tierra.

working with African American domestic workers and her central role as a labor reformer with the New York Department of Labor.[67] She knew the New York case had connections with the US Women's Bureau and was known for participating in national forums on the reform of domestic work. Phillips was to oversee collaboration among her office, the Puerto Rican government, the Women's Bureau, and local agencies like the YWCA that helped place workers. The Puerto Rican government charged her with creating a training and placement program to professionalize Puerto Rican domestic contract labor along lines that she had developed for African American women's work. Training would occur in Puerto Rico before the

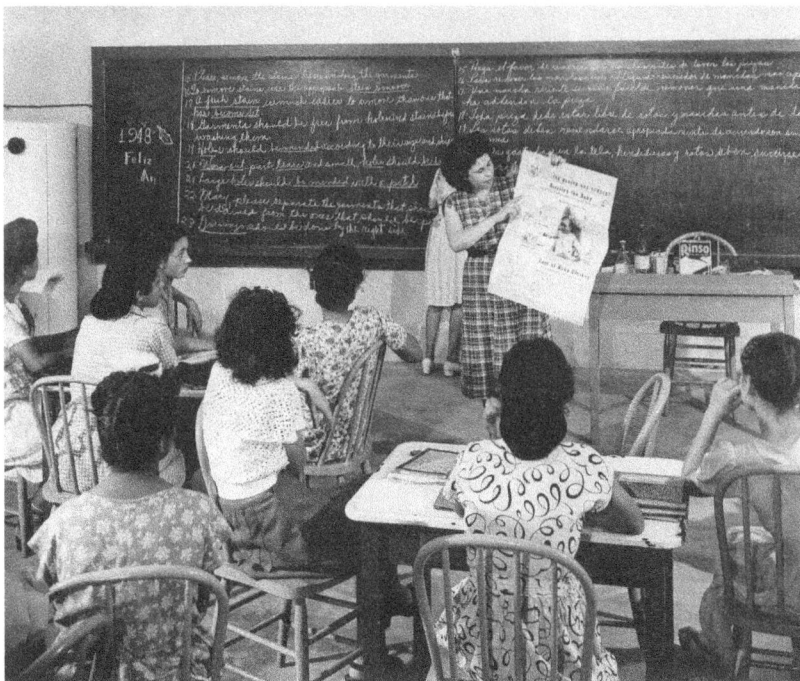

FIGURE 4.3. "Household Workers who are planning to work in the United States taking a course in English and childcare at the school run by the Department of Education"; Caguas, Puerto Rico, January 1948. Photograph by Charles E. Rotkin. Courtesy of the Collection of the Office of Information of the Puerto Rican Government, Archivo Fotografico, Archivo General de Puerto Rico, Puerta de Tierra.

women were placed in homes in New York City. Phillips's official title was assistant to the commissioner of labor of Puerto Rico in the United States. Phillips also worked alongside professional Puerto Rican women in home economics, education, and social work. These women made up an expanding network of reformers eager to develop the program and showcase their expertise (see figure 4.3).[68] All the Puerto Rican instructors who developed the program were trained in the United States. These programs allowed professional Puerto Rican women to claim new roles in state institutions that regulated the lives and labors of working-class women and not merely monitor labor migration to the United States.

Phillips's work for the Puerto Rican government began with a trip to Caguas, where she helped establish a new training program for household workers, grafting it onto an older home economics program. Puerto Rico already had vocational education programs within the public education system that provided training to girls and women in home economics.[69] Students learned about US concepts of domesticity and standards for housework and were instructed in the performance of caring labor. These programs drew on contemporary ideas about scientific motherhood that were also a central component of the archipelago's ongoing modernization and development program. The household worker program, which opened in October 1947, was similar in many ways, though it specifically prepared women for employment in the United States. It provided language classes in English and vocational classes about domestic and family life in the United States, both of which were meant to prepare students for placement in US homes. It would "help mature houseworkers improve their skills and give younger workers a sounder methodical approach to housemaid's tasks."[70] Students attended classes on the use of appliances like washing machines, on infant and childcare, and on female grooming, which included instruction in how to do one's hair and nails and how to dress for work (see figure 4.4).[71]

Upon placement of contract workers in jobs in the United States, the Puerto Rican state turned to developing a positive public relations campaign about labor migration, though migrant women were still largely unhappy working as domestics, and many quickly abandoned their jobs. When the first group of twenty-one women traveled to Scarsdale, New York, on their labor contracts, Phillips met them at Newark Airport, along with Commissioner Sierra and a group of social workers who would become leaders of the Migration Division.[72] Shortly thereafter, the Puerto Rican government reported that the "Pilot Project of Training and Placement of Household Workers" was going well and that the plan was to expand the program.[73] However, the employers and workers involved in the newly regulated program were not as enthusiastic about its outcome. Domestic workers still complained of generally poor conditions, and many of the women left jobs after short periods.[74] In the end, the government decided to suspend further professional training of domestics. Despite its short life, the Puerto Rican government still judged the program a success because it had portrayed the state and Puerto Ricans positively in the US press. Migration Division agents also had succeeded in establishing themselves as experts who would continue to work to regulate and organize Puerto Rican migration through vocational training programs in Puerto Rico and by providing assistance to workers in the United States.

While the program only lasted for a brief time, it provided a bridge for a number of women to migrate to the United States, forging communities

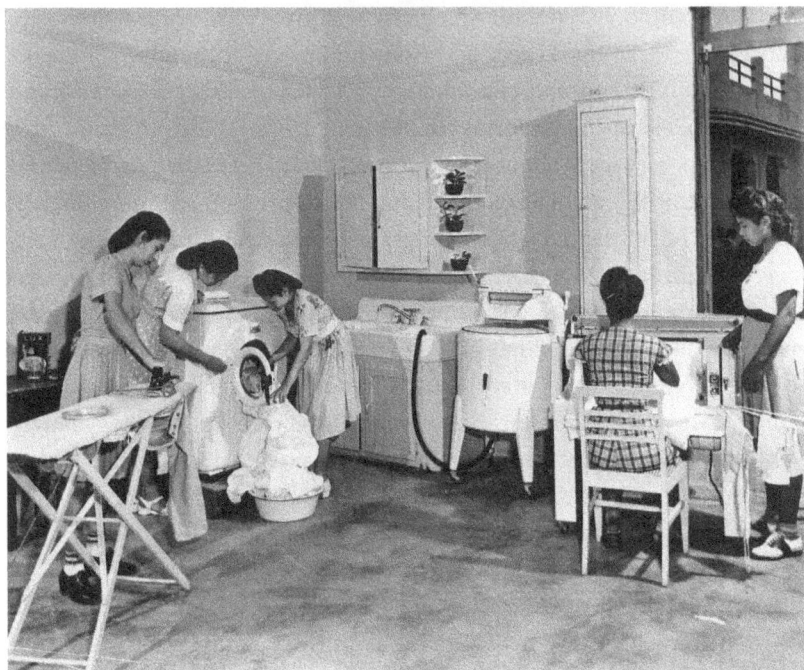

FIGURE 4.4. Household workers being trained by the Department of Education in Caguas, Puerto Rico, January 1948. Photograph by Charles Rotkin. Courtesy of the Collection of the Office of Information of the Puerto Rican Government, Archivo Fotografico, Archivo General de Puerto Rico, Puerta de Tierra.

that would grow in US cities. The fact that women did not stay in these jobs suggests how undesirable most live-in situations were; this work provided women with little time off or personal freedom and left them vulnerable to exploitation by their employers. Like African American women in the United States before them, Puerto Rican women sought to move out of household labor into more flexible occupations.[75] The contract workers additionally took issue with the deductions from their wages to pay for transportation costs as well as clothing, food, and other items provided by employers. In leaving such jobs, they deployed a weapon of the weak to protest unsatisfactory and degrading conditions. The abandonment by Puerto Rican domestic workers of live-in contract labor positions and their refusal to continue to have wages deducted from their pay for transportation costs was a form of resistance and rejection of the conditions workers faced in the United States.[76] Their actions also suggest that despite attempts at regulation, the Department of Labor contract program failed to create jobs in domestic work that Puerto Rican women wanted. Instead of a sustainable form of employment, the programs provided a pathway for women to migrate and, in turn, seek opportunities outside of state control.

Even though the training program in household work was short-lived, the Puerto Rican government's Migration Division offices in the United States expanded after 1948. The agency continued to place workers in jobs and help migrants facing discrimination and lack of access to good jobs, housing, education, and social services. Even as it built other offices dedicated to employment services, agents of the Migration Division in Chicago and elsewhere worked specifically to place former domestic workers in new jobs—some still in domestic work but for different families. In New York City, Petroamérica Pagán de Colón, one of the Puerto Rican social workers who had overseen the household worker program, headed a revamped New York Employment Division.[77] The Migration Division kept a list of open positions in domestic work that were sent to them by potential employers who had heard that the agency provided referrals. The agency continued placing women as the employment agencies had done in the 1930s. However, now placement was under the direction of social workers with experience in regulating labor migration, many of whom had helped develop the domestic work training program.

In the long history of Puerto Rican women's roles as domestic workers, the creation of the contract labor programs represents one moment among many when Puerto Rican women organized for better labor conditions in the United States. If we look for only traditional labor organizing, however, we miss their protest. Workers in Chicago, along with professional allies, protested conditions of a privately run, for-profit contract employment scheme and pressured the Puerto Rican government to establish its own household worker program and employment service. Still, this path to migration proved unsatisfactory, and Puerto Rican workers continued to seek other forms of employment, walking away from jobs when they faced exploitative conditions. Even with regulation and reform, these workers could not escape the legacy of racialized occupational segregation by sex that had linked them with African American women at the lowest levels of an expanding care work economy.

NOTWITHSTANDING THE SPOTTY record of success for the Household Worker Program, the Migration Division agents who worked on the project were successful in establishing themselves as migration experts who continued to work to regulate and organize Puerto Rican labor migration through programs that combined vocational training in Puerto Rico and assistance to workers in the United States. The intervention of Isales in the situation in Chicago sparked the concern of the Puerto Rican government over the conditions faced by domestic workers in the United States. One suggestion was that the Puerto Rican government needed to make more services available to migrants. Therefore, the late 1940s moment of Puerto Rican labor migration documented in this chapter was a dramatic and vital one in the history of the Puerto Rican diaspora. The migrants who arrived to work in US communities became some of the founders of new Puerto Rican communities throughout the United States and significantly expanded the ranks of long-standing communities like that in New York.

The outsized role of Puerto Rican women care workers in the history of the Puerto Rican diaspora cannot be overlooked. From the start, projects of gendered reform profoundly shaped the Puerto Rican community in the United States. Many migrant women were integrated into US economies as care workers, domestic workers, and maids. The funneling of Puerto Rican women and girls into these positions slotted them into raced and gendered racial hierarchies in US society that shaped their rights and belonging there. This was not new for Puerto Rican women, who had already experienced gendered and racialized occupational segregation in Puerto Rico, which had resulted in many women of African descent being pushed into care work. In the United States, these working-class women faced terrible conditions and were often separated from their families and communities. However, despite these challenging conditions, many resisted against all odds. Often alone and far from home, some young Puerto Rican women refused the labor terms imposed on them. They formed alliances with Puerto Rican students and household workers in the United States, who helped them advocate for labor standards. Their story eventually also garnered them the recognition of social worker activists like Isales, who, like a long line of labor-reforming social workers before her, began to work to make their caring labor count to state agencies and to advocate for labor protections for Puerto Rican migrant workers more broadly.

This historical moment of political organizing around welfare would result in more regulation and reform of labor migration by the Puerto Rican government. Social workers would continue to play critical roles in shaping how this reform was administered. However, the problems faced by workers would not be alleviated as they continued to face terrible work conditions and discrimination. But they would also continue to resist, walking away from low-paying and abusive jobs as they tried to make a better life. For working-class Puerto Rican women care workers and social workers in Puerto Rican communities in the United States, this was just one moment in a shared history of tension and struggle that would continue over the decades that followed.

Women's Leadership in Struggles over Welfare, Citizenship Rights, and Decolonization in the Puerto Rican Diaspora

In 1948, Flor M. Piñeiro, a Puerto Rican social worker in the United States, wrote an article about labor migration in which she noted that Puerto Ricans in the United States were struggling against an "unjust, bad intentioned, and prejudiced campaign of rejection."[1] She linked this struggle to racism in the United States and within the Puerto Rican community itself. According to her, such racial prejudice was spurred on by "fantastical statistics" about the number of Puerto Ricans traveling to the United States, which focused on juvenile delinquency and crime, and accused migrants of "consuming city assistance funds." To illustrate her point, Piñeiro recounted a story from her experience working in the New York City Department of Welfare as a graduate student. The case involved a Puerto Rican father with his two children who had been found sleeping on the street in the winter because they were unable to contact their family members. The family was temporarily accommodated in a hotel while the social workers began to work on the case and help them locate their family in the Bronx.

For Piñeiro, the family's case was just one of many "that caused a scandal in New York City." The incident "demonstrated the disorientation and lack of knowledge that many migrants had" upon arriving in the United States. She was clear that those who experienced such hardships comprised only a small group within a much larger migrant community, most of which was doing fine in the city and had thus never come to the attention of the authorities.[2] Even so, Piñeiro used the incident to argue that there should be an office to help orient Puerto Rican migrants to the city to prevent such extreme cases. Piñeiro's call for regulation and reform of Puerto Rican labor migration also occurred while working-class Puerto Rican migrants demanded that the state intervene to help them assert their rights as US citizens, workers, and clients of social welfare programs in the United States. As the Puerto Rican government continued to sponsor labor migration to the United States, the voices of social workers and working-class people would join a chorus demanding change.

In the postwar period, Puerto Rican women became important political leaders in the diaspora who played central roles in struggles over rights and demands for decolonization. This chapter tells the story of Puerto Rican women's political leadership through a focus on social workers whose role developing social welfare policies and programs for migrants provided them with a platform to craft new state institutions and political agendas. In doing so, it builds on scholarship on Puerto Rican migration that has emphasized the importance of state regulation and state-sponsored labor migration to the formation of communities in the United States.[3] It also expands this literature by focusing on women's leadership within these projects, which has not been at the center of most previous studies.[4] It examines how social workers employed by migration agencies played important roles in debates over "welfare" benefits and coverage of Puerto Rico under the US Social Security Act, as well as how they linked this work to their broader participation in struggles over Puerto Rican rights. Their stories also reveal how social workers with disparate political views used these projects to advocate for diverse visions of Puerto Rico's future. Some supported gradual change that aligned with the Puerto Rican populist state's "commonwealth" agenda; others joined nationalist uprisings for independence while a new generation sought fresh opportunities to organize diasporic communities. This chapter shows how, for all, the world was something that could be remade through political organizing and action.

When the Puerto Rican government created an expanded agenda to regulate and manage migration, it called on Puerto Rican women who were professional social workers to help develop these programs. In part, this was because social workers were already considered experts on migration because, over the previous decades, they had been actively building migration-oriented programs.[5] In addition, many had been trained in the United States or had close relationships with government officials and agencies stateside. After 1947, when the Puerto Rican government created the Employment and Migration Bureau offices in the United States, it staffed the agency with numerous social workers. When the bureau's office opened in New York City, it soon came to be known simply as the Migration Division.[6] In the 1950s, the bureau expanded to have main offices in New York City and Chicago and branches operating in numerous other US cities. Between 1951 and 1961, the agency oversaw the placement of 113,664 Puerto Rican migrants within the United States, and its work continued in the following years.[7] In each of these agencies there were social workers participating in the placement of workers and other activities.

While the work of Puerto Rican social workers in the Migration Division began with a focus on regulating labor migration, much of their day-to-day work centered on advocating for migrant rights. As social workers wove together US and Puerto Rican social welfare programs through interagency casework, they linked social welfare agencies in both locations and changed the role of the state in the lives of migrant citizens. Between 1948 and 1954, Migration Division social workers managed 12,415 visits to the agency about social cases and opened 7,562 cases that were followed more extensively.[8] Their casework with migrants also brought them face to face with the difficulties of displacement and harsh discrimination faced by Puerto Ricans in the United States. They encountered Puerto Rican migrant "clients" in great need who came to the agency's offices in search of help finding housing, food, childcare, jobs, and assistance contesting discrimination. These working-class migrant "clients" put pressure on the agency and social workers to listen to their stories and to acknowledge the devastating impact that labor migration had on many lives. Social workers responded in some cases by serving as advocates of migrants' rights, which included traveling with their clients to appointments at US social service agencies where they contested the racism they faced.

The work of Migration Division social workers was also closely tied to that of the expanding Department of Public Welfare in Puerto Rico, which had been created on the archipelago in 1943 and which expanded rapidly in the years that followed. While the Interagency Services Bureau of the Department of Public Welfare in Puerto Rico had already been corresponding directly with US social welfare agencies, the expansion of the Migration Division offices also helped them to organize and manage the circulation of information about Puerto Rican migrant clients between US cities and the archipelago.[9] Social workers Luisa Iglesias de Jesús and Rosario Nevares de Rodríguez noted that nearly all cases referred to the agency came from New York City, with about 60 percent pertaining to health issues faced by migrants, 25 percent being requests from the US Department of Welfare for background information on clients, and nearly 10 percent being cases where these agencies were seeking authorization to pay for transportation costs to return migrants to the archipelago. Much of the paperwork they processed had to do with determining and verifying residency status, which often determined access to benefits in the United States.[10]

This chapter considers how the work of Puerto Rican social workers on projects as migrant advocates in the United States also dovetailed with their participation in broader struggles over Puerto Rican citizenship rights and decolonization. It examines a few demonstrative examples of how social workers' political activism developed during this period. In some of these projects, social workers challenged prevailing notions of Puerto Rican dependency and exposed the exclusions that migrants faced as second-class citizens. This work included participating in public relations efforts on behalf of the Puerto Rican government—a project that enabled them to produce alternative social scientific knowledge that would be instrumental in partially reforming the colonial governance of Puerto Rico and laying the foundation for the creation a new commonwealth relationship with the United States after 1952. This work was connected to their organizing and lobbying for the inclusion of Puerto Rico and Puerto Ricans under federal social policy with increasing, albeit partial, success. However, while many social workers used their migration expertise to aid the colonial state, others challenged the Puerto Rican government, instead advocating for full independence as a means to decolonization. These nationalist social workers forged radical paths forward, sometimes taking up arms to challenge US colonial authority. Taken together, these divergent stories of political organizing for Puerto Rican rights by social workers who worked with migrants and on social policy reveal the dynamic political work of Puerto Rican women as agents of social change during this formative moment in Puerto Rican history.

The Puerto Rican Government's Employment and Migration Bureau as a Social Service Agency

After 1948, Puerto Rican social workers became central figures in organizing and managing the archipelago's labor migration, thanks to the expansion of the Employment and Migration Bureau, a Puerto Rican government entity operating in the United States. As the previous chapter outlined, in response to problems like those posed by the migration of Puerto Rican domestic workers to Chicago, the Puerto Rican government decided to augment the work of the bureau's New York City branch in regulating and managing migration by establishing the Migration Division. This development reflected one of the main ways that the Puerto Rican state came to act increasingly in the United States as a result of the labor migrations they had sponsored.[11] The Migration Division was intended to help migrant Puerto Ricans "adjust" and "assimilate" to living in the United States by serving as an employment agency and providing referrals to social services. Although the staff was small, the agency played an important role in developing a new relationship between the Puerto Rican government and migrant citizens in the United States.

In New York City, the Employment and Migration Bureau was headed by Manuel Cabranes, a social worker with long-standing ties to both Puerto Rican social welfare institutions and the US settlement house movement.[12] But while Cabranes and most of the agency's leadership were men, women social workers from the archipelago performed much of the bureau's work, managing day-to-day operations, developing migration-oriented programs, and working closely with migrant clients through individual casework (see figure 5.1).[13] Petroamérica Pagán de Colón, for example, initially managed labor migration at the bureau, but her role extended well beyond this arena when she became one of the Migration Division's primary representatives in public dialogues and campaigns surrounding migrant rights.[14]

The Social Service Section was an important section of the Migration Division in New York that expanded significantly in the postwar period, providing not only valuable services and information to migrants but also opportunities for social workers to be politically engaged. The Social Service Section was developed by Puerto Rican women who had been trained in the United States and had then cultivated social welfare programs in Puerto Rico in the early 1940s. US-based social work expert Mary Antoinette Cannon was also an instrumental organizer.[15] Cannon taught for many years at the New York School of Social Work and mentored many of the Puerto Rican students who studied there. After spending a year at the University of Puerto Rico's School of Social Work as a visiting professor, she became increasingly involved in social service projects targeting Puerto Rican migrants in New York City. Soon after, the Puerto Rican government recruited Cannon to help establish the social service section of the Migration Division, where her status in the local community and centrality as an expert

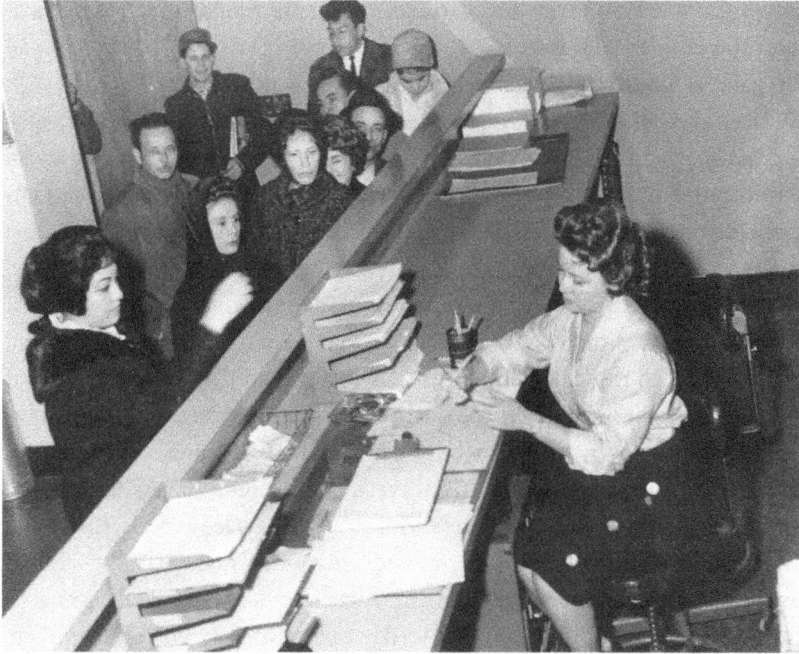

FIGURE 5.1. "Men and women waiting at the Migration Division office." Courtesy of the Offices of the Government of Puerto Rico in the United States Records, Archives of the Puerto Rican Diaspora, Center for Puerto Rican Studies, Hunter College, City University of New York.

within the social work profession helped the agency attain more power and recognition within the New York political landscape.

Over time, the Social Service Section became a crucial intermediary between Puerto Rican migrants and US social service agencies. In order to deal with the growing requests for assistance, the Social Service Section began to recruit more social workers from Puerto Rico, seeking bilingual professionals who understood both Puerto Rican and US social welfare programs. The first two recruits to be transferred from Puerto Rico to work with migrant clients in the United States were seasoned social workers. Francisca Bou, who went by the nickname "Paquita," had extensive experience in medical social work and had been trained in the United States and worked as a social worker in Puerto Rico before being employed by the Migration Division.[16] Matilde Pérez de Silva was also a founder of the social work profession in Puerto Rico with long connections to social work and public health agencies.[17] Bou and Pérez de Silva would both work for the

Migration Division for many years, seeing clients and also managing various other aspects of the agencies' work. They brought the authority of social work expertise from the archipelago to their new posts in New York.

They and other social workers from the archipelago worked alongside Cabranes, Pagán de Colón, and Cannon to help migrants navigate US social service institutions. In the 1950s, in the New York City office, there was generally a social work supervisor working in the office, three or four full-time social workers processing cases, a secretary helping with correspondence, and two social workers who worked most of the time traveling to the airport to work with cases there.[18] These social workers were often overwhelmed, and there was much more demand for their services than they were able to provide. Agents worked along three tracks: interventions via casework to solve individual problems, participating in community work, and sometimes addressing larger economic and social reasons for migration. As they linked the agency's employment programs with its social service aspects, they often found themselves serving as advocates for migrants who faced issues related to both, such as labor exploitation and social services refusals in US agencies. In this way, the division's day-to-day operations placed social workers directly on the front lines of the fight for migrants' rights.

The expansion of the Social Service Section was also foundational in connecting all of the Migration Division's different sections, as social work experts transferred clients and files among the agency's subdivisions. Having a shared office made it easy to send a client from the desk of one agent to that of another. The social workers' ability to function as a unit became one of the program's crucial strengths, as many migrants faced multiple problems related to housing, work, and discrimination when seeking state benefits. The Social Service Section's case files reveal that clients seeking help with applications to social service programs were often funneled toward the agency's employment programs as well. This frequent passing of files back and forth reflects the ways that labor and social welfare were intimately intertwined in the strategies that social workers developed throughout the Migration Division. These strategies ultimately worked to create a new model for conducting casework, one that prioritized multiple and connected issues facing migrants.

As social welfare became increasingly important for integrating Puerto Rican migrants into the United States, it opened up a space for Puerto Rican women in particular to expand their role as state agents. Utilizing their new approach to casework, social workers in the Migration Division began to connect social welfare initiatives in the United States with those in Puerto

Rico. They developed a robust Interagency Services Bureau that circulated clients' information between the archipelago and the United States. The program was run by social worker Aurora Garriga de Baralt out of the San Juan offices, and it utilized the services of a variety of social workers on the archipelago.[19] As the social welfare programs developed in Puerto Rico in the 1930s and 1940s, the agency created a means of transferring information about internal migrants between the burgeoning public welfare clinics.[20] Thus, having already mastered the bureaucratic circulation of information and case files on the archipelago, the bureau now extended these practices to their colleagues in the United States. Migration Division social workers corresponded with interagency services about numerous cases, requesting that all pertinent information about their clients be mailed to them in the United States. They charged social workers in Puerto Rico with collecting this data and often asked them to conduct fieldwork or interviews with clients' family members. Puerto Rican social workers in turn began writing to the Migration Division for information about their clients on the archipelago. These investigations became collaborations among social workers in different locations, as bundles of documents about clients were mailed between Puerto Rico, New York, Chicago, and other US cities. For clients who sought assistance, the social work practices developed within the Migration Division represented new forms of engagement with the Puerto Rican state in the United States.

Clients of the Migration Division

The social workers of the Migration Division worked during the period with numerous migrant clients who were facing extremely difficult conditions in the United States. For example, on August 26, 1951, one such client, María Cruz, arrived at the Migration Division offices in New York City seeking assistance when facing a crisis.[21] Her two-year-old son was sick in the Greenpoint Hospital and she had been referred to the agency by a medical social worker. Cruz had been living in the home of Claudia Baez for ten months since arriving in Brooklyn from San German, Puerto Rico. Baez was also a single mother, and she had agreed to help pay for Cruz's ticket and her room and board when she arrived in New York in exchange for childcare for her own baby. However, the agreement later soured after Cruz's own child got sick, which made living in the tiny apartment difficult and left Baez without childcare. Cruz had previously applied for public assistance to help support her child, and her application had been denied; she received a second rejection when she reapplied after the baby was hospitalized. When she arrived at the social service section of the Migration Division offices, she brought a formal denial letter from the Department of Welfare for Aid to Families with Dependent Children. Her conversation with social workers in this office would begin an investigation into her eligibility for benefits over the ensuing months.

Cruz's story illuminates how poor and working-class Puerto Rican women experienced migrating to the United States and navigated interactions with Puerto Rican and US social welfare agencies. After Cruz visited the Migration Division, a social worker named Carmen D. Nogueras initiated a casework process.[22] Nogueras conducted a series of interviews with both Cruz and Baez, corresponded with the social worker at the hospital caring for the child, and discussed the housing situation faced by the two women. In the end, it was determined that the conditions of the case had changed since the first denial that Cruz received, and Nogueras believed that Cruz should be eligible for assistance now. Representatives of the Migration Division corresponded with US social welfare agencies and increasingly served as intermediaries between US social welfare agencies and Puerto Rican clients, particularly those who were denied assistance.[23] In particular, they communicated with US social welfare agencies that were specifically created to work with recent arrivals to New York and migrant clients without residency. Over time, the Migration Division was increasingly called on to intervene in such cases.

When poor and working-class Puerto Rican women migrated to the United States they encountered many challenges. The first of these was finding housing and employment in cities that were increasingly hostile to Puerto Ricans.[24] They faced discrimination when seeking apartments and were funneled into the most low-paying and exploitative occupations. The clients were often single women with children who were trying to support themselves and their families.[25] The circumstances that these women faced sometimes led them to seek assistance from social welfare institutions, like the Department of Welfare. In some instances, these claims were made when women faced extreme duress, such as the story of Cruz, which highlights the experience of a woman whose child was sick, or Baez, who needed to work to support not only her own child but also her elderly mother. Stories like this one also included the experiences of women who lost the support of family members, who were unemployed, who were disabled, who couldn't find childcare, and who were caring for numerous other people in their familial networks.[26] Struggles over survival and managing care frame the stories of Puerto Rican migrant social welfare clients during this period.

Puerto Ricans in the United States often encountered intense discrimination when seeking social welfare benefits. In the offices of US social welfare agencies, they were sometimes treated as undeserving of benefits and as potential welfare dependents or "cheats."[27] As chapter 4 discussed, the stereotypes about Puerto Ricans and welfare that cast them in this way were both racialized and gendered and rooted in generalizations about Black and Latinx people having a proclivity toward welfare "dependency" in the United States.[28] This was despite the fact that the group with the highest percentage of welfare recipients was white women, not women of color. Puerto Rican clients also often encountered welfare agencies without Spanish-speaking employees who were unprepared to help them.[29] This combination of prejudice and ignorance created increasingly difficult conditions for migrants who were already facing difficult situations.

After facing discrimination or challenges seeking social welfare benefits, some Puerto Rican migrants sought assistance at the offices of the Migration Division of the Puerto Rican Department of Labor. They may have been referred to the agency by social workers at the Department of Welfare or they could have heard about the work of the organization from a friend or advertisements in the press. When the potential client arrived, they would encounter a receptionist who would then refer them to the Social Services Division of the organization to begin the intake process. Images from the Migration Division offices show Puerto Rican clients arriving at the agency's offices and meeting with secretaries and social workers who processed their cases (see figure 5.2). One of the social workers in the agency would interview them about the reason they were at the office and begin a case file that recorded information about the case. In some instances, copies of documents from other organizations, such as referral letters or benefit denials, would be slipped into the case file alongside the notes taken by the social worker. Some of the cases were remedied in a day, sometimes with a quick translation of a document, while others could span years of multiple visits by the client to the Migration Division and letters that were sent between dozens of agencies.

The case files of the social services section of the Migration Division map the variety of different challenges faced by Puerto Ricans as they sought social services. Among the most common difficulties faced by these clients were issues relating to language and cultural understandings about Puerto Ricans. In one case a woman who was working as a domestic worker in New

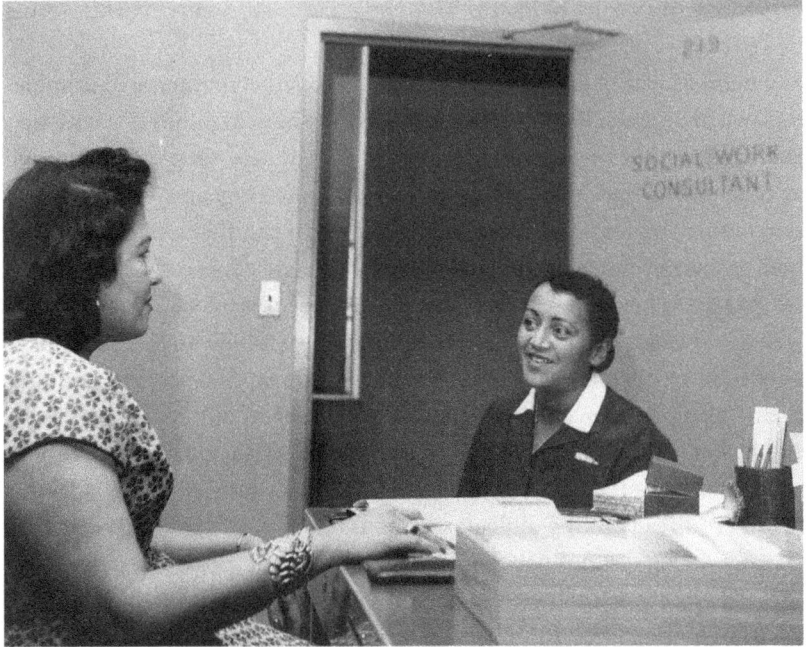

FIGURE 5.2. Social worker and client at the Migration Division. Courtesy of the Offices of the Government of Puerto Rico in the United States Records, Archives of the Puerto Rican Diaspora, Center for Puerto Rican Studies, Hunter College, City University of New York.

York specifically asked Migration Division social workers for help navigating residency requirements and dealing with the means-testing she faced in the United States.[30] In this case the social worker played a crucial role in serving as a translator, using their bilingualism to help the client. In addition, there were incidents where Puerto Ricans were denied services because officials didn't understand that they were US citizens and eligible for benefits.[31] The earlier version of the Migration Division had issued identification cards to prove that Puerto Ricans were US citizens.[32] However, over time the Migration Division was more likely to call up organizations that did this or investigate specific cases, while at the same time continuing their broader educational campaigns about Puerto Ricans being US citizens. Over time, the Migration Division was more likely to be dealing with questions about residency status, because of the tighter restrictions on benefits to people around residency that were passed during the period.[33] Questions about residency were also entangled with the larger desire of US social welfare agencies wanting "background information" to confirm "facts" about Puerto Rican clients as a part of means-testing.[34]

The type of information circulated by social workers included things like an arrival date from Puerto Rico, birth certificates, information about family members' possible financial contributions, marriage status, proof of parentage, and "advisability of return to Puerto Rico." Social workers had long corresponded with other cities and states about clients, but they now sought more information about clients who were in Puerto Rico.[35] In some instances the "return" to Puerto Rico was something that was being considered by US Department of Welfare officials; however, in other cases there were Puerto Ricans who came to the office specifically to try to get help paying the cost to return home.[36] The Migration Division came to be the main agency that would provide a conduit to this information—and connection to social workers at the rapidly expanding Department of Public Welfare in Puerto Rico.[37] What these cases show is that discrimination against Puerto Rican clients took many forms. The information that they provided that could be used by clients as they were being means-tested was also expansive. This included researching and organizing information that was available in the United States. However, the main thrust of this work was connecting the US social agencies with those in Puerto Rico.

The Migration Division responded by further developing interagency services between Puerto Rico and the United States. The social workers in the agency also expanded the types of casework with Puerto Rican migrants that resulted in connections between Puerto Rican and US agencies. Some of the most important interventions they made were helping migrants by accompanying them to contest denials in social welfare offices.[38] Despite the fact that the number of people working in the agency was small, the social workers would sometimes go with clients to the social welfare offices to advocate on their behalf. Sometimes they would make phone calls or write letters on behalf of clients that would serve similar purposes. Sometimes the letters were mailed, and in other cases the clients were given documents and materials that they could bring with them to welfare offices. Services in the offices included translation of documents as well as serving as interpreters in some cases.

While many of the referrals were made to the Department of Welfare, the Migration Division also served as a referral hub to a much more expansive body of social services that were available to migrants. They kept lists of social service organizations and built connections with those that provided services for migrants. The social workers knew about the places that Puerto

Rican migrants could be referred to, which were not always the places that the Department of Welfare would send them. This included the settlement houses that were open to Puerto Rican migrants and that provided different kinds of services to migrants.[39] It also included private charities that had services open to Puerto Ricans. In particular, many of these were religious services and included the Catholic Church agencies. One of the most important of these was Casita María, a Catholic organization with Puerto Rican leadership.[40] These types of organizations provided increasingly important services to Puerto Rican migrants as the years went on and often filled in to give assistance in instances where public organizations did not.

The expansion of social work as part of the Puerto Rican government's work with migrants in the postwar period opened up a larger space for social workers' political activity. As the Migration Division developed and established specialized departments like the Social Services Division, Puerto Rican social workers in the United States participated in a variety of political projects that stretched the role of the Puerto Rican state beyond its boundaries and into the diasporic communities in US cities. These social workers were instrumental in creating migrant offices throughout the United States during the Migration Division's early years of operation. They also developed a variety of approaches to casework with migrant clients, which included advocating for access to benefits and social services, linking the agency's multiple departments, and expanding interagency service programs that circulated client information between the United States and Puerto Rico. In the years to come, they were soon pulled into other projects sponsored by the Puerto Rican government, where they would find an even larger platform to continue their struggle for Puerto Rican migrants' rights.

Social Workers, Public Relations, and Social Scientific Knowledge

As increasing numbers of Puerto Rican social workers joined the Migration Division and US agencies, their work investigating and writing about migration would bring them into a number of political debates, particularly around whether or not Puerto Ricans were welfare dependent. Arguing that they were not, these social workers countered commonplace assumptions circulating in the press and within US government institutions that Puerto Ricans were a "drain" on US urban resources. Moreover, with the goal of challenging such racist discourse and shifting popular opinion about Puerto Rican migration, the Puerto Rican government called on social workers

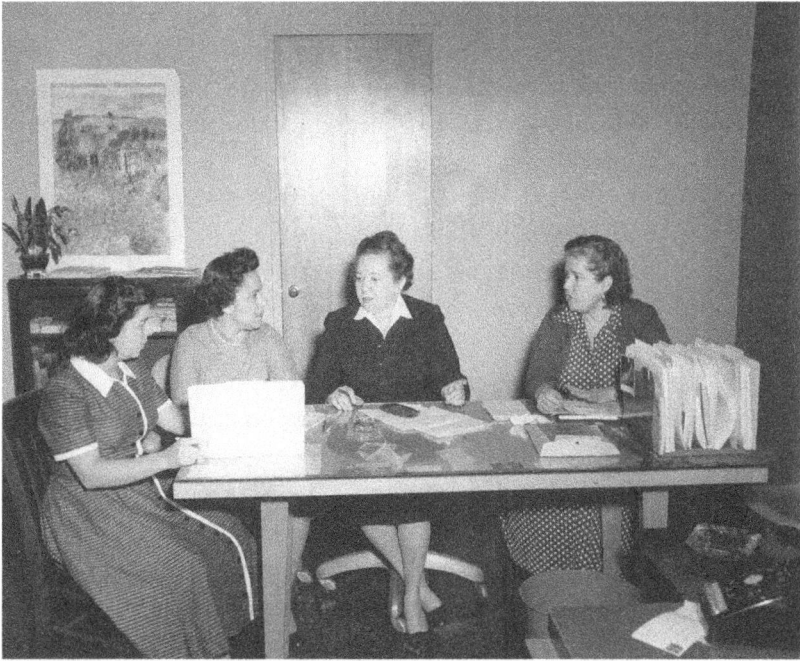

FIGURE 5.3. Social service section of the Migration Division. Matilde Pérez de Silva is in the middle, wearing a black jacket. Courtesy of the Offices of the Government of Puerto Rico in the United States Records, Archives of the Puerto Rican Diaspora, Center for Puerto Rican Studies, Hunter College, City University of New York.

as migration experts.[41] In this capacity, Puerto Rican women in both the United States and on the archipelago were tasked with producing and distributing social scientific knowledge about migration (see figure 5.3).

Social workers' participation in the production of social scientific knowledge about poverty would become one of the crucial spaces in which they were able to intervene in political discourses about Puerto Rican migration. Studying migration and creating social welfare programs led some to mobilize their role in social scientific studies about poverty to carve out a space in broader political debates. As active researchers and scholars in social scientific studies about poverty in both Puerto Rico and the United States, these social workers contributed to the creation and dissemination of what historian Alice O'Conner has called "poverty knowledge."[42] The knowledge culled from their investigations was used to write state policies that impacted the lives of countless Puerto Ricans. In addition, social workers' participation in the production of this knowledge was framed by their evolving politics and experiences living and working in colonial and migrant communities. As social workers increasingly worked in the United States, they began to see their participation in the creation of knowledge about Puerto Rican communities and poverty as something that took on new political meanings in the diaspora.

The role of social workers in producing poverty knowledge was particularly important in debates about Puerto Rican welfare dependency in New York, where numerous articles and references to the "Puerto Rican Problem" stirred up anti–Puerto Rican sentiment. In response to such animus, the Employment and Migration Bureau developed a public relations campaign to assert that Puerto Ricans were not a drain on the city's resources, as had been reported in the press for decades. Studies conducted by the Welfare Council of New York with the collaboration of Manuel Cabranes and other Puerto Rican representatives were instrumental in shaping this campaign.[43] The Migration Division was also involved in the creation of the Mayor's Advisory Committee on Puerto Rican Affairs (MACPRA), which was founded in 1949 during Mayor William O'Dwyer's reelection campaign in an attempt to win Puerto Rican votes. The MACPRA conducted its own research about Puerto Rican communities and welfare, with Migration Division social workers at the helm.[44]

The MACPRA's results and ensuing report were very important to the Employment and Migration Bureau as well as the Puerto Rican government in their campaign to educate the United States about Puerto Rican migrants and show that they were not like the demonizing portrayals circulating in popular media.[45] The report revealed to the public that the number of Puerto Rican migrants who received public assistance was remarkably small, only 10 percent in comparison with 4.5 percent of all New Yorkers.[46] The study also highlighted the social workers' research, making it clear that it was they who provided the data to contradict damaging popular opinions. The MACPRA study also served as a corrective to the narratives circulating in popular media about Puerto Rican migrants and welfare. The results demonstrating that most Puerto Ricans were not welfare dependent were widely publicized in the press, and numerous city representatives made statements that the "Puerto Rican Problem" had been exaggerated. The study challenged New Yorkers to think of Puerto Rican migrants as recent arrivals to the city, still navigating social service programs but largely migrating in search of work.

This was a great victory for the Puerto Rican government and the Migration Division, who capitalized on this new knowledge about Puerto Rican migrants to continue their public relations campaign. Efforts included circulating educational pamphlets about Puerto Rican migrants that argued that Puerto Ricans faced similar problems regarding assimilation and integration as other immigrant groups of previous generations. These materials also emphasized Puerto Ricans' US citizenship status to assert their belonging. The larger aim of this project was to provide an alternative current of understanding about Puerto Ricans that would make the United States more welcoming, one supported by social scientific evidence. By providing that evidence, Puerto Rican social workers not only produced positive and more accurate knowledge about migrants—knowledge that would certainly improve migrants' experiences in the United States—but also expanded their own political action.

The Social Security Act and Puerto Rican Migration

As the Employment and Migration Bureau developed, social workers also worked to expand Puerto Ricans' social citizenship rights. They argued, as Puerto Rican social workers had done already for fifteen years, that although Puerto Ricans were US citizens and thus entitled to the same benefits available to other US citizens, colonial relations had resulted in unequal forms of citizenship that disenfranchised Puerto Ricans, particularly those who remained on the archipelago. They demanded that Puerto Rico be covered fully by federal social policies developed in the United States. Moreover, they suggested that these limitations on citizenship had created social inequalities that would result in increased migration to the United States, where Puerto Ricans' citizenship had more value.

The Employment and Migration Bureau's work on citizenship came to a head in 1949, when the US government held a series of hearings about the possibility of extending the Social Security Act to Puerto Rico.[47] During these hearings, a number of Puerto Rican representatives spoke about the benefits of extending the act, or at least some of its provisions, to the archipelago.[48] Chief among them were Puerto Rican social workers who highlighted the limitations of the current programs developed by the insular government. While at first it seemed that they would be unsuccessful in obtaining broader coverage for Puerto Rico under the act, their political action would ultimately help facilitate major transformations in social policy.

The struggle for Puerto Rican coverage under the Social Security Act was not new, but this moment offered new ways for social workers to argue for its expansion. As earlier chapters have shown, Puerto Rican social workers had already been working diligently for over fifteen years to extend the

Social Security Act. Some advocated for coverage while working on New Deal projects and were somewhat successful. In 1939, the US government extended partial coverage under the act to Puerto Rico but limited funding to levels lower than those granted to US states. In addition, Puerto Rico was only included under particular parts of the act, such as the child welfare and public health provisions, which further marked the archipelago as a territory with distinct social policy. Throughout the 1940s Puerto Rican social workers had worked consistently and diligently to raise the issue of further expansion of the Social Security Act in Puerto Rico.[49] In 1946, María Pintado de Rahn stated in a radio broadcast in Washington, DC, that she and other social workers were lobbying for fuller coverage and that "the great needs and rights of American citizens of Puerto Rico . . . not being forgotten."[50] She argued that if the United States wanted "to make real the freedoms and rights that it . . . championed so gallantly in war and so forcefully in peace," it was essential to provide full social rights to Puerto Rico. She noted that in recent years France had expanded fuller social rights to its Caribbean territories and called upon the United States to invest in Puerto Rican social welfare. Despite numerous petitions and delegations to Congress in the years that followed, Puerto Rico had never been granted full coverage under the Social Security Act.

However, revamping the Employment and Migration Bureau to launch the Migration Division in 1948, and the creation of the MACPRA in 1949, opened up a new opportunity to discuss the possibility of extending Social Security benefits to Puerto Rico. These organizations argued that it was the federal government's responsibility to provide social services and support to Puerto Rican migrants as well as Puerto Ricans on the archipelago. Social workers played an important part in spreading this message by serving as educators to US officials about the history of US governance in Puerto Rico and the partial social rights available to Puerto Ricans. They began to target city officials in particular as a means of advocating not only for Puerto Rican migrants in the United States but also for the archipelago as a whole.[51] Despite continued restrictions on Puerto Rican representatives in US Congress due to the archipelago's colonial status, social workers sought to use migrant communities' electoral power in US party politics to open up a space for Puerto Rican representation.

During the 1949 hearings on Puerto Rico and the Social Security Act, Puerto Rican constituents articulated clear demands for broader coverage under social policy. Social workers submitted reports on the status of poverty on the archipelago and explained how the infrastructure that they had been developing under the Department of Public Welfare since 1943 could serve as the scaffolding through which to distribute further assistance to those in need. With input from US-based social service experts, these social workers had created the first archipelago-wide social welfare department, modeled on US programs. Their efforts expanded the reach of Puerto Rican social welfare programs into the lives of Puerto Ricans in unprecedented ways. During the 1949 hearings, those testifying sought to highlight Puerto Rico's expertise and existing capacity for managing the federal funding that would become available through the act's expansion.[52] However, despite the enthusiasm of the social workers and other Puerto Rican constituents, the idea of extending the Social Security Act to Puerto Rico continued to face criticism from US policymakers who did not want to take on the cost of creating a full benefits program for the archipelago's citizens. At the start of 1950, the result of the inquiry remained uncertain.

In response, the Puerto Rican government, the US-based Migration Division, and the MACPRA mobilized to gain support for the Social Security Act from US officials in cities with large populations of Puerto Rican migrants. It was an opportune time to address the issue, as recent increases in migration led US policymakers to newly consider Puerto Ricans' lack of rights. City officials began to see that improving conditions on the archipelago by extending social welfare could potentially reduce migration to the United States, since living in the United States enabled Puerto Ricans to access Social Security benefits. Social workers capitalized on the notion that migration was propelled in part by the lack of adequate work and social services in Puerto Rico. They explained that current insular social welfare programs had been developed under Partido Popular Democrático (PPD) leadership and were limited due to lack of funding. They argued that more federal assistance in Puerto Rico would easily enable them to use the infrastructure already in place to further develop social welfare programs and transform Puerto Rican society.

Social workers' message that more robust social benefits in Puerto Rico might help reduce migration to the United States helped create a change in opinion among US officials and the public. They revealed the ways in which Puerto Ricans not only received differential citizenship rights based on location but also that these discrepancies often created an impetus to move.[53] Emphasizing this inequity, they argued that the very need to migrate in order to collect benefits in the United States could be reduced if the archipelago's citizens received the same coverage under the Social Security Act as citizens living in the United States.

In addition to concerns about migration, Puerto Rico began to take on increased political importance for the United States in the postwar period.[54] In juxtaposition to the leftist and communist-inspired social movements taking place in other areas of Latin America and the Caribbean, Puerto Rico was described in US postwar discourse as having had a "peaceful revolution" with a gradual transition toward a new territorial status under the United States, a "showcase of democracy" due to US intervention and modernization. This narrative was strategically important to the United States as the Cold War continued and Puerto Rico became known as a "social laboratory" for studying social and political transformations in Latin America.[55] Such discourse not only served the US agenda of keeping Puerto Rico as a territory, but also erased the archipelago's long political struggle for independence. However, this political moment also facilitated the increased training of social workers in Puerto Rico, and numerous social workers and social scientists traveled between the archipelago and the United States. From the US perspective, the intention was that they would serve both on the archipelago and in other areas of Latin America in order to spread US social welfare ideologies. But Puerto Rican government officials used this circulation of people and ideas as an opportunity to work toward their own political agenda. They infused social worker training and other social scientific knowledge production with Puerto Rican understandings of social welfare as well as their own ideas about political organizing for social transformation.

To that end, the Migration Division organized educational conferences for US policymakers in Puerto Rico, sponsoring US mayors, social service agents, welfare administrators, and teachers to visit, travel, and learn about the archipelago. When they arrived, Manuel Cabranes, director of the Migration Division, was there to meet them. In discussions about the "inadequacies of the archipelago's relief program" and "easing the economic pressure on migration from Puerto Rico," Cabranes suggested "that Puerto Rico be used as a demonstration and training area for United States technicians who later would help the underdeveloped areas of the world under President Truman's Point Four program."[56] In doing so, he linked the expansion of federal social benefits to Puerto Rico to the US government's broader political agenda. Thus, providing social assistance to Puerto Rico could now be understood as a means of aiding US political control in Latin America and the Caribbean.

The Migration Division's educational initiatives expanded after the 1950s, as the agency brought hundreds of US government representatives, teachers, and political figures to Puerto Rico to introduce them to the modernization projects being developed by the PPD. Social workers from the Migration Division, including leader Matilde Pérez de Silva, oversaw these visits in collaboration with Puerto Rican government agencies on the archipelago.[57] In Puerto Rico they met with high-ranking leaders in the field of social work, such as Emma Purcell de Hernández, Felicidad Cátala, Celia Núnez de Bunker, and Mercedez Vélez de Pérez. Even the retired social work leader Beatriz Lassalle participated in some of these activities with the visitors.[58] As one of the founders of social welfare programs in Puerto Rico in the 1920s, she could draw on over forty years of experience working alongside US officials to develop social welfare initiatives.

These educational programs in Puerto Rico became a project that educated the US government about both the archipelago and about migrants now living in the United States. Participants not only engaged in seminar discussions, watched presentations, and met with Puerto Rican officials, but also were sometimes placed in homestays with Puerto Rican families and conducted fieldwork in poor Puerto Rican neighborhoods. By showing US officials the poverty that many citizens faced on the archipelago and the limited assistance they received because of the restrictions on social policy to Puerto Rico, these programs provided much-needed context for discussions about social services. The social workers also shared stories about the long history of their attempts to get more extensive coverage under the Social Security Act.[59] In these ways, social workers were able to make strong arguments about the need for substantive change to social policy—change that, due to Puerto Ricans' lack of political representation on the archipelago, could be achieved in the United States.

In the years that followed, the limitations of US social welfare for Puerto Ricans became the subject of numerous articles in US newspapers, enabling advocates as well as critics to weigh in with their opinions. Officials in New York and other US cities who still believed that Puerto Rican migrants were a drain on local resources welcomed such discourse.[60] For example, one article on the MACPRA noted that the group sought the "liberalization of the Federal Social Security Law," which "forbids use of Federal grants-in-aid for the aged, the blind, and dependent children in Puerto Rico."[61] The article went on to argue, "Without Federal aid from the continent, relief allotments in Puerto Rico are now limited to $7.50 a month per family, regardless of its size." The funding cap, so often bemoaned by social workers on the archipelago in their work to petition Congress, was described and then compared to what was available in New York. The article stated, "The average in New York City for all assistance payments in August was $81.31 per case, and

$40.73 per individual." Thus, US officials and the press now drew on Puerto Rican officials' knowledge about social welfare inequality.

In addition, advocates used the press to argue that it was the federal government's responsibility to address their concerns and provide Puerto Ricans on the archipelago with access to Social Security. An article published in the *New York Times* in 1950 about the MACPRA stated, "[All] the members of the committee headed by Mr. Hilliard had recommended passage of the Social Security provisions affecting Puerto Rico." According to the article, a broad coalition of New Yorkers, including "leaders of the Puerto Rican community here as well as religious and civic leaders interested in Puerto Rican affairs and the heads of all the city's departments affected by the recent large immigration of Puerto Rican[s] to this city" were all in agreement about the immediate necessity of this change. The article even quoted Mayor O'Dwyer as adamantly stating, "[It] would be manifestly unfair for Congress to refuse this aid both to Puerto Rico and to New York City" and that "failure to extend such equal treatment to Puerto Rico would be considered unfair by Puerto Ricans."[62] Only a few years earlier, such a statement issued by a US city official about extending the Social Security Act to Puerto Rico would have seemed impossible to the social workers who had lobbied Congress.

But the tide had shifted in their favor, and that year an entire delegation of US city representatives, primarily from New York City and Chicago, lobbied Congress to expand the Social Security Act to the archipelago. In 1950, largely due to their influence, a significant albeit still-restricted portion of the Social Security Act was extended to Puerto Rico. This resulted in startling transformations to the archipelago's social welfare status. The Puerto Rican government, with the help of its social workers, had established a system of social welfare and Social Security that, although limited by colonial restrictions, had changed the archipelago's relationship to the United States by weaving together social welfare programs. On both the archipelago and in the United States, many social workers who had worked tirelessly to achieve these results welcomed this new, more connected relationship.

Radical Alternatives: Social Workers and the Independence Movement

In Puerto Rico, not all social workers were happy with the way that social welfare policies were being developed as part of a larger political project to ensure a continued colonial relationship with the United States. On

November 1, 1950, the Puerto Rican social worker Blanca Canales was arrested in her hometown of Jayuya for her participation in a nationalist uprising.[63] Canales was one of the social workers first trained at the University of Puerto Rico at Río Piedras in 1928, and she had worked to create social service programs in the years that followed.[64] The uprising that she led was part of an island-wide campaign organized by Puerto Rican leader Pedro Albizu Campos protesting the continued colonial governance of Puerto Rico, as well as the proposed creation of a new territorial commonwealth status, the Estado Libre Asociado (Free Associated State). Canales and a group of other independence activists gathered in the center of Jayuya, raised the Puerto Rican flag, and held the town by force for three days before the Puerto Rican National Guard arrested them and put them in jail. Photographs taken after her arrest reveal a middle-aged woman in a nice dress, the picture of respectability as she stands surrounded by Puerto Rican police, her defiance written all over her face. In one such image (figure 5.4) she is shown surrounded by male figures and police officers who are interrogating her while in custody.

Blanca Canales was part of a cohort of social workers who were active in the Puerto Rican independence movement from the 1930s through the 1950s, many of whom participated in armed insurrections against US governance. As discussed in chapter 2, these nationalist women were trained in early social work programs at the University of Puerto Rico and managed to navigate their work for the Puerto Rican government while opposing US colonialism. As historian Olga Jímenez Wagenheim and other scholars of the history of the women in the independence movement have illuminated, such women's stories and sacrifices have only recently been the subject of formative historical analysis despite the fact that they were instrumental in shaping the nationalist movement throughout the twentieth century.[65] Social workers like Blanca Canales, Carmen Rivera de Alvarado, and Isabel Rosado Morales would go on to become some of the most important women leaders in the Puerto Rican independence movement.[66] Both Canales and Rivera de Alvarado were active in professional social work organizations from the early 1930s through the period covered in this chapter. These social workers would participate in political organizing at the same time as they continued their day-to-day activities as social workers.

For Blanca Canales, the route to a better future for Puerto Rico would be achieved through radical political action.[67] She and like-minded social workers collaborated closely with Albizu Campos and other nationalists throughout the 1930s and 1940s, even as they helped develop social welfare

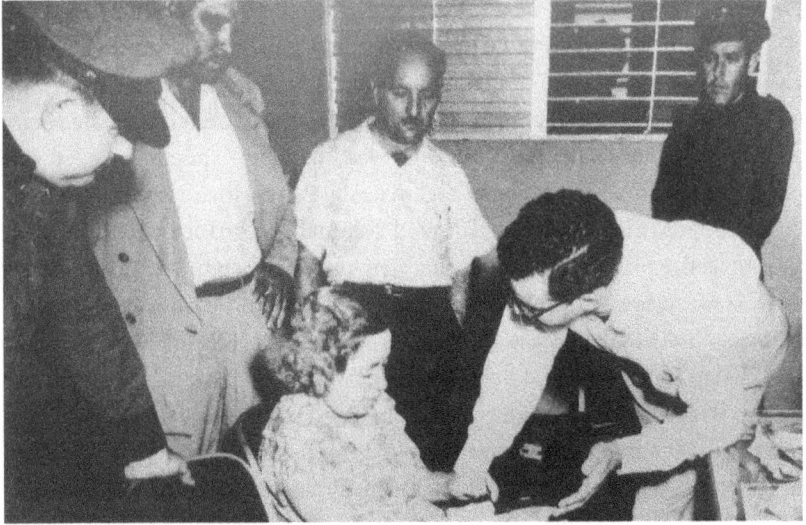

FIGURE 5.4. Blanca Canales after her arrest for participating in the Jayuya Uprising on October 30, 1950. Source: Nilsa M. Burgos Ortiz, *Pioneras de la profesión de trabajo social en Puerto Rico* (Hato Rey: Publicaciones Puertorriqueñas, 1998), 53. Originally published in *Claridad*, August 8, 1996.

programs on the archipelago for the Puerto Rican government. Canales would later describe how while she was working as a social worker she was also helping found nationalist groups, including the women's group Hijas de la Libertad (Daughters of Liberty).[68] But such organizers faced political persecution as the PPD oversaw an ongoing purge of independence leaders from government institutions. This became particularly difficult for social workers after the 1948 passage of the Ley de la Mordaza, a gag law that made it illegal for Puerto Rican citizens to criticize the government and speak out in favor of independence. However, Puerto Rican nationalists, among them social workers, continued to organize and plan actions despite this crackdown. It seems that one of the main holdouts of radical political vision within the Puerto Rican state was within professional programs that employed women social workers.

But political mobilization for independence would come to a head in 1950 with the passage of Public Law 600, which authorized Puerto Rico to create its own constitution but maintained its colonial relationship with the United States. In response, independence supporters, led by Albizu Campos, began developing plans for coordinated action around the archipelago to challenge US authority and proclaim a free Puerto Rico.[69] In 1950, the Independence Party launched a series of armed actions against the US government. It was at this time that Canales was placed in charge of the movement in her hometown of Jayuya. She took up arms alongside a group of other independence supporters. They seized the town, declaring that it was now part of an independent Puerto Rico, free from US governance. Shortly afterward, she was arrested along with a larger group of independence organizers, which included other nationalist women. Canales was convicted of a federal crime for destroying the Jayuya post office and sentenced to life in prison. She would serve out her sentence between West Virginia and Puerto Rico but was ultimately pardoned in 1967.[70] She became well-known on the archipelago as a political prisoner, embraced by activists who sought to free those who had participated in the uprisings. Her organizing and action marked a decisive protest against the PPD agenda.

The lives and radical activism of social workers like Canales reveal complex political allegiances during a moment of significant social transformation. Social workers who were active in campaigns to overthrow US colonialism also played key roles as state agents in social welfare programs. Even as they engaged in radical political actions that challenged colonial authority, they were committed to trying to expand social rights for Puerto Ricans under US governance. Consequently, they worked in coalitions with people with whom they disagreed politically to advocate for the extension of the Social Security Act and develop social welfare programs on the archipelago.[71] Despite their radical political vision, their goal was pragmatic—to create a system that would allow Puerto Ricans access to social services. In fact, their work in the field as social workers often enabled their broader organizing efforts. For example, as Canales and Rivera de Alvarado traveled between welfare offices on the archipelago, they used their mobility as an opportunity to meet with various independence supporters and spread their political message.[72]

But despite nationalist efforts for independence, the sweeping tide of the PPD could not be halted, and Puerto Rico's colonial status remained through a reworked commonwealth arrangement. In 1952, the Estado Libre Asociado was formally created, and the PPD won a decisive victory in the Puerto Rican polls. In response, independence organizing took on more drastic forms, and, in 1954, a group of independence supporters led by nationalist Lolita Lebrón attacked the US House of Representatives, wounding five congressmen and demanding that Puerto Rico be liberated from US colonial rule.[73]

Shortly afterward, Albizu Campos was sent to a federal prison in Atlanta, and the PPD government continued its crackdown on independence organizing with the support of the US government.

As political persecution against Puerto Rican nationalists increased, a number of organizers began working in exile in the United States.[74] Social workers were important members of the political coalitions that traveled to New York to build networks with other radical organizers and activists. Carmen Rivera de Alvarado, in particular, traveled extensively throughout the United States as well as Latin America to advocate for decolonization, socialism, and Puerto Rican independence.[75] She also continued to establish herself as a leader in the field of social work in the United States and by the 1970s began to articulate and write about a new form of Puerto Rican social work practice focused on decolonization. She wrote specifically about the ways that in Puerto Rico a particular variant of social work practice had developed among some social workers, which she described as "authentically Puerto Rican." According to Rivera de Alvardo, social work should be a "vocation of freedom," one that focused on the liberation of the individual, of groups, and of the communities in which one worked. She noted in her writing that only "those that are free can help liberate others." She argued that the "function of the social worker was not based on exercising their personal power over the individual" but rather to "recognize the right of the other to exercise their self-determination."[76] Writing later in life, she would emphasize that she believed that the main goal of social workers should be to help create communities that were empowered and that social workers should be engaged with political questions and party politics. She also wrote that social services should be in the hands of the working class who receive benefits from these programs, and that social workers themselves were also "workers" and should see themselves as such.[77] Her ideas, and those of other radical social workers who had organized for independence, would ultimately circulate throughout the United States and inform the development of new social work practices in the coming years.

Thus, at the same time that the Puerto Rican government and many social workers worked to create a more intertwined relationship between US and Puerto Rican welfare programs, other social workers proposed alternative visions of the archipelago's future. Those who organized with the independence movement represented a significant challenge to the agenda established by PPD leadership in these years. However, women like Carmen Rivera de Alvarado and Blanca Canales participated in these political developments in interlocking and complex ways. They and other Puerto Rican social workers used the professionalization of social work as political leverage to agitate for radical goals. In this way, they transformed the field of social work into an even more important space for women's political organizing.

Expanding the Migration Division of the Puerto Rican Government

Puerto Rican social workers' political work in the United States continued during the 1950s as the Migration Division expanded. Major transformations began in 1951 when PPD leadership reorganized migration offices in the United States, which included significant personnel changes. Clarence Senior, a social scientist from the United States, was appointed director of the Migration Division.[78] Senior published a number of studies that reflected his view that social scientific experts should manage migration from Puerto Rico, and he had been working with the PPD on a variety of ongoing modernization projects.[79] His appointment displaced Manuel Cabranes, who had first developed the agency.[80] Puerto Rican social worker Joseph Monserrat was hired to run the Migration Division's New York branch in a position that he would hold until 1960 when he was promoted to direct the entire agency.

Monserrat's leadership would have far-reaching consequences for the Migration Division. He drew on his own experiences as a Puerto Rican migrant raised in the United States, particularly those of racial discrimination, as well as his knowledge and investment in the forms of group work that were prevalent in the settlement house movement, in which he had a long professional history.[81] His fluency in discussing social service policies led the Migration Division to support varied community-oriented initiatives to help Puerto Rican migrants in New York City, including organizing for access to housing, education, and other social services and new social justice orientation programs.

But while the Migration Division's leadership remained male dominated, it was still women who largely oversaw the agency's daily operations (see figure 5.5). In particular, social worker Matilde Pérez de Silva worked closely with Monserrat on the Migration Division's social service aspects during these formative years. Others continued to collaborate with local social welfare agencies and developed new forms of casework in response to migrants' needs. The programs they established changed the discourse about migration, slowly showing city officials that Puerto Ricans were not foreigners who could be deported or denied social services simply on the basis of not having citizenship. In essence, in Puerto Ricans' attempts to make claims to social services in the United States, they tested the rights and benefits of US citizenship.[82] Migration Division agents intervened in cases to back up these claims, providing proof that they were legitimate. While agents and migrants still faced discrimination, such as framing Puerto Ricans as potential dependents, these debates did begin to rework the discussion of Puerto Ricans' access to social services in the United States.

In addition, the Migration Division worked to draw attention to the lack of Puerto Rican and Spanish-speaking social workers in US social welfare agencies. A survey conducted by the Welfare Council discovered that there were only thirty-eight Puerto Rican social workers employed in the ninety-nine social welfare agencies in New York City that responded. The organizations suggested that they would be interested in hiring more Puerto Rican and Spanish-speaking staff, but they had a hard time finding those with the necessary training in social work. Consequently, there were large numbers of unfilled positions for bilingual social workers. In response, the Welfare Council determined that promising Puerto Rican students should be recruited in high school and college by providing social work scholarships. They note in their report that such financial assistance was set to begin immediately. For their part, the MACPRA was able to negotiate the end of a three-year residency requirement for social workers, which also allowed for a rapid demographic change in the field.

In the years to come, these efforts would result in the creation of additional scholarship programs for Puerto Rican youth to study social work, including one named after Marie Antoinette Cannon, which provided support for students to study at the New York School of Social Work. The scholarship's first recipient was Antonia Pantoja, a young community organizer who would go on to become a central figure in the field of social work and a prominent activist in Puerto Rico.[83] The next chapter will examine how Pantoja and other Puerto Rican social workers built on the organizing of earlier social workers and took the field in new directions, connecting their work with grassroots organizing and developing a new community-oriented form of social work practice.

As the demand for Puerto Rican social workers grew alongside the migrant community itself, the Migration Division helped facilitate social workers' arrival from the archipelago, recruiting and placing them in jobs through its own employment services agency.[84] The placement of these workers was also something that became a more pressing political issue and reality, with increasing social pressure from US welfare agencies. The social mobility available to social workers also diversified the field, as growing numbers

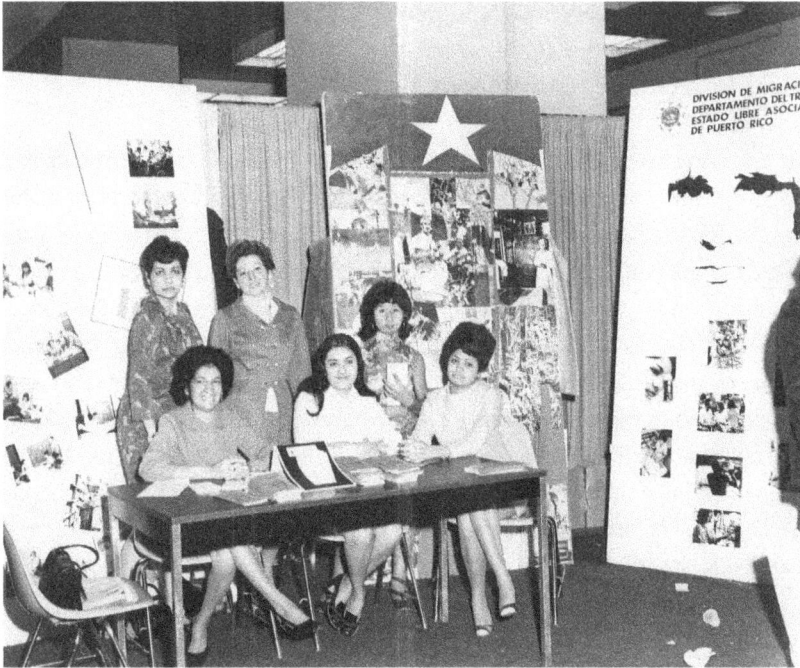

FIGURE 5.5. Women in a Migration Division booth. Courtesy of the Offices of the Government of Puerto Rico in the United States Records, Archives of the Puerto Rican Diaspora, Center for Puerto Rican Studies, Hunter College, City University of New York.

of students applied for scholarship programs in social work education programs in Puerto Rico and the United States.[85] Over time, the composition of the agency would also shift, as the division hired more social workers like Monserrat who were born or raised in the United States.

In addition to creating jobs for Puerto Rican social workers in the United States, the agency's efforts to increase their numbers functioned to improve services to migrants. As bilingual professionals, agents were able to navigate between different languages as translators of state structures. Seeking to promote "integration" and change practices within US agencies, they were charged both with making migrants legible to social service agencies and with linguistically and conceptually interpreting US institutions for their clients. They had firsthand experience with migrants' needs as well as with state agencies' treatment and understandings of Puerto Ricans in the United States. They used their position to establish themselves as experts on migration, challenge the perception that migrants were potential drains on US cities, and fight for social citizenship and access to social services, both in the United States and on the archipelago.

IN THE POSTWAR PERIOD, as migration to the United States expanded and sped up, the work of social workers became increasingly important in the Puerto Rican diaspora. In part, this was because the Puerto Rican working-class migrant community continued to demand that the Puerto Rican government respond to the terrible conditions that they faced in the United States. The Migration Division became a central hub of organization around migrant rights as migrants came to its offices when faced with discrimination and lack of resources. While some of the Migration Division social workers' work was about welfare, most became about Puerto Rican civil rights and human rights issues more broadly. Within this space, Puerto Rican women social workers became leaders in the community, and the profession expanded in significance and clout in the following years.

Between social workers there were diverging views about the best path forward for social change in Puerto Rican society on the archipelago and in the diaspora. The 1950s marked a time of great political division among women in the profession over how their work as social workers intersected with their commitments to broader political causes and to the future of the archipelago's political status. For some Puerto Rican social workers, political action through mobilization within the PPD or the statehood party meant following along organizing routes already well traveled. These social workers used their social scientific skills to compile "poverty knowledge" they believed would correct the racist ideas about Puerto Ricans that persisted in the United States. Many believed colonialism could be reformed or ended by further adaptation of the commonwealth status of Puerto Rico or by advocating for statehood. However, social worker activists also played outsized roles during the period in the Puerto Rican independence movement.

The radical legacy of Puerto Rican women social workers in independence organizing and in socialist organizing was the outcome of decades of previous political struggles. The activist leaders who had come of age in the late 1920s and cut their teeth on reform projects during the New Deal had dreamed of a future beyond US colonialism. They had agitated and worked alongside fellow nationalist women in a long struggle to advocate for an end to US imperialism. They had forged their particular ideas about social work, linking the goals of social welfare institutions with ideas about how decolonization could be achieved in Puerto Rico. They were sorely disappointed by the continuation of colonialism. These women took different paths forward through the radical actions of the independence movement in the 1950s. For Blanca Canales, the struggle for freedom from US colonialism was worth putting her life on the line as she took up arms to declare a free Puerto Rican nation. For others, it meant continuing to agitate in independence organizations while facing political persecution, blacklisting, and state surveillance. Nevertheless, these activists persisted and would become icons for later generations of Puerto Rican activists in the 1960s and 1970s who continued to fight for the independence of Puerto Rico on the archipelago and in the diaspora.

During the period, tensions were also emerging within the Puerto Rican community in the United States over the work of the Migration Division and other Puerto Rican agencies. The diasporic population was frustrated with the continued sponsorship of migration by the Puerto Rican government without ample or adequate reform of the conditions faced by Puerto Rican migrants in the United States. In addition, a new generation of Puerto Rican activists were becoming deeply involved in US-based civil rights organizations and social movements. This included many Puerto Ricans from working-class backgrounds who were trained in social work or were involved in increasing community-oriented activism in settlement houses and beyond. They would take up some of the same methods and causes as earlier generations of social work activists, but some would also push the movement in new directions that would further emphasize collaborations with working-class communities.

Community Organizers, Civil Rights Activism, and Demands for Care in Puerto Rican Communities in the United States

On May 2, 1989, Puerto Rican civil rights leader Antonia Pantoja gave a speech at Hunter College titled "Voces de Mujeres: Puerto Rican Women and Community Development in New York."[1] In this searing commentary on the history of Puerto Rican political organizing in New York City, Pantoja took scholars and political organizations to task for not remembering the historical contributions of Puerto Rican women to social justice and civil rights work in the United States. She spoke about "the group of Puerto Rican women who held leadership in New York City during the years 1945–1960s," and noted that throughout this period, the "leadership of the Puerto Rican community was heavily feminine" and that "this feminine leadership acted with a distinct style and philosophy."[2] Pantoja highlighted how these women's efforts centered on community organizing and working collaboratively toward social justice. However, despite the centrality of women's activism in Puerto Rican political history, Pantoja pointedly noted that Puerto Rican New York women were largely missing from "written and published work on Puerto Ricans."[3]

Antonia Pantoja was a social worker and community organizer in Puerto Rico and New York who founded numerous social organizations to help Puerto Rican communities in the United States (figure 6.1).[4] Pantoja's political activism was shaped by her own experiences growing up in a working-class family and later identifying as Afro-Puerto Rican and a lesbian. She had faced racism and structural inequality as a young person in Puerto Rico and as a migrant in the United States. While Pantoja became a social worker, she had a tense and critical relationship with the field. She later noted that she knew from the start of her training as a social worker that she "did not want to be a caseworker, since [she] believed caseworkers participated in making people adjust to situations that they should fight against, situations that hurt them or rendered them powerless."[5] Instead, inspired by grassroots activism in New York City and the civil rights movement, Pantoja would work to forge a new kind of social work that made community organizing its central aim.

This chapter tells the story of the "feminine leadership" in Puerto Rican communities in the United States that Pantoja describes in her speech, tracing women's political activism in community-oriented projects through a focus on professional care workers. Scholarship on the history of Puerto Rican communities in the United States has begun to document the activists' participation in struggles for civil, economic, and political rights. This chapter focuses on the Puerto Rican women who were professional care workers in this history, showing their vital contributions to Puerto Rican political organizing through community-oriented work. It shows how these activists politicized their roles as professional care workers as they worked to create social services programs and institutions in Puerto Rican communities that were under community control. It also emphasizes how this work intersected with their participation in social movements like the US civil rights movement, the Black freedom struggle, feminist organizing, and the Puerto Rican independence movement. The chapter concludes by considering the role of these women in shaping intellectual knowledge about the Puerto Rican diaspora through scholarship that contributed to the academic study of social work, community organizing, education, and Puerto Rican studies. These stories shine a light on the lasting intellectual legacy of these women activists.

The Puerto Rican social worker activists whose stories are told in this chapter were from working-class backgrounds and later worked as community organizers in New York City during the 1950s through the 1970s. Alongside Pantoja, the chapter considers the activism of other community

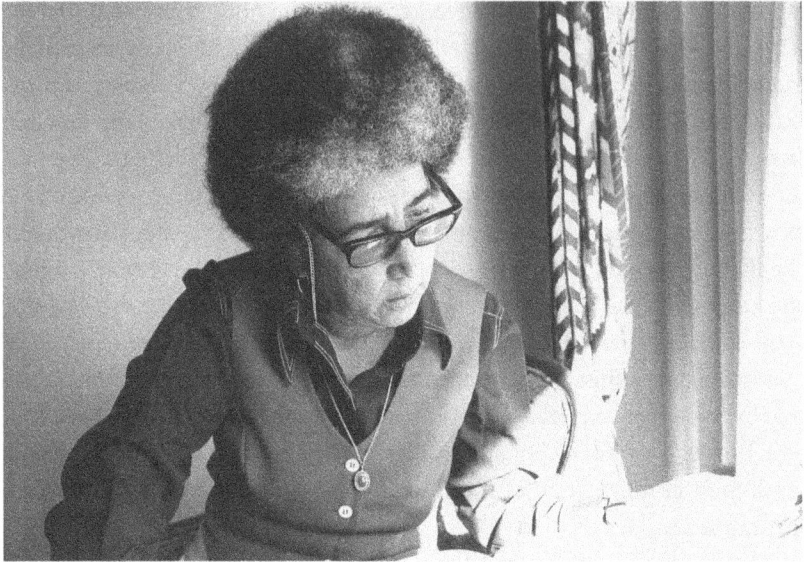

FIGURE 6.1. Antonia Pantoja reading a book. Courtesy of the Antonia Pantoja Papers, Archives of the Puerto Rican Diaspora, Center for Puerto Rican Studies, Hunter College, City University of New York.

activists, including women like Yolanda Sánchez, Esperanza Martell, and Josephine Nieves. These women represented new generations of social work activists, most of whom were raised in the United States or identified as New Yorkers. These women also took advantage of the opportunity to professionalize as social workers to advance their participation in struggles for civil, economic, and political rights. Among these activists were also women who identified as Afro-Puerto Rican and Black and whose work was also profoundly connected to activism within the Black freedom movement.[6] For many, their work was also related to their participation in leftist, socialist, feminist, and independence-oriented activism. As their life histories show, there were various and divergent ways that Puerto Rican social worker activists organized in New York, and their stories shed light on how their work as community organizers was influenced by their participation in social movements.

As community organizers in New York, this group of Puerto Rican social worker activists fought for community and working-class control over social service and public health institutions. In doing so, they developed social work practices that both built on and diverged from earlier generations of social work activism. This work included their participation in social service programs created during the US civil rights movement, programs that emphasized community control and self-help.[7] It also included more radical organizing for social welfare and health care rights that intersected with the struggle of social movements to demand care for working-class communities. In some instances they joined forces with other activists and care workers in struggles over social services and public health in Puerto Rican communities during the 1960s and 1970s.[8] Central to this generation of social workers was thinking about ways that their work could be created in unity with working-class communities. The community-oriented social work of these activists would also launch them into roles as educators and producers of knowledge with lasting intellectual legacies. This chapter shows how their work would help support new generations of Puerto Rican youth to take pride in their identities and fight for a better future for all Puerto Ricans.

Antonia Pantoja, Puerto Rican Social Workers, and Political Activism after 1950

Antonia Pantoja's life story exemplifies how, during the 1950s, a new generation of social workers was able to transform social work into a form of political activism. Like Pantoja, many of these social workers' life experiences and work were shaped by their migrating to or being raised in the United States. Pantoja wrote that her primary identity was as a "Nuyorican"—a Puerto Rican New Yorker—because her experience in the city had so deeply transformed her life.[9] Pantoja further noted that "as a member of the group that had left the island," she "knew that we could build new lives in the city while preserving our culture in our institution-building to create our community life." Social work provided an avenue to do this work, but she also noted that she didn't want to be a part of a "profession that implied or indicated a separation from [her] community."[10] As a Nuyorican and migrant, her approach to social work was conditioned by her early experiences in Puerto Rico and her new life in New York.

Pantoja was born in 1922 in Puerto Rico and grew up in the poor neighborhood of Barrio Obrero. During her early years, she was raised by her maternal grandfather, an urban tobacco worker, and by her grandmother, a household worker and laundress, both of whom were of African descent.[11] She grew up poor in the city amid the labor union organizing in Puerto Rico's tobacco industry during the 1920s and 1930s. Pantoja had seen her grandfather cruelly hurt by anti-union and US government operatives after he participated in a tobacco workers strike. Afro-Puerto Ricans like Pantoja's grandfather were crucial figures in this labor movement.[12] Though Pantoja recalled that her relatives were often fearful of expressing nationalist sentiment themselves, they did shelter a nationalist who had been hurt during the Ponce Massacre. Her experiences bearing witness to the political organizing in her family, as well as the harsh political violence that her community experienced, made her aware of pervasive injustice from an early age. She later wrote that these experiences shaped her interest in social justice, as did her experience as an Afro-Puerto Rican.[13]

As a child, Pantoja and her family were also impacted by ongoing transformations in the Puerto Rican state, specifically the intervention of social welfare and public health programs in the lives of poor communities. Her family received relief from the New Deal agencies created as a part of the Puerto Rican Relief Administration (PRERA).[14] As this agency brought relief in the form of unfamiliar foodstuffs imported from the United States, her family had to learn how to cook differently.[15] Pantoja's life would also be impacted by the expansion of public health programs in Puerto Rico when, after her first year in high school, she was diagnosed with tuberculosis. She spent three months convalescing in a sanatorium in Aibonito, one of the clinics created as a part of the regional development of health care infrastructure after the New Deal.[16] Here, she also encountered social workers tasked with overseeing the health care program. In the 1940s, after her health improved, she took advantage of expanding public education opportunities on the archipelago to achieve a significant amount of social mobility. She trained to become a teacher at the Normal School at the University of Puerto Rico and began working in the public education system.

During her first experiences teaching in rural schools, Pantoja began to realize the power and significance of education as a space of social transformation. Pantoja first traveled by horseback to a school in the mountain town of Cuchillas and later was transferred to a Segunda Unidad Rural in Padilla. In these schools, she would likely have worked alongside Puerto Rican social workers and participated in the cultural nationalism that brewed in this community.[17] She later described this experience as one of her best as an educator because of the freedom that she was given to experiment with new forms of teaching and community organizing. In her classroom and those of her colleagues, Puerto Rican students and teachers often stood in opposition to the pedagogical norms enforced under US colonialism, teaching in Spanish and offering critical interpretations of the colonial order. When Pantoja was later transferred to an urban school where the teachers were not as involved in the institution's governance, she became quickly frustrated by the work. However, her experiences developing grassroots education in rural Puerto Rico shaped her understanding of knowledge production as a collaborative effort and the radical potential of educators' work in social transformation.

After teaching for a short period in Puerto Rico, Pantoja migrated to the United States. In Puerto Rico, teachers were not paid regularly, and she waited for months for her wages even as she struggled with the financial burden of caring for her family. She also later observed that the social restrictions that she faced because of her gender and race in Puerto Rico were overwhelming, and her decision to leave was a form of resistance.[18] Pantoja's sexuality also likely impacted these decisions as she joined a queer diaspora in the United States.[19] She migrated, seeking freedom to build her life and start fresh. However, her first experiences in the United States were also marked by racism and xenophobia. She witnessed and experienced racial and ethnic discrimination and was unable to find work as a teacher because of her accent. When her professional skills did not translate into a teaching job in the United States, she sought alternative work in needleworking and lamp-making factories. There, she became involved in labor organizing with her fellow workers, the beginning of a process of reinventing herself as an activist and as a New Yorker.

Pantoja's first years in New York were also full of adventure as she entered a bohemian world of artists and intellectuals and she found she could express herself in new ways. During these years, she read voraciously, wrote poetry, and joined heady discussions of politics and philosophy. It was at this time that Pantoja also had her first long-term romantic relationship with a woman and became a part of a broader lesbian and queer community in New York City. And, while her writings offer little details about these experiences, she nevertheless noted that they were formative, and she talked about how she was able to live a life that had not been possible for her in Puerto Rico.[20] She later reflected that she was lucky to have learned about the city from "the artists."

The social world she entered in New York then was also an exciting place to engage with various political organizations and viewpoints. During this period, Pantoja participated in a class at the Jefferson School called "The Marxist Interpretation of the History of Puerto Rico," in which she was the only Puerto Rican student.[21] In this class, she learned much about US imperialism and the colonial history of Puerto Rico. She wrote, "I had never heard this type of information spoken publicly, nor had I seen it documented in print before."[22] She noted, "This information was a great discovery for me, but it made me afraid. I was afraid of such ideas."[23] She would later reflect on the fact that these experiences were transformative because they gave her a new perspective on the relationship between Puerto Rico and the United States and the radical potential of learning about Puerto Rican history. She began to see access to a critical education about Puerto Rican history and culture as a central need in the Puerto Rican community. Her political advocacy in the years to come would often center on advocating for Puerto Rican history to be taught in migrant communities.

During this period, Pantoja also had her first formative experience working in a New York institution dedicated to community organizing. She was hired as a youth worker at the 110th Street Community Center and, in this position, worked with Puerto Rican families and children. She later wrote that this job "would reconnect me to my Puerto Rican roots."[24] The goal of this organization was to bring together the ethnic communities in the rapidly changing area by creating new community projects. In this space, Pantoja worked with organizers who, she said, "held a radical perspective, were active in the labor movement, and held ideas about how to organize and move for action."[25] This exposure to community organizing shaped her later trajectory, and she participated in the political fermentation happening in New York City. The people she met through her work in the community center also encouraged her to return to school to get her BA degree, and she enrolled in Hunter College, City College of New York.

As an undergraduate at Hunter, Pantoja would meet other Puerto Rican students interested in community organizing work. This included Maggie Miranda and Marta Valle, who also wanted to create institutions of service for Puerto Rican New Yorkers.[26] Because many of them had grown up poor or living in New York, they also represented a new generation keenly aware of the challenges faced by poor Puerto Ricans who sought health care, education, and social welfare benefits from New York institutions. These students were also particularly interested in taking a more holistic approach toward assisting Puerto Rican families. They saw that access to housing, education, health care, and social welfare services were interconnected and needed to be addressed simultaneously.

For these Puerto Rican women students, social work offered both a career path and an avenue to pursue social justice work in the Puerto Rican community. In part, becoming a social worker was a practical choice, as the profession continued to be a primary avenue for women to get a professional degree. Yet the field also continued to be a space where some women could enter a realm of political organizing and action.[27] While social work was not the profession Pantoja envisioned for herself when she began her studies, it offered a clear road to working within her community. Alongside other Puerto Rican students she met at Hunter, she would pursue a degree at the New York School of Social Work, which later became the School of Social Work at Columbia University. Outside the classroom, Pantoja's cohort gathered to discuss issues they faced as social workers and ways to help their communities, and they began to imagine new ways to organize within Puerto Rican neighborhoods.

Social Workers, Civil Rights, and Community Organizing

The informal gatherings that Antonia Pantoja organized with her fellow students at Hunter College blossomed into more regular meetings to discuss the situations faced by Puerto Ricans in the United States. Over time, the students also began meeting with other Puerto Rican organizers, some of whom worked for the Migration Division of the Puerto Rican government. They discussed the need for leaders who understood the experience of the Puerto Rican community in New York. According to Pantoja, they also "began to formulate [their] own philosophy," one that was rooted in the idea that "organizations should be held accountable to the community, governed and managed by Puerto Ricans, and that the city government should be held accountable for offering services to [the Puerto Rican] community."[28] The meetings of these young people, many of whom were social workers, would soon lead to the foundation of several Puerto Rican–led civil rights organizations in New York.

The students gathered at the same time as Puerto Rican communities in New York were struggling for civil rights, and many of the leaders in this political organization were women who focused on grassroots mobilization. Pantoja would later note that Puerto Rican women were leaders in the diaspora because of their experiences as migrants and labor organizers.[29] Puerto Rican activists collaborated and worked alongside a wide range of community organizations led by other groups in the city, and this work would produce collaborations—as well as tensions—in the years to come.[30] In particular, their work would end up being tied to the emergence of the war on poverty.[31] Many Puerto Rican women leaders who emerged during this period were social workers, including Antonia Pantoja, Marta Valle, Yolanda

Sánchez, and Josephine Nieves.[32] In these roles, Puerto Rican women leaders were fundamental in developing the field of community organizing both within and outside of social work.

The grassroots political organizing that Puerto Ricans spearheaded increasingly conflicted with the work of the Migration Division of the Department of Labor of the Puerto Rican government. The agency was created in 1948 to regulate labor migrations, and its main focus was on the integration and assimilation of Puerto Ricans into US economies and society. Much of the work of the agency was conducted by social workers and other professionals who worked to help advocate for Puerto Rican migrant workers who faced harsh labor conditions and discrimination in the United States.[33] While in the beginning, most of the social workers were professionals from Puerto Rico, the agency increasingly hired Puerto Rican social workers who were raised or born in New York. The changing demographics within the agency and its continued attention to migrant rights transformed the kind of work it performed.[34] The new generation of activists who emerged during this period, including Pantoja, wanted to create institutions run by Puerto Ricans in New York and attuned to the needs of the local community. Critics of the Migration Division argued that, as a Puerto Rican government organization, it was primarily accountable to the archipelago's government rather than to Puerto Ricans in New York. Tensions emerged both within the agency as well as between the agency and the Puerto Rican New York community. Nevertheless, the Migration Division continued to play an essential role as a hub where the community gathered and a source of support for Puerto Rican youth interested in professional opportunities.

The network of Puerto Rican students and social workers Antonia Pantoja met after she attended college began to gather more frequently, and they discussed creating a formal group composed of Puerto Rican professionals. In 1953, they formed the Hispanic Young Adult Association (HYAA) to address the inequality and struggles faced by Puerto Ricans in New York (see figure 6.2).[35] While this group was initially connected to the Migration Division, where they would meet, its members were also critical of the agency's unwillingness to give New York Puerto Ricans autonomy in organizing. They were also critical of the government's continued role in sponsoring labor migration. Pantoja noted that the agency continued to promote an agenda of assimilation, which she argued could only be achieved by white or light-skinned Puerto Ricans.[36] As an Afro-Puerto Rican woman, she underscored that this agenda was failing the broader community by overlooking the reality of racial and class differences within the Puerto Rican community

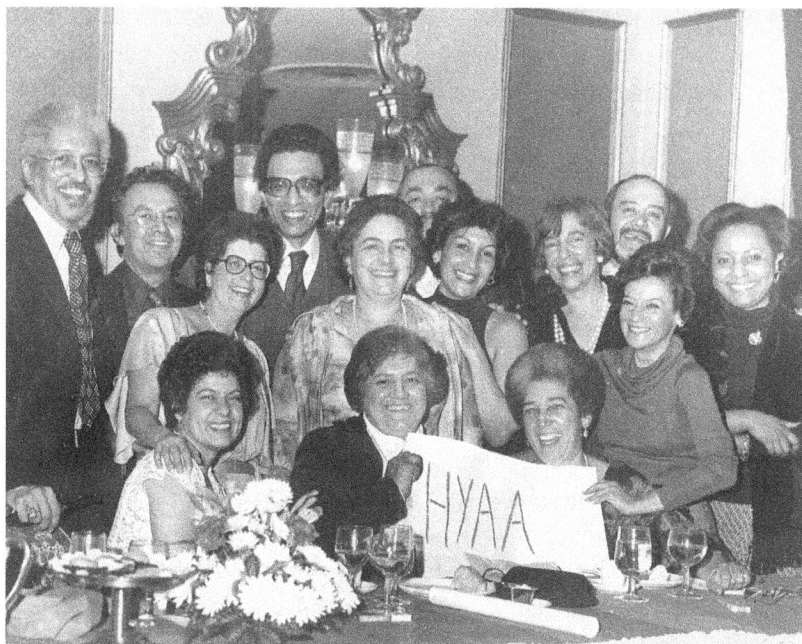

FIGURE 6.2. Former Hispanic Young Adults Association members with Antonia Pantoja (*left*) and Alice Cardona, who hold a sign. Courtesy of the Antonia Pantoja Papers, Archives of the Puerto Rican Diaspora, Center for Puerto Rican Studies, Hunter College, City University of New York.

and promoting passage into "white middle-class" US society. She believed that HYAA could contribute by seeking to empower all Puerto Ricans by celebrating Puerto Rican culture, recognizing Afro-Puerto Rican heritage in the community, and centering efforts promoting economic equality. Some of HYAA's first initiatives were establishing a homeless shelter in a church and creating a Puerto Rican Youth Conference that provided another space for youth to connect. Over time, the group would also change as the youth increasingly organized around their ethnic identity. The organization renamed itself the Puerto Rican Association for Community Affairs (PRACA) and continued developing new initiatives in the community in the years to come.

During the period, the Migration Division provided funding for some Puerto Rican students to attend college to strengthen the number of Puerto Rican professionals in the United States. Pantoja received a scholarship from them to attend the School of Social Work at Columbia University. This scholarship was named in honor of Marie Antoinette Cannon, who had been a key figure in developing social work practice in Puerto Rico, worked in Puerto Rico and the United States, and helped develop the Migration Division.[37] The person in charge of giving the scholarship, Matilde Pérez de Silva, was herself a social worker who had participated in building the social services section of the agency. Pantoja had met Pérez de Silva as a teenager while in the tuberculosis sanatorium in Puerto Rico, and the older woman remembered her and provided a glowing recommendation for the scholarship.[38] It was one of many scholarships the Migration Division and Puerto Rican social agencies explicitly administered to support students in professional careers.[39] The scholarships funded Puerto Rican students, including those studying social work, who later became civil rights leaders, community organizers, and political figures in their communities. Through these initiatives, the earlier efforts of Puerto Rican activists and government officials to diversify the field of social work began to come to fruition.

While the field of social work opened up a space for Pantoja to become a professional, from the start she was ambivalent about becoming a traditional social worker or doing casework. As she later noted in her memoir, she was instead interested in the possibility the field provided to become a community organizer and leader. When she began her studies at Columbia, she immediately sought courses and conversations around community organizing, social policy, and administration. However, she soon discovered that these fields were primarily dominated by men who were being trained to become leaders and policymakers.[40] While Pantoja felt pressure from the advisors in her program to train as a caseworker who would work with individual clients, she nonetheless pushed back against the recommendations of her counselors. She took as many courses in community organizing as she could. Later, she would seek to address the gendered educational tracking and discrimination that she faced herself as a student. Throughout her studies, she fought to be seen and trained to be a leader.

After she graduated from Columbia in 1954, she further distanced herself from more traditional forms of social work by engaging in the growing field of community organizing. In part, this occurred through her participation in the growing and rapidly transforming work of settlement houses in New York. Pantoja was recruited to work at the Union Settlement House overseeing programs for adults, and she later said that it was then that she "stopped being a social worker in the traditional sense of the word."[41] According to historian Sonia Lee, the work of Puerto Rican social workers in settlement houses served as "laboratories" for the training of future civil rights leaders.[42] At the settlement house, Pantoja worked alongside other Puerto Rican and African American activists. Among them was Manny Díaz, a fellow Afro-Puerto Rican social worker who became a civil rights leader.[43] Both Díaz and Pantoja were hired when settlement houses sought to diversify their ranks and their roles in the community. While earlier work in these settlement houses had focused on the integration and assimilation of ethnic white immigrants, the agencies began to shift their focus toward providing services to the growing African American and Puerto Rican communities in their changing neighborhoods.[44] The settlement house provided another education to Pantoja, exposing her to new forms of community organizing developed by social service providers of color.[45] This work also strengthened her relationships with other Puerto Rican social workers and activists she continued meeting with to discuss the possibility of creating community-led institutions. The training and relationships she forged during this period would help provide the foundation for further community organizing and civil rights projects in the coming years.

Not long after Pantoja began working at the Union Settlement House, she was chosen to participate in New York City's Commission on Intergroup Relations (COIR), which would later become the New York Commission on Human Rights. First established in 1955 by Mayor Robert F. Wagner, COIR investigated and reported on discrimination on the basis of race, ethnicity, and religion.[46] COIR was composed of individuals from various racial and ethnic backgrounds, and Pantoja was selected to represent the Puerto Rican community. Seasoned African American civil rights leader Dr. Frank S. Horne led the group.[47] Horne would become a mentor to Pantoja, encouraging her to develop projects addressing the conditions faced by Puerto Ricans in the city. Pantoja was keenly aware of the racial diversity within the Puerto Rican community and the fact that many Puerto Ricans were of African descent, so her work pushed back against that of other Puerto Rican leaders who often silenced race and focused on assimilation.[48] During this period, she was also deeply inspired by the work of Horne, who had helped create civil rights organizations led by African American youth, and she began thinking about how she could use the models she was learning about in her own work. At COIR, she developed the Puerto Rican Project that would emphasize organizing youth to become community advocates and civil rights activists.

Pantoja's collaborations during this period resulted in the creation of a new group called the Puerto Rican Forum. Pantoja continued meetings with friends and fellow social workers who were members of the ongoing efforts of the Puerto Rican Association for Community Affairs (PRACA).

While they had previously had the support of the settlement houses and the Migration Division, these initiatives had been limited by the visions of each group, and they now sought to create more robust independent projects. The Puerto Rican Forum emerged from these collaborations, and the Puerto Rican scholar Frank Bonilla became its first president.[49] The group was invested in the creation of self-help organizations, promoting community development, and learning and teaching about Puerto Rican history and heritage.[50] One of the main projects organized by the Puerto Rican Forum was the Puerto Rican Community Development Project (PRCDP), created in 1963 and led by Pantoja. The group worked broadly as a civil rights organization and formed alliances with numerous other community organizations in the city.[51]

The organizing within the Puerto Rican forum also led to the creation of the group ASPIRA, which Pantoja would later list as her most outstanding organizing achievement. The main work of ASPIRA was as an educational initiative to provide guidance counseling and programs for Puerto Rican youth and help them apply to college.[52] The project began in the Puerto Rican Forum, and soon after, it became an independent organization. Shortly after it was founded, numerous ASPIRA clubs were operating throughout New York, and the group continued to expand. Youth in the program were trained to be organizers who brought people together and sought to foster dialogue and instigate social change. Another essential part of the education that ASPIRA provided was teaching Puerto Rican youth about the history and culture of their community, and the youth later reflected that this education had a transformative impact on their lives.[53] While the work Pantoja oversaw in this organization was connected to earlier practices in the field of community organizing, it also represented something new in the Puerto Rican community by focusing on the education of the next generation. Thus, a new generation of young people were given opportunities that allowed them to become leaders in their community.

Due to its emphasis on training a group of community leaders—in essence, an elite—the work of ASPIRA was sometimes controversial. Some activists suspected such an elite would inevitably become disconnected from its communities instead of spurring broad social change and political transformation. Participants pushed back against these criticisms by arguing that the group mainly assisted poor and working-class Puerto Rican youth and fostered leadership in various fields. Historian Sonia Lee argues that over time, members of ASPIRA "experienced a political radicalization" and that the "program facilitated the political development of a Puerto Rican coalition of youth that was invested in transforming public education as well as addressing other spaces in the community where Puerto Ricans faced discrimination and marginalization."[54] The lasting impact of ASPIRA was the cohorts of young people from poor families who later went into public service careers, including many who became interested in community organizing and social work.

While ASPIRA engendered political action and radicalization, the group's respectability politics may have also been restrictive to its members. Like other civil rights organizations of the period, ASPIRA intentionally presented a normative image to the public.[55] While students noted that they felt pride in presenting themselves as group members, there were also moments when this respectability could be stifling. This emphasis on respectability impacted Pantoja herself, shaping her work and political legacy. She never ran for public office because she feared having her personal life and particularly her sexuality scrutinized. When Pantoja wrote a memoir later in her life, she struggled with how to write about her sexuality and romantic relationships with women, seeking at first to leave out these personal experiences and then later choosing to include them in her own way.[56] Literary scholar Lourdes Torres has highlighted how Pantoja's memoir shows how she focused on "passing" as heterosexual—even though, if one reads between the lines, her life as a lesbian woman and her relationships with women are central to her memoir.[57] However, those who knew her well and worked with her in organizations like ASPIRA would later note that she was not "in the closet" and that colleagues generally knew about her sexuality and her partners.[58] Nevertheless, silences and erasures about sexuality were part of the politics of respectability in the civil rights movement, and they constrained how Pantoja presented herself and later wrote about her life.

In the years that followed, the forms of community organizing work that Pantoja and her cohort of social worker activists created would have long-lasting impacts on the community. When Pantoja departed ASPIRA, she left in charge Yolanda Sánchez, an Afro-Puerto Rican social worker activist whose legacy as a community organizer mirrored that of Pantoja. The work of these women would continue to focus on community organizing within the field of social work as well as an emphasis on building Puerto Rican–led political and social organizations. In the years to come, there would also be increased participation of a new generation of Puerto Rican social workers, some of whom had been mentored by women like Pantoja and Sánchez, in other radical social movements that erupted in the later 1960s. The history of social worker participation in these projects reveals the intergenerational connections forged between social worker activists who participated in struggles for civil rights and social justice.

Social Work and Social Movements in the 1960s and 1970s

In 1970, Afro-Puerto Rican activist Esperanza Martell joined the group El Comité, which emerged from tenants' organizing and housing rights activism in New York City (see figure 6.3). Martell later noted that she was inspired to become a community organizer by the example set by her mother and by growing up amid a "strong community of women."[59] She recounted how her mother, who "took care of children and was the neighborhood nurse," was also a "hotel maid for twenty-five years" as well as "an active union member." She also said that her childhood role as an intermediary between people in her community and the state influenced her life. As a child, she "was the community translator at the welfare center, schools, and hospitals."[60] These experiences would shape her approach to community organizing and engagement with feminist organizing and participation in forming the Latin Women's Collective, a foundational Latina feminist organization in the 1970s.[61] Later in life, this work also drew her to social work, and as a social worker and teacher, she continued her work with people in need. Martell's story shows how a new generation of youth activists in the 1970s took up the mantel of community organizing, sought social transformation through creating more revolutionary social movements, and continued to transform the field of social work in the years to come. While this generation of activists would embrace a more radical agenda than Pantoja—primarily through their advocacy for a Puerto Rican nationalist agenda—their work often built on that of the Puerto Rican social workers who came before them.

Martell was one of many Puerto Rican youth activists in New York who became involved in the vibrant world of leftist political organizations in New York in the late 1960s and 1970s.[62] Among other groups, this included the establishment of El Comité and the creation of the New York branch of the Young Lords Party, which was composed of young people organizing for the rights of their community.[63] These groups were mainly composed of youth of color, including Puerto Rican, Dominican, Latinx, and African American youth, some of whom had already gained experience as political organizers in the growing student movements of the 1960s. Their activism was marked by their dedication to providing community-led social services in their communities and by the strong presence of women within their

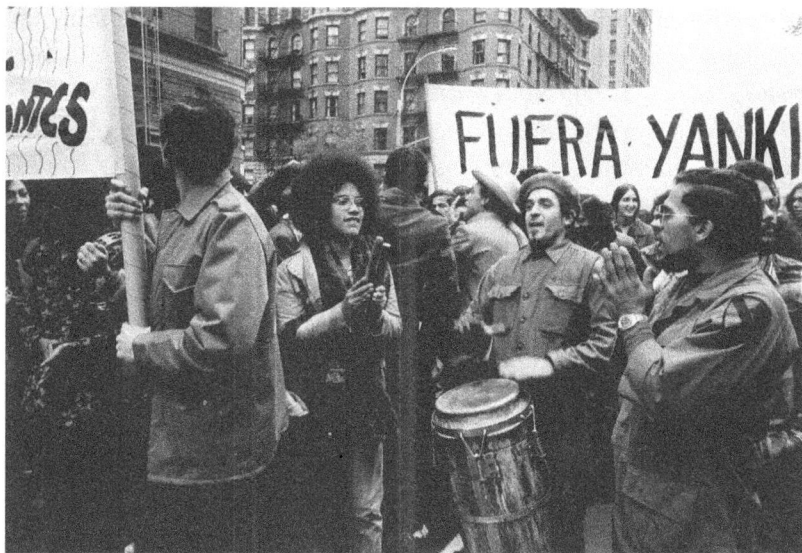

FIGURE 6.3. Esperanza Martell (*center*) at a protest gathering. Courtesy of Máximo Rafael Colón. © Máximo Rafael Colón.

leadership. Indeed, over time these organizations also became more and more explicitly feminist in their outlook.

While the activists and organizers involved in some of these movements saw themselves as offering a revolutionary, rather than reformist, path forward for the Puerto Rican community, some—including Martell—would be social workers who would take the field in new directions. Thinking about the longer trajectory and context of the work of this generation can challenge narratives about the decline or end of these movements, instead emphasizing the long-lasting significance of the community-oriented work they did in the 1970s and the decades that followed.

As the youth organizers of this generation began to come together, they discovered that many needs in the community were not being fulfilled, including essential social and health services. Historian Johanna Fernández has highlighted how youth organizing during the period, particularly within the Young Lords, was marked by its attention to providing social services.[64] Such activism was in part rooted in the student activism developed by youth of color, in New York City and around the country, which had gained strength in higher education institutions. Also, the civil rights movement and groups like ASPIRA paved the way for these political mobilization and protest forms.

In 1969, when students occupied City College of New York to demand the admission of more students of color and a curriculum that addressed their history, there were numerous ASPIRA members in their ranks. Pantoja herself would later reflect with pride on the activism of former protégés whose forthright radicalism, in some sense, descended from her reformist style.[65]

This organizing also moved toward more radical Puerto Rican youth activism in the 1970s. This activism was inspired by organizing around the country and the world, including that of the African American, Latinx, Native American, and Asian American youth who confronted racial injustice, colonialism, and white supremacy in the United States.[66] Puerto Rican youth also drew inspiration from the movement for Puerto Rican independence, as nationalist groups from the archipelago continued to organize branches in the United States.[67]

Creating Puerto Rican-led social movements in New York went hand in hand with the broader community organizing projects. This was the case of El Comité, which formed in 1970 and was specifically linked to tenant organizing on the West Side of New York in response to "urban renewal" projects displacing poor Puerto Rican communities.[68] This work began with tenants squatting to protest the demolition of housing in the area. Soon after, the group's work expanded to encompass a wide variety of programs addressing the conditions of poor and working-class people, including health care and social services.[69] While El Comité imagined a broadly transformed society that would meet such needs, they were also notably invested in having community control over the institutions and programs that served the community. Over time, the work of the group became more integrally involved in seeking independence for Puerto Rico—a shift encoded in a change of name from El Comité to El Comité–Movimiento de Izquierda Nacional Puertorriqueña (Puerto Rican National Left Movement).

Perhaps the most well-known Puerto Rican–affiliated youth group of the period, the Young Lords had similar origins in community organizing efforts.[70] The group was first formed in Chicago. Like the Black Panthers who inspired it, the Young Lords sought to "protect and serve" their community.[71] In 1969, a newly created New York City–based branch had taken as its first major project a "garbage offensive": a concerted effort to address widespread sanitation problems in their neighborhoods. These problems were due to the municipal government's dereliction in garbage collection and related duties in poor communities of color. The Young Lords were also critical of social service agencies, and member Juan González noted that "while those agencies sought assistance from the government for Puerto Ricans, the

Young Lords *demanded* that assistance as a right."[72] Shortly after the garbage offensive, the group occupied a local church and began administering a social services program, including free breakfast programs for children and tuberculosis testing. The Young Lords understood that such social programs were sorely needed in neighborhoods with few health services.[73]

As activism among Puerto Rican youth expanded within groups like El Comité and the Young Lords, tensions emerged over allowing participants who were already involved in social service or government work to participate. In the case of El Comité, the role of professionals became a cause for concern early in the organization's formation. Some leaders feared that a more reformist community organizing approach would co-opt the movement. They sought to distinguish themselves from previous organizations in the Puerto Rican community—such as the Puerto Rican Forum, which was mainly organized by social workers.[74] Still, while they were critical of this work, many of El Comité's leaders had connections to the work of earlier social service agencies. Esperanza Martell later wrote that she saw herself "as a real product of the University Settlement House Movement" because these groups "developed leadership skills in poor working-class Puerto Rican and African American youth."[75] Carmen Vivian Rivera was an ASPIRA member who later became a member of the Young Lords and eventually pursued a career in electoral politics and advocated for health care rights.[76] Their frustration with the limitations of the work done by earlier social worker activists led them to seek alternative forms of organizing. For Martell, this meant a long career where she worked "with every age group from nursery school to seniors, advocating and organizing as a social worker."[77] This work would help contribute to the transformation of the meaning of social service reform and social work in the Puerto Rican community over the years to come.

During this period, Puerto Rican professionals and working-class youth and students who became leaders in social movements sometimes came together as they organized around health care access and rights. One example of this collaboration can been seen in protests around Lincoln Hospital in the Bronx after 1969. The Young Lords became deeply involved in drawing attention to the conditions faced by patients and workers in Lincoln Hospital. Their activism was connected to other workers and activists who protested the conditions in which they worked and who demanded accountability for how poor people were treated in these facilities. They shed light on how the care provided in the worn-down and decaying hospital was not adequate and that many patients faced various forms of discrimination.

The organizing that happened at Lincoln Hospital was led by a broad co-alition of Puerto Rican and African American organizers and hospital employees who formed the Lincoln Collective and a group called the Health Revolutionary Unity Movement (HRUM).[78] The group demanded "total self-determination of all health services" and well-paying, safe jobs for community members who found employment in the hospital.

At the time, many women of color, including Puerto Rican women, were working in Lincoln Hospital in low-paying occupations, especially as nurses and hospital aides. The hospital activism was connected to broader organizing around the labor rights of care workers during the period. The boundaries and lines between professionals and nonprofessionals within this movement were changing as large numbers of poor women, especially women of color, entered the caring professions as home care aids. Historians Eileen Boris and Jennifer Klein have shown how recruitment into this labor force was seen as providing work for potential dependents on welfare and the state.[79] The continued feminization and racialization of these caring fields also led to low wages for health care workers. These women organized to protest their work conditions, and their organizing became connected to that of the Puerto Rican–led social movements of the period.

The organizing at Lincoln Hospital also became essential to a broadening movement for reproductive justice. Puerto Rican doctor Helen Rodríguez Trías and other activists created the Committee to End Sterilization Abuse (CESA). This organization shed light on the large numbers of Puerto Rican women who were sterilized in the hospital.[80] The Young Lords also took up this cause and advocated for reproductive justice in part because of their participation in the organizing at Lincoln Hospital. Historian Jennifer Nelson has shown how the Young Lords Party argued that women should have control over their bodies and also that "institutions that provide health care to Puerto Rican women needed to be collectively controlled by Puerto Rican communities to ensure that they were safe from medical abuses."[81] Community control of institutions was one of the main demands of organizers as a part of their broader struggle for health care access. Moreover, reproductive rights organizing in the Young Lords also demonstrated the growing feminist politics that emerged in these social movements.

In the 1970s, women within El Comité and the Young Lords also came together to make feminist discourse an important intellectual touchstone for their movements. They held consciousness-raising sessions where they talked critically about gender roles, patriarchy, and their experiences as women within these emerging movements. According to member Sandra Trujillo, some of these women formed the Latin Women's Collective (LWC), which "focused on the issues facing working-class Latina women in the areas of education, day care, health, and labor."[82] Within the Young Lords, women also began organizing around their experiences, and they created a Women's Union in 1971 to address the needs of working-class women. The group published the newspaper *La Luchadora*. According to former member and historian Iris Morales, this publication "featured stories about women workers in factories and hospitals, and in other people's homes as domestics, as well as women who were homemakers or who received public assistance."[83] They were particularly interested in discussing gender discrimination, workplace inequality, and the need for employee-provided day care services. The end result of this organizing was significant transformations within the Young Lords, including rewriting the organization's manifesto to include feminist goals.[84] This feminist work also meant a continued focus on community organizing efforts, particularly on thinking about women's experiences.

The feminist organizing within these social movements also led to more interest among activists in learning about the history of Puerto Rican women, particularly nationalist women.[85] This interest only intensified after the Young Lords began to send delegations to Puerto Rico to meet with leading figures in the Puerto Rican independence movement. The newspaper of the Young Lords published an interview with Blanca Canales on September 25, 1970, conducted by members Juan González and Juan "Fi" Ortíz.[86] In this interview, they noted that "Doña Blanca was a social worker then, which put her in touch with many of the social problems of the island, problems which were then, as well as they are now, symptoms of yanqui colonialism in Puerto Rico." In Puerto Rico, the young organizers encountered the radical history of women social worker activists who were leaders in the independence movement. When the interviewers asked Canales, "What is the role of the woman in the revolution," she replied, "The role of woman is as important as of the man. The revolutionary woman must act accordingly with the demands of the revolution, be it to arm herself, educate her people or whatever necessary."

Through the recovery knowledge about the history of Puerto Rican women who supported the independence movement, a new generation learned of the radical history of social work in Puerto Rico. Some young activists encountered social workers from Puerto Rico who had come to the United States because of connections and affiliations with political organizations and US universities.[87] For example, the social worker and independence organizer Carmen Rivera de Alvarado traveled between the archipelago and the United States throughout her career. She spent significant time in New York as one of the founders of the Movimiento Pro-Independencia in Puerto Rico and as a leader of the Partido Socialista Puertorriqueño (Puerto Rican Socialist Party).[88] Rivera de Alvarado also spent 1972 as a distinguished visiting professor at the School of Social Work at Hunter College and was later honored by the Department of Puerto Rican Studies at Lehman College.[89] She learned and taught alongside younger social worker organizers and activists in this capacity. This work would later result in her speaking and writing more extensively about how social workers could advocate for the decolonization of Puerto Rico.[90] In this way, an earlier generation of social workers from Puerto Rico became involved in reconceiving the history of the development of social work in Puerto Rico as a foundation for the ongoing struggle for decolonization in Puerto Rico.

In the late 1970s and early 1980s, social movements like El Comité and the Young Lords ended. However, the decline in these organizations did not stop the types of community organizing work they had fostered. Their declines resulted from various factors, including the fact that groups had spread themselves too thin as they attempted to create branches in Puerto Rico. However, the most devastating factor was the surveillance, infiltration, and counterintelligence tactics inflicted on the groups by the FBI and New York City police.[91] Facing these challenges, many activists left the organizations but continued to work toward social transformation in their communities. Some former members remained working as community organizers while others entered the fields of labor organizing, public health, social work, and education. Minerva Solla would become a labor organizer, recalling that the "Young Lords Party inspired [her] in fighting for social justice in the health care system."[92] Likewise, Gloria M. Rodríguez continued organizing feminist women's groups, having discovered that her "purpose was the higher cause—about service."[93] These are just some examples of how members of these groups continued their work in the community. When one listens for these echoes of the Young Lords and El Comité as they resounded into the future through the ongoing endeavors of former members, it becomes difficult to judge these movements as having failed.

The legacy of 1970s organizing for social services was also kept alive by El Comité member Esperanza Martell, who would continue to serve as a social worker and teach community organizing.[94] Martell's work in social work shows how radical women social workers of a new generation envisioned new possibilities within the profession. While this vision differed from social workers who came before them, it was nevertheless connected to previous generations' work. This work built on that of Puerto Rican so-cial workers in the settlement house movement in the 1950s, including civil rights leaders like Pantoja, and on the more radical work of independence leaders like Blanca Canales and Carmen Rivera de Alvarado. Through these changes, social work remained a space where women took leadership in ad-vocating for their communities and demanding societal transformations. The activists and organizers of the 1970s would continue agitating around these is-sues long after the movements they participated in had disbanded. They also came to have a sense of their place in history, becoming unofficial archivists who worked to preserve the memory of the organizations they helped build and to ensure the legacy of women across social work, political organizing, and radical activism.

The Intellectual Legacy of Puerto Rican Social Workers

Reflecting on her career as a community organizer, Antonia Pantoja high-lighted that she was motivated to continue this work because of a desire for social justice. She looked forward to the "possible achievement of a just society where we can all live with our differences—racial, cultural, age, sexual preference, and religion—without having to suffer punishment and where we can develop to our fullest potentials."[95] She also emphasized that having women in leadership was a prerequisite for enacting progressive so-cial change. Puerto Rican women leaders had surrounded Pantoja as she organized and believed that while "you cannot generalize about differences between males and females," she had herself witnessed how women leaders tended to eschew "power simply for personal gains" and instead were "more concerned with using power to acquire resources to improve the life of our community."[96] The history of community organizing work within these in-stitutions, much of which was done by social workers, was something she sought to highlight and preserve for a younger generation. Through her educational and scholarly work starting in the 1970s, she sought to record the history of these women. She was not the only member of her cohort of social workers who also became involved in producing knowledge about community organizing and Puerto Rican history within and outside of aca-demia. These social workers' educational and intellectual contributions kept their vision of social work alive for the next generation.

In the 1970s, Pantoja continued her work as an educator by working in various higher education institutions and teaching community organizing. First, she became a professor at Columbia University's School of Social

Work, teaching courses on community organizing. Years before, some of the faculty still teaching had discouraged her from taking these sorts of classes when she returned to the school as a professor.[97] In 1972, Pantoja received her PhD from the Union Graduate School and immediately helped create Universidad Boricua, later called Boricua College. This institution is still in operation and continues to focus on community organizing and student-led curriculum design. After dealing with health challenges, she moved to California in 1978, where she worked at the School of Social Work at San Diego State University and created the Graduate School for Community Development. In San Diego, she worked alongside her long-time partner, Wilhelmina Perry, an African American activist and fellow social worker.[98] Herself a social worker and activist, Perry participated in the civil rights movement, and the two of them would go on to organize, write, and teach together for the rest of Pantoja's life. The social workers and community activists Pantoja and Perry mentored would continue to take social work, community organizing, and the arts in new directions.

Antonia Pantoja's scholarly work from the 1980s onward focused on community organizing within schools of social work. Students in social work programs were increasingly interested in learning how to develop projects in concert with local communities, not merely "for" them. Pantoja also drew on her expertise in community organizing to write about inter-cultural relationships and social inequality. At Columbia, she participated in the Cultural Pluralism Committee, which produced a study on undergradu-ate education. In this study, she highlighted that in the United States, "[the] model for successful assimilation is racially white, English speaking and Anglo-Saxon in cultural behavior" and that those who were different were punished.[99] She then examined the notion of "cultural pluralism," where "individuals and groups and communities can function in one, two, or more language and cultural styles; where individuals and groups can abide by and function successfully adhering to different customs and religions adhering to less crippling class and sexual stereotypes than those accepted today, and where no one race, culture, sex or class is preferred over another."[100]

In the study on so-called cultural pluralism, however, Pantoja critiqued how the term was used in public education discourse, arguing that these goals could never be achieved without a more precise analysis of social inequality. She protested, "Cultural pluralism does not exist," and instead, "[What] does exist is institutional racism and inequality operating against non-whites, women, homosexuals, and those that dare to be different." The study argued that the only way to achieve the goal of putative cultural pluralism was through "cultural socio-economic pluralism" that itself would only be possible through the "radical commitment to pursue social and economic policies which would result in an equal distribution of the life-enhancing and life-sustaining resources to all ... citizens."[101] For Pantoja, education was an essential part of social transformation. Still, the need for a transformative redistribution of economic resources became an increasingly important focus of her intellectual and political work.

The scholarship produced by Puerto Rican social workers in the United States during the 1970s was also in dialogue with the work of Puerto Rican social workers on the archipelago who supported the independence movement. During this period, these social workers traveled to New York City to participate in nationalist activism.[102] They also continued to advocate both for transformations in colonial US social policy toward Puerto Rico as well as for the end of the US colonization in Puerto Rico. Among these social workers was Carmen Rivera de Alvarado. In the 1970s, Rivera de Alvarado held residencies at US schools of social work while also speaking and writing about the history of Puerto Rican social workers and welfare politics. She advocated the idea that social work and social workers could play an essential part in the work of decolonizing Puerto Rico. While she recognized traditional modes of social work as conservative, she nonetheless saw social work as a "vocation of freedom,"[103] a way of helping people become self-sufficient and providing them with basic services to better control their destinies. Through her work as a scholar and educator in Puerto Rico and the United States, Rivera de Alvarado helped institutionalize knowledge about the radical potential within the field of social work. In Puerto Rico, the long connection between social work, independence activism, and visions of decolonization would continue to be transmitted through a new generation of social workers who were also nationalist intellectuals.[104]

In 1984, Pantoja's journey also brought her back to Puerto Rico; she and Perry decided to retire there. However, upon her arrival on the archipelago, she became immediately involved in new community organizing projects, and her plans to retire were left behind. She first began teaching at the School of Social Work at the University of Puerto Rico, Río Piedras. Here, she worked alongside social workers from the archipelago and fostered these connections, yet she soon felt frustrated by the hierarchical leadership style at the school. When she proposed new courses, she found that her ideas were stifled, and she decided instead to seek out organizing opportunities outside the school. Soon after, she became involved in creating an economic development project in the towns of Cubuy and Lomas, returning to

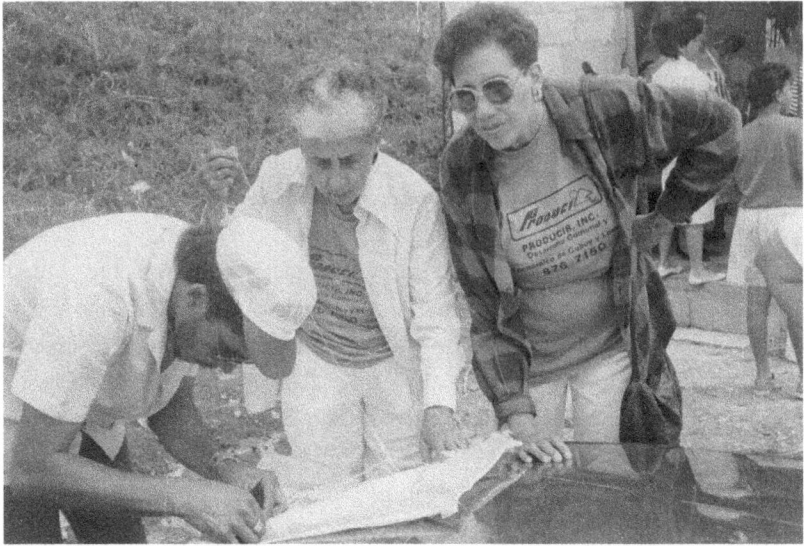

FIGURE 6.4. Antonia Pantoja (*center*) and Wilhelmina Perry (*right*) in Puerto Rico wearing Producir shirts. Courtesy of the Antonia Pantoja Papers, Archives of the Puerto Rican Diaspora, Center for Puerto Rican Studies, Hunter College, City University of New York.

the mountains where she had taught so many years before. The project was developed in collaboration with Perry and named Producir (see figure 6.4). The main focus of the work was to address the question of economic justice in Puerto Rico by promoting the creation of locally owned community businesses.

Producir began with developing agricultural projects and farming initiatives owned by the community. Pantoja remembered that the "work was very important in realizing that to change a condition of poverty and dependency a community could begin a process of restoration of its basic function."[105] The products that were produced collaboratively by local farmers were sold in town, and an economic cooperative that was owned by all those who participated was created. Pantoja and Perry also documented their work in this organization through their scholarly work, writing that "social work professionals, on the front lines of community work, have to become knowledgeable about economic processes" and that "although we may not be able to do all the work that is needed, [social workers] remain a profession vital to the processes of development, and the challenge is before us."[106]

Social workers could serve as "community development workers" who helped develop projects in the community, but equally important was that they needed to let these organizations go, allowing them to be run entirely by community collectives. Pantoja and Perry left behind Producir when they returned to New York in 1998. In her memoir, Pantoja wrote that while the work she was doing in Puerto Rico was important, she had come to terms with the fact that she was a Nuyorican and that her true home was in New York.[107]

When she returned to New York, Pantoja reconnected with social workers she had worked with in projects like the Puerto Rican Forum and continued their work as community organizers and leaders in the field of social work. For example, Pantoja's colleague Josephine Nieves, whom she knew from the Puerto Rican Youth Conference and ASPIRA, had become an essential social work leader. Nieves began her career working for the New York Department of Welfare before becoming frustrated with casework and getting more involved in community organizing projects.[108] She had worked alongside Pantoja and others in forming Puerto Rican–run organizations and then working for the government. Nieves also became closely involved in creating Puerto Rican studies at the City University of New York (CUNY). The development of Puerto Rican studies had come out of the student organizing of the 1960s and 1970s, activism that demanded the admission of Puerto Rican students, hiring of Puerto Rican faculty, and teaching Puerto Rican history and culture. Nieves was uniquely poised as a professional social worker and government official to be hired to direct the newly designed Puerto Rican studies program at the university.[109] According to Nieves, "Puerto Rican Studies was an organizational form through which we challenged the university and created space to test and develop our own educational agenda."[110] For Nieves and others who forged Puerto Rican studies, the goal was to have cultural representation and "examine the critical connections linking our political, economic, social, and cultural realities within the broader socio-economic context of American society."[111] In other words, the aim of these programs was to transform knowledge through an investigation of the Puerto Rican experience.

Josephine Nieves would also carry on the community organizing of Puerto Rican social workers in new directions through her continued work as a leader in the field of social work. Nieves was elected the first Latina director of the National Association of Social Workers (NASW). Her tenure during the 1990s coincided with immense political challenges in the field as the social welfare provisions created under the Social Security Act were dismantled by "welfare reform." In her role as leader of the NASW, Nieves spoke out against the reform policies that devastated poor communities by chipping away at funding for welfare programs. She traveled around the country, decrying the reforms and highlighting how they were particularly devastating to communities of color.[112] Through this work, the legacy of Puerto Rican social work activism became a part of mainstream dialogues about social welfare policy and practice.

This history also reveals the linkages between community organizing and the development of educational initiatives focused on teaching Puerto Rican history and culture. These demands for what would become a full-fledged academic discipline originally came in part from small study groups within ASPIRA, from the critical consciousness-raising sessions in El Comité, and from students at the City University of New York whose intellectual lives had already been shaped by legacies of organizing. The intellectual legacy of Puerto Rican social workers continued as they wrote about their experiences in social movements, theorized about community organizing, and led Puerto Rican studies initiatives in higher education. Pantoja's work and vision of social work continue because she emphasized empowering youth, sharing knowledge, and connecting people through community organizing.

THE HISTORY OF PUERTO RICAN social worker activists in the 1960s and 1970s illuminates their intellectual and political contributions to the Puerto Rican community and their connections to broader social movements. Pantoja's life offers a unique window into this story, from her earliest years experiencing the social transformations underway in Puerto Rico under the New Deal, through her youthful years as a civil rights activist, to her later years pushing the boundaries of community organizing work in Puerto Rico and the United States. The stories of Pantoja and her fellow social workers also highlight the importance of "feminine leadership" in the fight for Puerto Rican rights in the United States and their instrumental role in establishing enduring institutions in the Puerto Rican community. Pantoja's story also illustrates how the field of social work transformed as it became more diverse, with growing numbers of working-class and Black Puerto Ricans joining the profession. While these social workers' activism built on nearly fifty years of Puerto Rican women's political organizing around social welfare, it also represented a new wave of activism for human rights.

During this period, the social work activism that emerged was deeply connected to broader struggles for civil rights and racial justice in the United States. Many of the most influential leaders in the profession were Afro-Puerto Rican women like Antonia Pantoja, Yolanda Sánchez, and

Esperanza Martell, who proudly claimed their identities as Black and Puerto Rican. These women fought against racism within the Puerto Rican community and against discrimination faced by Puerto Ricans of African descent more broadly in society. Their activism was closely linked to local and national social movements that aimed to critique structural racism in society. They joined coalitions and built relationships with other Black and African American activists and organizers. Pantoja's intellectual and romantic partnership with Wilhelmina Perry was one example of such a connection, demonstrating a vital connection between Black women of different backgrounds in the social work field. Together, Black women social work activists of this generation organized relentlessly to address how racism impacted health, social services, housing, and education in their communities.

The social work activism discussed in this chapter revolved around creating and promoting community-oriented social services. These social workers strongly believed their work should be accountable to the people they served. Their ideas were drawn from a long history of organizing social welfare programs in the United States and Puerto Rico. However, this period was also unique because growing numbers of social workers were from the communities they served and had firsthand experience of poverty. Within the organizations they created, they emphasized a praxis, a way of *doing* things that prioritized collaboration and dialogue. These dialogues were closely linked with social workers' feminist views and were sometimes associated with criticisms of gender roles and patriarchal social structures. The social work organizing that emerged was community oriented, committed to addressing racial injustice, and often feminist. As a result, social workers further developed and reworked the social work project as collaborative and envisioned new possibilities for the profession and their communities.

Epilogue
Envisioning Caring Futures

This book charts how debates over social welfare and the creation of so-cial welfare programs for Puerto Ricans on the archipelago and in the dias-pora became important locations of political organization. Its story begins shortly after the US colonization of Puerto Rico, and it ends in the 1970s with a discussion of Puerto Rican activism for social and economic jus-tice in the United States. During this final period, social workers like An-tonia Pantoja and Yolanda Sánchez politicized care as they developed new community-oriented approaches within social work. Their organizing drew on their experiences growing up in working-class communities, identifying as Afro-Puerto Rican, and witnessing their families and friends applying for social welfare benefits. These social workers believed that working-class communities should have control over the institutions that served them. They also linked their work to the civil rights movement and Puerto Rican, Latinx, feminist, and labor rights groups. Their work also specifically sought to help migrant communities by bringing together political action in the diaspora with that on the archipelago. These efforts show how the political worlds of Puerto Ricans on the archipelago and in the United States remained intertwined. The types of political action they forged remain potent models of community action as Puerto Ricans have continued to face increasingly difficult economic conditions, attacks on social provisions, and continued displacement and migration.

The stories told in this book center on the importance of Puerto Rican women's organizing around care work and social reproduction. In each chapter, I emphasize how debates over care labor, social welfare, and social policy became arenas of class struggle, where fights for women's rights and racial justice often occurred.[1] The history of Puerto Rican women's activ-ism that emerges from these moments of political mobilization is complex and includes moments of more reformist and regulatory forms of social welfare state–building in Puerto Rico, the fight to access social rights and

US citizenship as migrant citizens in the United States, and the rise of new forms of social welfare practice dedicated to the creation of community-controlled social institutions. The book also shows how working-class women who performed much of the reproductive labor in Puerto Rican society became the targets of social welfare policies and government programs that funneled women into paid household labor. I emphasize how welfare recipients and domestic workers sometimes fought back against how their care work was valued, by contesting the value of their labor in means-testing schemes, and by demanding that society value and fairly compensate women for their reproductive labor. Together, these histories of political mobilization around social reproduction underscore the robust and diverse legacy of Puerto Rican women's activism and mobilization over the twentieth century.

Contemporary political organizing in Puerto Rican communities has also continued to be shaped by struggles over social reproduction and care work as well as by the impact of displacement and migration to the United States. In the late twentieth and early twenty-first centuries, Puerto Rico underwent the largest wave of emigration to the United States in history, a movement of people that exceeded the earlier waves discussed in this book. These migrations highlight the continued relevance of thinking about writing histories of Puerto Rico that grapple with communities on the move. In this book, I have drawn on the methodologies developed by scholars of migration, immigration, and transnational communities. These approaches can help us understand current Puerto Rican migrations by shedding light on how US colonialism has conditioned these movements. They also can help us understand the impact of circular migration that has occurred continually over generations. These migrations have also shaped Puerto Rican communities and politics, as Puerto Ricans in the diaspora continue to be involved in and connected to the archipelago at the same time as they organize to combat ethnic and racial exclusion in the United States. When migrants arrive in the United States, they often become involved in these long, ongoing struggles. Within this context, political organization that links Puerto Ricans on the archipelago and in the United States is more important than ever.

After the 1970s, the arena of social welfare politics became even more politically charged. As attacks on social welfare resulted in a major dismantling of the policies created under the New Deal, Puerto Rican activists contested the push toward austerity and changes in social policy. Still, cuts accelerated under President Ronald Reagan, who advocated for means-testing and work requirements for welfare recipients. The arguments made to justify these policy changes relied on public discourse that demonized women on welfare, especially women of color, who were portrayed by the media and policymakers as undeserving of assistance. Puerto Rican women on the archipelago and in the United States, alongside African American women and other women of color, were described as "welfare queens." Over time, Puerto Rican women became increasingly associated with persistent racist stereotypes. In response, Puerto Ricans organized in different ways, including by joining other poor people in the United States in coalitions that demanded "welfare rights."[2] During this period, nationwide struggles around access to welfare benefits contested restrictions on welfare benefits and agitated for the rights of poor women and their families to economic justice and human rights.

At the same time, Puerto Ricans on the archipelago were also profoundly impacted by economic policies that cut social provisions from the 1960s through the 1990s. Facing the ravages of an ever more extractive colonial economy, they continued contesting the partial forms of federal social benefits extended to the US territories. Debates over the extension of federal food stamp programs became one of these sites of struggle. The initial Food Stamp Act of 1964 excluded Puerto Rico, but in the 1970s, parts of the program were gradually extended, and by 1977, over 56 percent of the population received benefits. In 1982, a separate block grant program, the Nutrition Assistance for Puerto Rico (NAP), was created to administer these benefits, but the unequal and provisional access Puerto Ricans were granted to these funds continued to result in second-class social welfare benefits for the archipelago.[3] The devastating impact of this inequality and austerity politics would continue in the 1990s with the passage of sweeping welfare reform under President Bill Clinton. The Personal Responsibility and Work Opportunity Reconciliation Act of 1996 (PRWORA) resulted in an "end to welfare as we know it" in the United States and Puerto Rico by cutting welfare benefits for low-income families.[4] Its immediate impact on Puerto Rican communities in the United States and the archipelago was catastrophic, as many families were denied assistance.[5] In the years that followed, many women, among them numerous heads of household, remained in poverty without a means to support themselves or their families.

At the start of the twenty-first century, Puerto Rico fell into an increasingly dire economic crisis resulting from previous colonial economic policies. This resulted from the end of corporate tax havens, and the 2008 economic recession deeply impacted the Puerto Rican economy. The migration that resulted was even larger than the mass migration of Puerto Ricans between the 1940s and 1960s, chronicled in this book. Between 2006 and 2016, over half a million Puerto Ricans—more than 14 percent of the archipelago's population—moved to the United States.[6] In response to the growing recession, the Puerto Rican government borrowed large amounts of money, and its debt ballooned quickly to over $74 billion, causing it to default on its payment. As a result, in 2016, the US government passed the Puerto Rico Oversight, Management, and Economic Stability Act (PROMESA). This law created a fiscal oversight board in Puerto Rico composed of unelected members charged with implementing austerity measures and cutting public services.[7] Puerto Ricans on the archipelago and in the diaspora staged numerous protests after the act's passage. The protesters included teachers, nurses, social workers, and other professionals in care work occupations who sought to highlight the devastation to education, health care, and social services resulting from these policies. Despite their efforts, the cuts to services continued and contributed to a deepening social and economic crisis.

It was only one year after the implementation of PROMESA that Hurricane Maria hit Puerto Rico in September 2017. After the deadly hurricane, the archipelago was devastated by major structural damage, and afterward, nearly the entire population was left without power and half without access to tap water. Recovery efforts were stalled by a slow response by the US government, and Puerto Rico's colonial status limited the terms of federal assistance.[8] The administration of relief programs was restricted by the colonial differences in funding that had already long plagued other federal assistance programs. This was particularly devastating when relief claims under the Federal Emergency Management Agency (FEMA) were not honored and left local communities unable to rebuild. After Hurricane Maria, there was a push in both Puerto Rico and the United States to argue that "as United States citizens," Puerto Ricans deserved a better response to the crisis on the part of the US government. However, popular media coverage after the hurricane also often failed to cover the ways that US colonialism had legally shaped differential second-class variants of social welfare programs in Puerto Rico with devastating consequences.

In the summer of 2019, the political organizing after Hurricane Maria culminated in massive island-wide protests in Puerto Rico. These protests demanded the resignation of the governor, Ricardo Rosello, and became known by their hashtag, #RickyRenuncia. Fueling these protests were journalists' revelations of corruption as well as the damning publication of computer messages sent between government officials.[9] During the protests, half a million Puerto Ricans marched in the capital and around the archipelago, demanding accountability for the failure of the state to respond to the needs of the people. The marchers and protesters were comprised of a wide range of individuals belonging to various political parties. The protestors challenged the undemocratic governance in Puerto Rico that was created under PROMESA, questioned the legitimacy of the debt, and called for an end to austerity policies.[10] Moreover, they sought accountability for the failure of federal assistance programs to help most Puerto Ricans. In response to these events, the governor resigned, but a full response to the demands of protestors has not yet manifested.

One of the other significant results of the hurricane was a dramatic outmigration to the United States, compounding the migration already underway during the preceding decades. During this period, growing numbers of Puerto Ricans left for the United States, many of them following the pathways that earlier generations of Puerto Rican migrants had created.[11] Scholars have highlighted how the exact number of migrants has been widely underreported, though they estimate that between 2017 and 2019, half a million people left Puerto Rico.[12] That would mean that between 2006 and 2019, the archipelago may have lost nearly 28 percent of its population. This migration has also resulted in the growth of the Puerto Rican community in Florida, which in recent years has received more Puerto Rican migrants than any other state.[13] As this migration occurred, Puerto Rican communities in the United States were very involved in organizing services for recent arrivals. Meanwhile, Puerto Ricans in the United States formed groups that traveled to the archipelago to assist. Their work illustrated the long-interconnected forms of activism that continue between the archipelago and the diaspora.

After Hurricane Maria, there was also a widespread flourishing of community organizing and feminist activism in Puerto Rican communities. This included the creation of grassroots organizations that sought to provide services to local communities in the absence of adequate state support. Some of this community-oriented work became known as the movement for *auto-gestión*—where grassroots organizers provided food and necessities to those in need.[14] This organizing included the creation of Centros de Apoyo Mutuo (Mutual Support Centers).[15] These projects were linked to the creation of local agricultural cooperatives that have advocated Puerto Rican self-sufficiency, and they were connected to a vibrant environmental movement—which has long existed on the archipelago.[16] Women organizers led many local community organizing projects, including those of Taller Salud, a feminist group that provided health care services and organized for gender and racial justice in Loíza, Puerto Rico.[17] Such local efforts coincided with a broader resurgence in feminist organizing on the archipelago, led by groups like La Colectiva Feminista en Construcción, which organized demonstrations and community-oriented projects.[18] Together, the actions of protestors, community activists, and feminists has provided growing energy to demands for political, social, and economic change in Puerto Rico.

These stories show how the twenty-first century has ushered in a new wave of political mobilization and organization led by Puerto Rican women activists. For organizers of social movements, the politics of care work has remained central to their mobilization. For example, in an article by journalist Sandra Guzmán, from the summer of 2019, "Meet the Women Leading Puerto Rico's Feminist Revolution," the author interviewed Zaida Robles, a nurse and activist who worked as a farmer while continuing her participation in the Puerto Rican environmental movement.[19] Robles said that, after Hurricane Maria, "women took charge and did what we have always done: take care of our families and take care of what needs to be done." She emphasized care work as central to Puerto Rican activism, and her vision of that care work was one that included many forms of political action. She went on to say, "We're being displaced and crushed. But women are putting our pants on and fighting back." Her words sound like an echo of the call to action made by many of the Puerto Rican women activists in this book. The struggle continues, with Puerto Rican women at the helm.

In the years that followed the organizing covered in this book, Puerto Rican women social worker activists have continued to protest US colonialism and the specific ways that it has limited social, economic, and political rights. On June 18, 2018, a Puerto Rican social worker named Vega Otero spoke out at a United Nations General Assembly meeting about the political status of Puerto Rico. According to the summary of her testimony, Otero noted that "the catastrophic financial and social situation of Puerto Rico could not be attributed to natural disasters."[20] She argued that the devastating Hurricane Maria in 2017 had only compounded poverty on the archipelago. According to Otero, "The island's financial crisis and burgeoning debt, and the subsequent imposition of austerity measures, had had a negative effect on basic rights such as health care, food, education, housing and social security." Furthermore, she said this resulted from "120 years of colonial rule." Her demands joined a chorus of other voices from Puerto Rico and Latin America in the hearing that called for the immediate decolonization of Puerto Rico. Otero's indictments of the unelected fiscal control board in Puerto Rico, PROMESA, were also echoed by her professional organization, the Colegio de Profesionales de Trabajo Social de Puerto Rico. The Colegio denounced the fiscal control board and issued a statement that the board represented a continuation of US colonialism on the archipelago.[21] These statements show how social workers continued to spearhead activism and advocacy around Puerto Rican rights in the wake of Hurricane Maria. The critiques of Otero and her colleagues represent just two moments of advocacy in a growing wave of political organizing around care, social welfare, and citizenship rights that has swept the archipelago and the diaspora during the early twenty-first century.

This book provides historical context for understanding Puerto Rican women's political organizing. It shows how social workers and clients of social welfare programs navigated the political and economic changes wrought by US colonialism throughout the early to mid-twentieth century. It simultaneously tells a history of care work and demands for collective care that were embodied in Puerto Rican women's lives across generations. After 2018, Puerto Rican activists like Otero have continued to organize to confront the persistence of US colonialism on the archipelago as well as to seek better rights and conditions for Puerto Ricans on the archipelago and in the diaspora. Responding to political disasters, this organizing has continued to center on the politics of care work and the importance of social reproduction in society as well as on broader struggles for collective care that seek the well-being of all Puerto Rican people. In these movements, both Puerto Rican women social workers and working-class care workers have continued to take up leadership roles in social movements demanding dignity and equity for their communities. Both groups follow in the footsteps of earlier generations of activists who found debates and discourses over social welfare to be an important place to agitate for the rights of Puerto Rican citizens.

Notes

INTRODUCTION

1. Paris-Chitanvis, "Yolanda Sánchez," 98.

2. Paris-Chitanvis, "Yolanda Sánchez," 93.

3. For more on the history of social work and community organizing during this period, see Pantoja, *Memoir of a Visionary*.

4. On the life and work of Yolanda Sánchez, see Alberto Maldonado, *Portraits of the Puerto Rican Experience*, 77–78. Also see the interview with Sánchez in Morales, *Puerto Rican Poverty and Migration*, 174–79; Bell, *East Harlem Remembered*; "CUSSW Mourns the Death of Alumna Yolanda Sánchez, Powerhouse in El Barrio," Columbia University, School of Social Work, accessed October 15, 2024, https://www.columbia .edu/cu/ssw/news/2012-june/cussw-loss-mourned.html; "PRdream Mourns the Passing of Yolanda Sánchez, 1932–2012," PRdream, accessed October 15, 2024, http://www. prdream.com/wordpress/topics/2012/06/3604/; "In Memoriam: Yolanda Sánchez, MS Social Work," National Association of Social Workers, New York City Chapter, September/October 2012, https://www.naswnyc.org/general/custom.asp?page=363.

5. Trips like this one meant to connect Puerto Ricans in the United States with the archipelago. Some of these trips were also sponsored by the Puerto Rican government. For more, see Pantoja, *Memoirs of a Visionary*.

6. For more on Yolanda Sánchez and tenants' rights activism, see Gold, *When Tenants Claimed the City*.

7. "Yolanda Sánchez, 1932–2012," Latino Education: National Latino Education Research and Policy Project, Northeast Region, accessed October 15, 2024, https:// opencuny.org/nlerap4ne/2012/06/yolanda-sanchez-1932-2012/.

8. Morales, *Puerto Rican Poverty and Migration*, 174–79. For more on Puerto Rican feminist organizing during this period, see Muzio, *Radical Imagination*; Carroll, *Mobilizing New York*; Morales, *Through the Eyes of Rebel Women*.

9. Paris-Chitanvis, "Yolanda Sánchez," 96.

10. For more on the history of social work in Puerto Rico, see Burgos Ortiz, *Pioneras de la profesión de trabajo social en Puerto Rico*. On the history of social workers in carceral fields, see Ortíz Díaz, *Raising the Living Dead*.

11. On the history of Puerto Rican citizenship, see Thomas, *Puerto Rican Citizen*; Sánchez Korrol, *From Colonia to Community*; Erman, *Almost Citizens*; McGreevey,

Borderline Citizens; Cabán, *Constructing a Colonial People*; Burnett and Marshall, *Foreign in a Domestic Sense*.

12. For more on the Puerto Rican economy and poverty levels, see Collins, Bosworth, and Soto-Class, *The Economy of Puerto Rico*.

13. Studies on the history of social welfare in the United States include Gordon, *Pitied but Not Entitled*; Abramovitz, *Regulating the Lives of Women*; Ward, *The White Welfare State*; Fox, *Three Worlds of Relief*. Studies of the history of social welfare in Latin America include Guy, *Women Build the Welfare State*; Sanders, *Gender and Welfare in Mexico*; Blum, *Domestic Economies*.

14. One notable exception is sociologist Marietta Morrissey, who has written about the history of the extension of social welfare policy to Puerto Rico. See Morrissey, "The Making of a Colonial Welfare State." The Puerto Rican government also commissioned a study of the differential payments made to Puerto Ricans under these programs. See Cabranes, *A Study of Federal Public Assistance Payments to Puerto Rico*.

15. For example, Puerto Rico and Puerto Ricans have not often been included in major studies on social welfare and social work in the United States, like Katz, *In the Shadow of the Poorhouse*; Gordon, *Pitied but not Entitled*; Walkowitz, *Working with Class*.

16. In the context of Latin America, studies of gender and the state have emphasized the importance of thinking about the connections between labor, citizenship, and social policy. See, for example, Dore and Molyneux, *Hidden Histories of Gender and the State in Latin America*; French and James, *The Gendered Worlds of Latin American Women Workers*; Macpherson, *From Colony to Nation*; Putnam, *The Company They Kept*; Tinsman, *Partners in Conflict*; Olcott, *Revolutionary Women in Postrevolutionary Mexico*; Rosemblatt, *Gendered Compromises*; Sanders, *Gender and Welfare in Mexico*; Putnam, "Citizenship from the Margins."

17. In recent years historians have examined how social welfare and struggles over social citizenship have shaped the experiences of colonized and migrant people within the context of European empires and colonialism. Many of these studies have been transnational and examined how imperialism and social welfare policies have impacted immigrants and migrants. See, for example, Bailkin, *The Afterlife of Empire*; Nasiali, *Native to the Republic*; Midgley and Piachaud, *Colonialism and Welfare*.

18. For more on the colonial history of social welfare, social work, and social policy in Puerto Rico, see Guardiola Ortiz, *El trabajo social en Puerto Rico*; Burgos Ortiz, *Pioneras de la profesión de trabajo social en Puerto Rico*; Reyes, *Sobrevivencia, pobreza, y "mantengo."*

19. Guy, *Women Build the Welfare State*, 3.

20. For more on the Archivo General de Puerto Rico, see Findlay, *We Are Left without a Father Here*, 13–23.

21. Here I look at the records of the Offices of the Government of Puerto Rico in the United States Records held at the Archives of the Puerto Rican Diaspora, Center for Puerto Rican Studies, Hunter College, City University of New York (hereafter cited as OGPRUS).

22. For more on the history of migration from Puerto Rico to the United States, see Duany, *Blurred Borders*.

23. I draw on the methods of migration scholars and those who have done transnational history. In the Puerto Rican context, the use of *transnational* is complicated because of the continued colonial status of the island. For more information, see Duany, *Blurred Borders*; García-Colón, *Colonial Migrants at the Heart of Empire*. For examples of transnational historical scholarship, see Hoffnung-Garskof, *A Tale of Two Cities*; Putnam, *Radical Moves*.

24. For more on the history of US colonialism in the Spanish Caribbean, see McCoy and Scarano, *The Colonial Crucible*. On the United States imagining its colonial endeavors in Puerto Rico as benevolent, see Findlay, "Love in the Tropics."

25. Findlay, "Love in the Tropics," 141; Findlay, *Imposing Decency*.

26. Briggs, *Reproducing Empire*. See also Flores Ramos, *Eugenesia, higiene pública y alcanfor para las pasiones*.

27. On the construction of Puerto Rican citizenship, see Erman, "Meanings of Citizenship in the U.S. Empire"; Erman, *Almost Citizens*; McGreevey, *Borderline Citizens*.

28. Burnett and Marshall, *Foreign in a Domestic Sense*.

29. Burnett and Marshall, *Foreign in a Domestic Sense*, 384.

30. Mathews, *Puerto Rican Politics and the New Deal*.

31. Building on historian Linda Gordon, this book considers the evolution of the definition of "welfare" in the United States as a set of state policies of social provision created for poor citizens—including specific public assistance programs—not the full spectrum of social provisions created by the state. See Gordon, "What Is Welfare?" in *Pitied but Not Entitled*.

32. See Morrissey, "Making of a Colonial Welfare State."

33. The reforms that they promised included ones that would regulate US sugar trusts and redistribute land to the working class. See, for example, García-Colón, *Land Reform in Puerto Rico*.

34. For more on the PPD during this period, see Dietz, *Negotiating Development and Change*; Findlay, *We Are Left without a Father Here*.

35. Grosfoguel, *Colonial Subjects*.

36. Despite protests, in 1953 the United Nations General Assembly decided that Puerto Rico would no longer be considered a colonial possession because it determined that the island met the standards of self-government outlined in its own agenda. Trías Monge, *Puerto Rico*, 124–27, 136–40.

37. Duany, *The Puerto Rican Nation on the Move*; Whalen and Vázquez-Hernández, *The Puerto Rican Diaspora*; García-Colón, *Colonial Migrants at the Heart of Empire*; Meléndez, *Sponsored Migration*.

38. Thomas, *Puerto Rican Citizen*.

39. Thomas, *Puerto Rican Citizen*; Sánchez Korrol, *From Colonia to Community*.

40. García-Colón, *Colonial Migrants at the Heart of Empire*; Meléndez, *Sponsored Migration*.

41. The Puerto Rican government had created the Puerto Rican Bureau of Employment and Identification in 1930, which helped Puerto Rican migrant workers; this effort

was later expanded in 1948 into the Employment and Migration Bureau, which finally became the Migration Division of the Puerto Rican Department of Labor in 1951. For more on this agency, see Thomas, *Puerto Rican Citizen*; Duany, *Blurred Borders*.

42. See, for example, Baerga, *Género y trabajo*; Silvestrini, "Women as Workers"; Whalen, *From Puerto Rico to Philadelphia*; Ortiz, *Puerto Rican Women and Work*; Findlay, *We Are Left without a Father Here*; Benmayor et al., *Stories to Live By*; Sánchez Korrol, *From Colonial to Community*.

43. For US history, see, for example, Hunter, *To 'Joy My Freedom*; Romero, *Maid in the U.S.A.*; Boris and Klein, *Caring for America*; Glenn, *Forced to Care*; Glenn, *Unequal Freedom*; Nadasen, *Household Workers Unite*; May, *Unprotected Labor*; Urban, *Brokering Servitude*; Ervin, *Gateway to Equality*. For Latin America and the Caribbean, see, for example, Matos Rodríguez, *Women and Urban Change in San Juan, Puerto Rico, 1820–1868*; Hicks, *Hierarchies at Home*; Chaney et al., *Muchachas No More*; Blum, *Domestic Economies*.

44. For example, see Nadasen, *Care*; Parreñas, *Servants of Globalization*; Parreñas, *The Force of Domesticity*; Wilkerson, *To Live Here, You Have to Fight*; Fraser, *Fortunes of Feminism*; Boris and Klein, *Caring for America*; Boris and Parreñas, *Intimate Labors*; Boris, *Making the Woman Worker*; Glenn, *Forced to Care*; Duffy, *Making Care Count*; Tungohan, *Care Activism*; Bhattacharya, *Social Reproduction Theory*; Ferguson, *Women and Work*; Francisco-Menchavez, *The Labor of Care*; Briggs, *How All Politics Became Reproductive Politics*.

45. Glenn, *Forced to Care*, 6.

46. Boris and Klein, *Caring for America*, 5.

47. Boris and Klein, *Caring for America*, 5.

48. Nadasen, *Care*, 15–16.

49. Boris, "The Racialized Gendered State"; Boris, "Force and the Shadow of Precarity."

50. Aruzza, Bhattacharya, and Fraser, *Feminism for the 99%*, 24. For more on social reproduction theory, see Fraser, *Fortunes of Feminism*; Bhattacharya, *Social Reproduction Theory*.

51. Wilkerson, *To Live Here, You Have to Fight*, 3.

52. Wilkerson, *To Live Here, You Have to Fight*, 14.

53. In thinking about the gendered labor of welfare state building, I draw on Donna Guy's work on Argentina. Guy, *Women Build the Welfare State*.

54. Here I draw on the perspectives of scholars writing about the history of welfare as well as welfare recipients organizing for "welfare rights." Orleck, *Storming Caesar's Palace*; Nadasen, *Welfare Warriors*; Williams, *The Politics of Public Housing*; Kornbluh, *The Battle for Welfare Rights*.

55. See, for example, D'Antonio, *American Nursing*; Threat, *Nursing Civil Rights*; Hine, *Black Women in White*; Reisch and Andrews, *The Road Not Taken*; Walkowitz, *Working with Class*; Bell, *The Black Power Movement and American Social Work*; Dowden-White, *Groping toward Democracy*.

56. Choy, *Empire of Care*.

57. Here I build on the scholars who have examined the role of professional women in Puerto Rican communities in the United States. See Sánchez Korrol, "In Search

of Unconventional Women"; Sánchez Korrol, "The Forgotten Migrant"; Rúa, *Latino Urban Ethnography and the Work of Elena Padilla.*

58. My use of biography and prosopography builds on the work of scholars writing about women's history, particularly those focused on African American and Latina women, who have used life histories as a means to examine the history of gender and race in the United States. Examples of such work include Ransby, *Ella Baker and the Black Freedom Movement*; Taylor, *The Veiled Garvey*; Schechter, *Exploring the Decolonial Imaginary*; Ruiz and Sánchez Korrol, *Latina Legacies*, Cotera, *Native Speakers*; Pérez Rosario, *Becoming Julia de Burgos*; Marino, *Feminism for the Americas*; Blain, *Set the World on Fire*; Wilkerson, *To Live Here, You Have to Fight.*

59. For an example of this type of work, see Bell, *The Black Power Movement and American Social Work.*

60. This idea was clearly articulated by Antonia Pantoja in describing her social work practice. See Pantoja, *Memoir of a Visionary.*

61. Glenn, *Forced to Care.*

62. For examples of powerful histories of the connection between caring labor, struggles for social change, and social rights in the United States, see Hunter, *To 'Joy My Freedom*; Boris, *Home to Work*; Boris and Klein, *Caring for America*; Nadasen, *Household Workers Unite*; Nadasen, *Welfare Warriors*; Orleck, *Storming Caesar's Palace*; Williams, *The Politics of Public Housing*; Kornbluh, *The Battle for Welfare Rights*; Wilkerson, *To Live Here, You Have to Fight.*

63. For more on the history of race and domestic labor in Puerto Rico, see Matos Rodríguez, *Women and Urban Change in Puerto Rico*; Crespo, "Domestic Work and Racial Divisions in Women's Employment in Puerto Rico, 1899–1930."

64. On the history of Puerto Rican domestic workers in the United States, see, for example, Whalen, *From Puerto Rico to Philadelphia*; Rúa, *A Grounded Identidad*; Toro-Morn, "Gender, Class, Family, and Migration."

65. For more on the history of race, people of African descent, and social work in Puerto Rico in the 1950s, see Del Moral, "'Una niña humilde y de color.'"

66. On the participation of Afro-Puerto Ricans in social movements, see, for example, Denis-Rosario, *Drops of Inclusivity*; Román and Flores, *The Afro-Latin@ Reader*; Hoffung-Garskof, *Racial Migrations*; Fernández, *The Young Lords*; Lee, *Building a Latino Civil Rights Movement*; Lloréns, *Making Livable Worlds.*

CHAPTER 1. WOMEN BUILDING SOCIAL WELFARE PROGRAMS
IN PUERTO RICO AFTER 1917

1. Bary and the Children's Bureau, *Child Welfare in the Insular Possessions of the United States, Part I.*

2. Bary and the Children's Bureau, *Child Welfare in the Insular Possessions of the United States, Part I.*

3. Beatriz Lassalle del Valle (who often published under the name Beatriz Lassalle) discussed her participation in the development of social welfare programs and the field of social work in various articles she published in Puerto Rican newspapers and social work journals. See, for example: Beatriz Lassalle, "Servicio Social: Un poco más

de la historia sobre el trabajo social en Puerto Rico," *El Mundo*, October 11, 1935, 9, 13; Lassalle, "Veinticinco años de servicios sociales públicos en Puerto Rico"; Lassalle, "El año del los niños"; Lassalle, "Breves Palabras." For additional information about Lassalle's life and work written by her contemporaries, see Angelis, *Mujeres puertorriqueñas*, 155; Negrón Muñoz, *Mujeres de Puerto Rico*, 170–73; Krüger Torres, *Enciclopedia grandes mujeres de Puerto Rico*, 295–98; Denoyers, "Servir, divisa de una vida: Entrevista con Beatriz Lassalle"; Angela Négron Muñoz, "Figuras sobresalientes del feminismo en Puerto Rico: Beatriz Lassalle del Valle," *Puerto Rico Illustrado*, May 18, 1929, 19; Silva, "Beatriz Lassalle y su obra para la Cruz Roja." For a resume of Lassalle's work up until 1935, see Bourne, *Professional Training for Social Work in Puerto Rico*, 13. For a brief biographical overview of Lassalle written after she passed away, see Mendoza Tío, "Beatriz Lassalle del Valle."

4. On social science and the history of Puerto Rico, see Briggs, *Reproducing Empire*.

5. Lassalle, "Servico Social"; see note 3 above.

6. During her life Lassalle was categorized as both "mulatta" and "white" in US federal census records. She was understood to be of "mixed" race by her US Children's Bureau colleague Helen Bary. However, as scholars of race in Puerto Rico have shown, it was common for people of African descent, especially those of families who were middle or upper class, to identify as white. The social construction of race and racial fluidity in Puerto Rico has been examined by historian María del Carmen Baerga. See, for example, Baerga, "Routes to Whiteness, or How to Scrub off the Stain"; Baerga, *Negociaciones de sangre*. For more on the history of racial whitening and racial silencing in Puerto Rico, see Lloréns, *Imaging the Great Puerto Rican Family*; Rodríguez-Silva, *Silencing Race*; Godreau, *Scripts of Blackness*.

7. Denoyers, "Servir, divisa de una vida," 114.

8. For more on economic history during this period, see Dietz, *Economic History of Puerto Rico*.

9. For more on Puerto Rican labor history at the time, see, for example, Baerga, *Género y trabajo*; Meléndez-Badillo, *The Lettered Barriada*; Sanabria, *Puerto Rican Labor History, 1898–1934*.

10. For more on the history of Puerto Rican citizenship, see Erman, *Almost Citizens*; McGreevey, *Borderline Citizens*; Cabán, *Constructing a Colonial People*.

11. *Public Protection of Maternity and Infancy—Porto Rico: Hearings on H.R. 6142 before the Committee on Interstate and Foreign Commerce*, 68th Cong., 1st Sess. (1924).

12. *Public Protection of Maternity and Infancy—Porto Rico*, 17.

13. Erman, *Almost Citizens*.

14. There is a wealth of literature on the history of maternalism in the United States and maternalists' role in imperial projects, particularly dealing with the formation of social welfare programs and policies. For example, see Koven and Michel, *Mothers of a New World*; Wilson, *The Women's Joint Congressional Committee and the Politics of Maternalism, 1920–30*; Klein, Plant, Sanders, and Weintrob, *Maternalism Reconsidered*.

15. For an in-depth history of Puerto Rican social agencies, charitable work, and liberal reform politics in Puerto Rico during the nineteenth century, see the work of Teresita Martínez-Vergne. Martínez-Vergne has demonstrated the ways that the

organization of charity in San Juan during this period unfolded after the abolition of slavery and how it focused on regulating the lives of Puerto Ricans of African descent. In her work she examines the records of the Casa de Beneficencia in San Juan. Martínez-Vergne, *Shaping the Discourse on Space*. Another important study that emphasizes the ways that social welfare agencies regulated working-class women workers was conducted by Félix Matos Rodríguez, who examined how working women, and particularly domestic workers, were targeted by liberal reformers during a similar period. See Matos Rodríguez, *Women and Urban Change in San Juan*. On the history of the development of social work between Spanish rule and the invasion of the United States, see Serra, "Bienestar público en Puerto Rico: Desarrollo historico." In this article, Serra outlines how under US colonial rule the separation of church and state and political reforms began a reorganization of charitable agencies in Puerto Rico. On the longer history of the development of social welfare organizations under Spain, see the series of articles on the history of the development of charity in Puerto Rico by Francisco de Goenaga in the 1940s, published in the Puerto Rican social work journal *Bienestar Público*. For example, de Goenaga, "Desarrollo historico del asilo de beneficencia de Puerto Rico."

16. On the history of the suffrage movement in Puerto Rico, see Barceló Miller, *La lucha por el sufragio femenino en Puerto Rico, 1896–1935*; Jiménez-Muñoz, "'A Storm Dressed in Skirts'"; Findlay, *Imposing Decency*.

17. Santiago-Valles, *"Subject People" and Colonial Discourses*; Carrasquillo, *Our Landless Patria*.

18. See, for example, Findlay, *Imposing Decency*; Briggs, *Reproducing Empire*; Go, *American Empire and the Politics of Meaning*.

19. Findlay, *Imposing Decency*.

20. Guy, *Women Build the Welfare State*.

21. Denoyers, "Servir, divisa de una vida"; Negrón Muñoz, *Mujeres de Puerto Rico*.

22. In the 1910 United States Census Record for the Francisco Lassalle Doval household the family is listed as living in San Juan, Puerto Rico. Francisco Lassalle Doval was born around 1858, and he was fifty-two years old at the time of the census. His race is listed as "mulatto" and his occupation as that of municipal judge. Beatriz Lassalle's mother, Estefanía Valle Rivera de Lassalle, is listed as "white." Beatriz is listed as "mulatta," and her sister is listed as "white." It is possible that her sister had a different father or that the family members were categorized as racially different by census takers. In addition to the main members of the family, a number of Black and white servants lived in the household, suggesting the family was well off. By the time the 1920 census was taken, Beatriz Lassalle's father had passed away and all the women in the household are listed as white.

Francisco Lassalle Doval was one of the first six lawyers admitted to the Supreme Court of Puerto Rico in 1901, and he was a member of the Republican Party; he may have previously worked as a typographer in Ponce. It is possible that he was a member of the cohort of artisan intellectuals of African descent discussed by Jesse Hoffnung-Garskof in "To Abolish the Law of Castes." For more on his experience becoming a lawyer and judge, see Robert H. Todd, "Primeros exámenes de revália se llevaron a cabo en 1901, participando seis abogados," *El Mundo,* August 31, 1947, 4, 13.

23. For more on the history of race, race-making, and racial silencing in Puerto Rico and the Puerto Rican diaspora, see Baerga, *Negociaciones de sangre*; Baerga, "Routes to Whiteness, or How to Scrub Off the Stain"; Hoffnung-Garskof, "To Abolish the Law of Castes"; Román and Flores, *The Afro-Latin@ Reader*; Hoffnung-Garskof, "The Migrations of Arturo Schomburg"; Rodríguez-Silva, *Silencing Race*; Findlay, *Imposing Decency*. On Afro-Puerto Rican history and archives, see Figueroa, "Afro-Boricua Archives."

24. Lassalle spent one summer at Harvard, where she took courses in "English and Nature Study." See Bourne, *Professional Training for Social Work in Puerto Rico,* 13. The students in these programs were segregated and funneled into educational institutions according to how colonial officials imagined their racial status. Some ended up at training schools dedicated to "racial uplift," like the Carlisle Indian School and Tuskegee Institute for African American students. Others enrolled at prestigious universities like Harvard and Yale alongside mostly white students. Around the same time that Lassalle arrived, there were simultaneously hundreds of other young women teachers who arrived in the city on military cargos sponsored by the Department of Education, bound for summer schools held at Columbia and Cornell. See Osuna, *A History of Education in Puerto Rico*; Osuna, "An Indian in Spite of Myself"; Navarro-Rivera, "Acculturation under Duress"; Negrón de Montilla, *Americanization in Puerto Rico and the Public-School System, 1900–1930*; Guridy, *Forging Diaspora*; Del Moral, *Negotiating Empire*; Navarro, *Creating Tropical Yankees.*

25. For an excellent discussion of domesticity, empire, and care, see Choy, *Empire of Care.* On intimacy and imperialism, see also Stoler, *Haunted by Empire*; Wildenthal, *German Women for Empire, 1884–1945.*

26. Denoyers, "Servir, divisa de una vida"; Negrón Muñoz, *Mujeres de Puerto Rico.*

27. She published a children's book during this period that was a translation of Greek mythology into Spanish. Lassalle, *Cuentos mitológicos.* The role of school inspectors in Puerto Rico during the period is discussed in Del Moral, *Negotiating Empire.*

28. On the history of the suffrage movement and women's political activism in Puerto Rico, see Barceló Miller, *La lucha por el sufragio femenino en Puerto Rico, 1896–1935*; Azize Vargas, *La mujer en la lucha*; Jiménez-Muñoz, "'A Storm Dressed in Skirts'"; Findlay, *Imposing Decency*; Roy-Féquiére, *Women, Creole Identity and Intellectual Life in Early Twentieth-Century Puerto Rico.*

29. Jiménez-Muñoz, "'A Storm Dressed in Skirts,'" 437–40.

30. The quote is from Krüger Torres, *Enciclopedia grandes mujeres de Puerto Rico,* 296. The two grew so close that Lassalle became her daughter's godmother. For more on the friendship of Beatriz Lassalle and Ricarda López de Ramos Casellas, see Enríquez Seiders, *Ricarda López de Ramos Casellas.*

31. Marino, *Feminism for the Americas.*

32. See, for example, Sklar, Schuler, and Strasser, *Social Justice Feminists in the United States and Germany*; Sklar, *Florence Kelley and the Nation's Work.*

33. Junior Red Cross, *The Junior Red Cross*; American Junior Red Cross, *A Program of Junior Red Cross Service, Outlined in Proceedings of the Educational Conference, January 7, 1918*; Serbía, "Historia de la cruz roja juvenil en Puerto Rico."

34. Training in scientific motherhood in the United States is discussed in Ladd-Taylor, *Mother-Work*; Mink, *The Wages of Motherhood*.

35. For more on the history of social feminism in the United States and how it changed over time, see Cobble, *The Other Women's Movement*.

36. Tyrrell, *Woman's World/Woman's Empire*.

37. Flores Ramos, *Eugenesia, higiene pública y alcanfor para las pasiones*.

38. Irwin, *Making the World Safe*; Jones, *The American Red Cross from Clara Barton to the New Deal*.

39. Lassalle, "Breves palabras."

40. These programs have remained unstudied in the Puerto Rican context. However, in the United States, historians have written about them as one of the main precursors to the creation of public welfare provision and the development of the welfare state.

41. On the early Puerto Rican migrant community in New York City, see Sánchez Korrol, *From Colonia to Community*; Thomas, *Puerto Rican Citizen*; Glasser, *My Music Is My Flag*; Hoffnung-Garskof, "The Migrations of Arturo Schomburg"; Hoffnung-Garskof, *Racial Migrations*; Colón, *A Puerto Rican in New York, and Other Sketches*.

42. For more on the development of the New York School of Social Work, see Meier, *A History of the New York School of Social Work*; Feldman and Kamerman, *The Columbia University School of Social Work*; Berengarten, Columbia University, and CUSSW Alumni Association, *The Columbia University School of Social Work*; Walkowitz, *Working with Class*.

43. For more on the history and development of social work practices of casework, see Richmond, *Social Diagnosis*; Agnew, *From Charity to Social Work*; Peel, *Miss Cutler and the Case of the Resurrected Horse*; Tice, *Tales of Wayward Girls and Immoral Women*.

44. For more on the history of the settlement house movement in the United States, see Trattner, *From Poor Law to Welfare State*; Crocker, *Social Work and Social Order*; Lasch-Quinn, *Black Neighbors*.

45. Denoyers, "Servir, divisa de una vida."

46. Denoyers, "Servir, divisa de una vida," 116.

47. On the history of the Children's Bureau and US empire, see Bullard, "Children's Future, Nation's Future"; Bullard, *Civilizing the Child*.

48. For a comprehensive history of the Children's Bureau, see Lindenmeyer, *A Right to Childhood*.

49. For a discussion of the impact of "Americanization" as a Children's Bureau policy, see Mink, *The Wages of Motherhood*; Glenn, *Forced to Care*; Bernstein, *Racial Innocence*; Ward, *The Black Child-Savers*.

50. Mink, *The Wages of Motherhood*.

51. In the United States, see Ladd, *Mother-Work*. On Latin American variations of these public health visions, which were closely tied to eugenics, see Stepan, *The Hour of Eugenics*.

52. For more on Puerto Rican suffrage leaders and maternalist politics, see Jiménez-Muñoz, "'A Storm Dressed in Skirts.'"

53. Bary and the Children's Bureau, *Child Welfare in the Insular Possessions of the United States, Part I.*

54. Lassalle, "Servico Social"; see note 3 above.

55. Lassalle, "Servicio Social."

56. There is an oral history of Helen Bary that discusses her work in Puerto Rico and the writing of the report; see Bary, Parker, and Leiby, *Labor Administration and Social Security.* Bary became one of the architects of Social Security legislation in the United States. As the oral history relates, Lathrop was one of her mentors, but she did not get along well with Grace Abbott or Katherine Lenroot, the other women who held leadership roles in the administration.

57. Bary, Parker, and Leiby, *Labor Administration and Social Security.*

58. Helen Bary published a number of articles under her pen name, Valeska Bari. The story with a character named Beatriz is: Valeska Bari, "Goddess of Liberty," *The Forum*, July 1927, 48–61. For more of her writing on Puerto Rico, for example, Valeska Bari, "Gift of Tongues," *The Atlantic*, September 1925, 389–94.

59. Bary, Parker, and Leiby, *Labor Administration and Social Security*, 119.

60. Bary, Parker, and Leiby, *Labor Administration and Social Security*, 120.

61. Children's Bureau, *Children's Year*, 5.

62. Children's Bureau, *Children's Year*, 5.

63. Children's Bureau, *Children's Year*, 9. Training in scientific motherhood in the United States is discussed in Ladd-Taylor, *Mother-Work*; Mink, *The Wages of Motherhood.*

64. Knowlton Mixer wrote a book about Puerto Rico after his visit. See Mixer, *Porto Rico.*

65. Dock, Pickett, and Noyes, *History of American Red Cross Nursing.*

66. This is similar to the process described in Kunzel, *Fallen Women, Problem Girls.*

67. Bary and the Children's Bureau, *Child Welfare in the Insular Possessions of the United States, Part I.*

68. For more on the history of this, see Martínez-Vergne, *Shaping the Discourse on Space*; Matos Rodríguez, *Women and Urban Change in San Juan*; Flores Ramos, *Eugenesia, higiene pública y alcanfor para las pasiones.*

69. Ladd-Taylor, *Mother-Work.*

70. Findlay, *Imposing Decency.*

71. Lindenmeyer, *A Right to Childhood.*

72. Silvestrini, *Los trabajadores puertorriqueños y el partido socialista.*

73. Baerga, *Género y trabajo.*

74. For more on the history of race and domestic labor in Puerto Rico, see Matos Rodríguez, *Women and Urban Change in Puerto Rico*; Crespo, "Domestic Work and Racial Divisions in Women's Employment in Puerto Rico, 1899–1930"; Martínez-Vergne, *Shaping the Discourse on Space.*

75. On the history of working women's resistance during this period, see Matos Rodríguez, *Women and Urban Change in Puerto Rico.*

76. Matos Rodríguez, *Women and Urban Change in Puerto Rico.*

77. On the resistance of women who were accused of being prostitutes, see Findlay, *Imposing Decency*.

78. For more on working-class and socialist women's organizing during the 1920s, see de Pagán, *El obrerismo en Puerto Rico*; Barceló Miller, "Halfhearted Solidarity."

79. Barceló Miller, "Halfhearted Solidarity."

80. Bary and the Children's Bureau, *Child Welfare in the Insular Possessions of the United States, Part I*, 31–32.

81. Bary and the Children's Bureau, *Child Welfare in the Insular Possessions of the United States, Part I*, 63–65.

82. Briggs, *Reproducing Empire*; Flores Ramos, *Eugenesia, higiene pública y alcanfor para las pasiones*.

83. Bary and the Children's Bureau, *Child Welfare in the Insular Possessions of the United States, Part I*, 3.

84. For more on reformers' emphasis as single motherhood as a problem, see Findlay, *Imposing Decency*.

85. Bary and the Children's Bureau, *Child Welfare in the Insular Possessions of the United States, Part I*, 64; Findlay, *Imposing Decency*, 64.

86. For more on the Puerto Rican diaspora in 1920, see Sánchez Korrol, *From Colonia to Community*; McGreevey, *Borderline Citizens*.

87. Bary and the Children's Bureau, *Child Welfare in the Insular Possessions of the United States, Part I*, 64.

88. Bary and the Children's Bureau, *Child Welfare in the Insular Possessions of the United States, Part I*, 64.

89. de Pagán, *El obrerismo en Puerto Rico*; Barceló Miller, "Halfhearted Solidarity."

90. Boria, *Cuidado diurno para niños de madres que trabajan*.

91. One such socialist feminist social worker and advocate for day care programs was Felicia Boria Fuentes, who later conducted a study of day care services on the archipelago. Boria, *Cuidado diurno para niños de madres que trabajan*, 13–14.

92. Bary and the Children's Bureau, *Child Welfare in the Insular Possessions of the United States, Part I*.

93. Bary and the Children's Bureau, *Child Welfare in the Insular Possessions of the United States, Part I*, 55.

94. The intersection of child domestic work and circulation and the formation of social work practices has been explored in the context of Latin America in Blum, *Domestic Economies*.

95. Bary and the Children's Bureau, *Child Welfare in the Insular Possessions of the United States, Part I*, 55.

96. Bary and the Children's Bureau, *Child Welfare in the Insular Possessions of the United States, Part I*, 60–61.

97. Bary and the Children's Bureau, *Child Welfare in the Insular Possessions of the United States, Part I*, 61.

98. Bary and the Children's Bureau, *Child Welfare in the Insular Possessions of the United States, Part I*, 55.

99. Bary and the Children's Bureau, *Child Welfare in the Insular Possessions of the United States, Part I*, 56.

100. Bary and the Children's Bureau, *Child Welfare in the Insular Possessions of the United States, Part I*, 60.

101. Bary and the Children's Bureau, *Child Welfare in the Insular Possessions of the United States, Part I*, 59.

102. Bary and the Children's Bureau, *Child Welfare in the Insular Possessions of the United States, Part I*, 60.

103. Bary and the Children's Bureau, *Child Welfare in the Insular Possessions of the United States, Part I*, 60.

104. Bary and the Children's Bureau, *Child Welfare in the Insular Possessions of the United States, Part I*, 62.

105. Bary and the Children's Bureau, *Child Welfare in the Insular Possessions of the United States, Part I*, 62.

106. Bary and the Children's Bureau, *Child Welfare in the Insular Possessions of the United States, Part I*, 61.

107. Lassalle, "Servicio Social"; see note 3 above.

108. Bary and the Children's Bureau, *Child Welfare in the Insular Possessions of the United States, Part I*, 74.

109. "Social Service Activities of the Department of Health," 25.

110. "Social Service Activities of the Department of Health," 25. See also, Lane, "Educational Activities of the Department of Health of Porto Rico."

111. "Social Service Activities of the Department of Health," 25.

112. "Social Service Activities of the Department of Health," 26.

113. "Social Service Activities of the Department of Health," 26.

114. "Social Service Activities of the Department of Health," 26.

115. "Social Service Activities of the Department of Health," 26.

116. Rodriguez Pastor, "Our Bureau of Social Welfare," 112.

CHAPTER 2. LABOR, WELFARE, AND GENDERED CITIZENSHIP
IN NEW DEAL PUERTO RICO

Portions of this chapter were first published in "'Women Ask Relief for Puerto Ricans': Social Workers, the Social Security Act and Puerto Rican Communities, 1933–1943," *LABOR: Studies in Working-Class History*, no 3. (December 2016). I would like to thank Julie Greene and Leon Fink for their feedback and encouragement along the way.

1. For more about the development of PRERA as a part of the extension of New Deal policies to Puerto Rico, see Mathews, *Puerto Rican Politics and the New Deal*; Rodríguez, *A New Deal for the Tropics*.

2. "Women Ask Relief for Puerto Ricans: Extension of Social Security Act Urged by Five Delegates to Convention," *New York Times*, June 1, 1936.

3. For more on the ways in which US empire in Puerto Rico was configured in racialized and gendered terms, see Findlay, *Imposing Decency*; Briggs, *Reproducing Empire*; Matos Rodríguez and Delgado, *Puerto Rican Women's History*; Ortiz, *Puerto Rican Women and Work*; Del Moral, *Negotiating Empire*; Macpherson, "Citizens vs. Clients"; Macpherson, "Doing Comparative Caribbean (Gender) History."

4. Mathews, *Puerto Rican Politics and the New Deal*; Rodríguez, *A New Deal for the Tropics*; Burgos Ortiz, *Pioneras de la profesión de trabajo social en Puerto Rico*; Cabranes, "El trabajo social en las segundas unidades rurales."

5. Morrissey, "The Making of a Colonial Welfare State"; Cabranes, *A Study of Federal Public Assistance Payments to Puerto Rico*.

6. Burgos Ortiz, *Pioneras de la profesión de trabajo social en Puerto Rico*; Rivera de Alvarado, *Lucha y visión de Puerto Rico libre*.

7. Canales, *La constitución es la revolución*; Rosado Morales, *Mis testimonios*.

8. For more on the history of Puerto Rican women's labor and labor organizing during the period, see Baerga, *Género y trabajo*; Silvestrini, "Women as Workers"; Whalen, *From Puerto Rico to Philadelphia*; Ortiz, *Puerto Rican Women and Work*; Matos Rodríguez and Delgado, *Puerto Rican Women's History*.

9. Baerga, *Género y trabajo*; Boris, *Home to Work*.

10. Rodríguez, *A New Deal for the Tropics*.

11. Silvestrini, "Women as Workers"; Silvestrini, *Los trabajadores puertorriqueños y el partido socialista*.

12. Mathews, *Puerto Rican Politics and the New Deal*; Rodríguez, *A New Deal for the Tropics*.

13. There were widespread economic problems on the archipelago that were addressed by reformers during this period and have been documented in histories of Puerto Rico. Historian Lillian Guerra examines the limitations and difficulties that occurred as a part of the Americanization project, which failed poor Puerto Ricans who were struggling with the impact of the Great Depression and US capitalist development in Puerto Rico. Guerra, *Popular Expression and National Identity in Puerto Rico*. Widespread landlessness, while a problem before US intervention, became a greater issue when people who had informal access to land were no longer able to move because property came under US ownership. See Ayala and Bernabe, *Puerto Rico in the American Century*; Carrasquillo, *Our Landless Patria*.

14. The *jíbaro* was also imagined over time in different ways and eventually would come to be a symbol of Puerto Rican whiteness and maleness. For more on the history of the *jíbaro* and education, see Guerra, *Popular Expression and National Identity in Puerto Rico*; Del Moral, *Negotiating Empire*; Del Moral, "Rescuing the *Jíbaro*."

15. On the history of social work education in Puerto Rico, see Burgos Ortiz, *Pioneras de la profesión de trabajo social en Puerto Rico*; Ramú de Guzmán, "Historia de la escuela de trabajo social de la Universidad de Puerto Rico."

16. Francisco Vizcarrondo and other Puerto Rican reformers wrote extensively about the transformation of the educational program in Puerto Rico and also presented information about this program in forums outside the archipelago. See, for example, Vizcarrondo, *The Second-Unit Rural Schools of Porto Rico*.

17. For more on the history of vocational education in Puerto Rico under US rule, see Negrón de Montilla, *Americanization in Puerto Rico and the Public-School System, 1900–1930*; Del Moral, *Negotiating Empire*.

18. Carmen Rivera de Alvarado wrote about her experiences as a social worker in essays and lectures that were published during her life and posthumously. See Rivera

de Alvarado, *Lucha y visión de Puerto Rico libre*, 113. For more on the life and work of Rivera de Alvarado, see Seda Rodríguez, "Legado de Carmen Rivera de Alvarado a la profesion de trabajo social en Puerto Rico."

19. Rivera de Alvarado later wrote about the history and development of Puerto Rican women's work within nationalist organizations. Rivera de Alvarado, "La contribución de la mujer al desarrollo de la nacionalidad Puertorriqueña." This article was originally published in the pro-independence newspaper *Claridad* on September 20, 1970.

20. Rivera de Alvarado, *Lucha y visión de Puerto Rico libre*, 112–13.

21. Rivera de Alvarado, *Lucha y visión de Puerto Rico libre*, 116–17.

22. Dorothy Bourne was an experienced social worker from the United States who moved with her husband, James Bourne, to Puerto Rico. She was hired soon after by the Puerto Rican government and went on to work for years on the archipelago. For more information, see Bourne and Bourne, *Thirty Years of Change*. On the development of social work training in Puerto Rico, see Burgos Ortiz, *Pioneras de la profesión de trabajo social en Puerto Rico*.

23. Dorothy Bourne notes that the social work participants helped develop the training program. Bourne, *Professional Training for Social Work in Puerto Rico*. She received a certificate in rural social work from Cornell University after working as a social worker for a number of years. The Bournes were likely in conversation about the possibility of their involvement in the administration of the archipelago before FDR won the presidential election, and shortly after this happened, James Bourne was chosen to oversee the creation of New Deal agencies on the island. Mathews, *Puerto Rican Politics and the New Deal*.

24. Vizcarrondo, *The Second Unit Rural Schools of Porto Rico*, 13.

25. Negrón de Montilla, *Americanization in Puerto Rico*; Del Moral, *Negotiating Empire*; Vizcarrondo, *The Second Unit Rural Schools*.

26. Vizcarrondo, *The Second Unit Rural Schools of Porto Rico*, 1. For more on the development of home economics in Puerto Rico, see Ferguson, *Home Making and Home Keeping*.

27. Vizcarrondo, *The Second Unit Rural Schools of Porto Rico*, 13.

28. Vizcarrondo, *The Second Unit Rural Schools of Porto Rico*, 5. For more on needlework during this period, also see González García, *Una puntada en el tiempo*.

29. Baerga, *Género y trabajo*; Boris, *Home to Work*.

30. Baerga, *Género y trabajo*; Boris, *Home to Work*.

31. On Boria's life and work, see Krüger Torres, *Enciclopedia grandes mujeres de Puerto Rico*, 91–92. For more on her work with the Women's Bureau, see Muñiz-Mas, "Gender, Work, and Institutional Change"; Felicia Boria, "El salario de la mujer," *El Mundo*, September 24, 1934.

32. Krüger Torres, *Enciclopedia grandes mujeres de Puerto Rico*, 91–92. US Federal Census records from the period have various racial categorizations for Felicia Boria and her family members. She was listed as "mulatta" as well as "white" in these records throughout her lifetime.

33. For more on the history of the Federacion Libre de los Trabajadores in Puerto Rico and the history of the Socialist Party in Puerto Rico, see, for example, Silvestrini,

Los trabajadores puertorriqueños y el Partido Socialista; Sanabria, *Puerto Rican Labor History*. For more on the Federacion Libre de los Trabajadores and Prudencio Rivera Martínez, see Rodríguez-Silva, *Silencing Race*; Meléndez-Badillo, *The Lettered Barriada*.

34. Cabranes, "El trabajo social en las Segundas Unidades Rurales."

35. Rivera de Alvarado, *Lucha y visión de Puerto Rico libre*.

36. Ramírez de Arellano and Seipp, *Colonialism, Catholicism, and Contraception*; López, *Matters of Choice*; Briggs, *Reproducing Empire*.

37. Briggs, *Reproducing Empire*, 98–102. See also Stepan, *The Hour of Eugenics*; Guy, *White Slavery and Mothers Alive and Dead*.

38. Rivera de Alvarado, *Lucha y visión de Puerto Rico libre*, 45–52.

39. Ramírez de Arellano and Seipp, *Colonialism, Catholicism, and Contraception*.

40. Briggs, *Reproducing Empire*; López, *Matters of Choice*; Córdova, *Pushing in Silence*.

41. Bourne and Ramos, *Rural Life in Puerto Rico*. The study that Bourne and Ramos conducted in the 1930s was the basis for a follow-up investigation that was published thirty years later. The second study was written during a moment when there was a widespread belief among liberal reformers in the positive influence of the "planned" development of the archipelago under the populist reforms of the Partido Popular Democrático (PPD). Bourne and Bourne, *Thirty Years of Change in Puerto Rico*.

42. Blanca Canales's cousin was Nemesio Canales, a well-known nationalist and feminist who had proposed a bill that first approved suffrage for women in Puerto Rico. Before passing away as a young man, Nemesio Canales had met and befriended Pedro Albizu Campos in the 1920s. When Blanca Canales met Albizu Campos, they spoke about her cousin. See the interview with Blanca Canales cited in Burgos Ortiz, *Pioneras de la profesión de trabajo social en Puerto Rico*, 57–63. For more on Canales, see Canales, *La constitución es la revolución*; Wagenheim, *Nationalist Heroines*; Power, "Puerto Rican Women Nationalists vs. U.S. Colonialism"; Materson, "Gender, Generation, and Women's Independence Organizing in Puerto Rico."

43. For the Jayuya Uprising of 1950, which Blanca Canales led, see Ayala and Bernable, *Puerto Rico in the American Century*, 167. Isabel Rosado Morales wrote a memoir that mentions her experiences and involvement in the nationalist organizing of Puerto Rican teachers and social workers. Rosado Morales served eleven years in prison for her nationalist activities; she was arrested shortly after the nationalist attack on the US Congress in 1954 led by her friend and fellow nationalist Lolita Lebrón. Rosado Morales, *Mis testimonios*.

44. Rivera de Alvarado, *Lucha y visión de Puerto Rico libre*.

45. Canales, *La constitución es la revolución*.

46. PRERA published two annual reports outlining the work that it completed. The agency was a branch of the Federal Emergency Relief Administration (FERA), created in May 1933. The goal of FERA was to reduce unemployment in the United States by creating job programs, including the Civil Works Administration. FERA programs ended in 1935, when the Works Progress Administration (WPA) and the Social Security Administration were created. For more, see Rodríguez, *A New Deal for the Tropics*.

47. Bourne, "Introduction to the First Annual Report," in Puerto Rico Emergency Relief Administration, *First Annual Report of the Puerto Rican Emergency Relief Administration*, 7.

48. Manuel Rodríguez has documented how PRERA impacted Puerto Rican communities during this period in *A New Deal for the Tropics*.

49. For more on the politics of development in Puerto Rico, see Santiago-Valles, *"Subject People" and Colonial Discourses*; Grosfoguel, *Colonial Subjects*.

50. Bourne and Bourne, *Thirty Years of Change*; Burgos Ortiz, *Pioneras de la profesión de trabajo social en Puerto Rico*.

51. Espino wrote the section of the PRERA report dedicated to the "Bureau of Social Services." Puerto Rico Emergency Relief Administration, *First Annual Report of the Puerto Rican Emergency Relief Administration*, 27.

52. Puerto Rico Emergency Relief Administration, *First Annual Report of the Puerto Rican Emergency Relief Administration*, 27–33.

53. While most social workers in Puerto Rico during this period were women, there was a small number of male social workers; they were overrepresented in leadership positions within social welfare organizations. For more on this, see Burgos Ortiz, *Pioneras de la profesión de trabajo social en Puerto Rico*.

54. Rodríguez, *A New Deal for the Tropics*, 57.

55. Puerto Rico Emergency Relief Administration, *First Annual Report of the Puerto Rican Emergency Relief Administration*, 65.

56. Quoted in Puerto Rico Emergency Relief Administration, *First Annual Report of the Puerto Rican Emergency Relief Administration*, 28.

57. The recruitment and training of social work "aides" allowed some people who were not elites to enter the profession of social work. See Burgos Ortiz, *Pioneras de la profesión de trabajo social en Puerto Rico*; Rodríguez, *A New Deal for the Tropics*, 65; Ayala and Bernabe, *Puerto Rico in the American Century*.

58. Puerto Rico Emergency Relief Administration, *First Annual Report of the Puerto Rican Emergency Relief Administration*, 395. In the United States, the women's work program of FERA, overseen by Ellen S. Woodward, gave jobs to many "white-collar" workers. Woodward went on to direct WPA programs for women. See Swain, *Ellen S. Woodward*.

59. Puerto Rico Emergency Relief Administration, *First Annual Report of the Puerto Rican Emergency Relief Administration*, 395. For more on the history of the needlework industry in Puerto Rico, see Baerga, *Género y trabajo*; Boris, *Home to Work*.

60. Baerga, *Género y trabajo*.

61. Silvestrini, "Women as Workers."

62. Baerga, "Puerto Rico: From Colony to Colony," 129–32.

63. Baerga, "Puerto Rico: From Colony to Colony," 120–32.

64. Puerto Rico Emergency Relief Administration, *First Annual Report of the Puerto Rican Emergency Relief Administration*, 395.

65. On the history of milk stations in Puerto Rico, see González, "Nurturing the Citizens of the Future."

66. For more on the birth control aspects, see Ramírez de Arellano and Seipp, *Colonialism, Catholicism, and Contraception*; Briggs, *Reproducing Empire*.

67. On the history of eugenics in other areas of Latin America, see Stepan, *The Hour of Eugenics*; Córdova, *Pushing in Silence.*

68. For an investigation of the history of race in Puerto Rico and its intersection with social reforms, see Rodríguez-Silva, *Silencing Race.* On the history of housing development as a site of race-making, see Dinzey-Flores, *Locked In, Locked Out.*

69. For Luis Muñoz Marín, the creation of the Chardón Plan and the reforms it instigated also provided a space to create a new political platform and party on the archipelago, the PPD. The party was officially created in 1938, and it would take only a few years for Muñoz Marín to consolidate political power, becoming first the president of the insular senate and soon afterward the chosen political figure of the US state. For more, see Ayala and Bernabe, *Puerto Rico in the American Century.*

70. Espino, "Trabajo social dentro de un programa de reconstrucíon."

71. Briggs, *Reproducing Empire*; Ramírez de Arellano and Seipp, *Colonialism, Catholicism, and Contraception.*

72. For more on the history of suffrage in Puerto Rico, see Findlay, *Imposing Decency.*

73. On the exclusions of Puerto Rican women of African descent from professional spaces, see Alegría Ortega and Ríos González, *Contrapunto de género y raza en Puerto Rico.*

74. Pastor, "History and Development of the Laws Licensing Social Workers in Puerto Rico."

75. Burgos Ortiz, *Pioneras de la profesión de trabajo social en Puerto Rico*, 39. The United States changed the name of Puerto Rico to "Porto Rico" in 1898, and it was not changed back to the correct spelling until 1932.

76. Burgos Ortiz, *Pioneras de la profesión de trabajo social en Puerto Rico*, 42.

77. Canales was also a member of the Nationalist Party that advocated for Puerto Rican independence. Burgos Ortiz, *Pioneras de la profesión de trabajo social en Puerto Rico*, 40.

78. Burgos Ortiz, *Pioneras de la profesión de trabajo social en Puerto Rico*, 40.

79. Rivera de Alvarado was one of the founders of social work in Puerto Rico. She was raised in a socialist household and went on to become an important supporter of the independence movement in Puerto Rico. Rivera de Alvarado, *Lucha y visión de Puerto Rico libre.*

80. Briggs, *Reproducing Empire*; Ramírez de Arellano and Seipp, *Colonialism, Catholicism, and Contraception.*

81. Bourne, "Puerto Rico's Predicament," 202. Bourne and Bourne, *Thirty Years of Change in Puerto Rico.*

82. Bourne, "Puerto Rico's Predicament," 201–2.

83. Mathews, *Puerto Rican Politics and the New Deal.*

84. Hanson, *Transformation*, 161.

85. Mathews, *Puerto Rican Politics and the New Deal*, 248.

86. Rivera de Alvarado, *Lucha y visión de Puerto Rico libre*, 117. The resident commissioner was a nonvoting representative of Puerto Rico in the US Congress.

87. For more on the social workers lobbying work in Washington, DC, during this period, see Rivera de Alvarado, *Lucha y visión de Puerto Rico libre*, 117.

88. Celestina Zaludondo Goodsaid was a social work leader in Puerto Rico for decades, who published extensively about the development of social policy. She was a strong advocate for inclusion of Puerto Rico under the Social Security Act during the period covered in this chapter and her work on this issue would continue into the 1950s. For more on Zalduondo's life and work see Pagán, "Celestina Zalduondo"; Lassalle, "Mi sentir sobre Celestina Zalduondo," 19. For examples of Zalduondo's writing about social welfare programs and social welfare policy in Puerto Rico, see Zalduondo, "Bienestar de al niñez en Puerto Rico"; Zalduondo, "El programa de asistencia pública del estado libre asociado de Puerto Rico." For a discussion of Zalduondos's experience working for Puerto Rican New Deal relief programs, see Rodríguez, *A New Deal for the Tropics*, 74–75.

89. Pintado de Rahn wrote about Abbott's role in her life. Pintado de Rahn, "Grace Abbott, Maestra." Abbott was the chief of the Children's Bureau of the US Department of Labor between 1921 and 1934 and a leader in the movement for the creation and expansion of social policy and the Social Security Act in the United States. For more on her life and work, see Costin, *Two Sisters for Social Justice*; Muncy, *Creating a Female Dominion in American Reform, 1890–1935*; Ware, *Beyond Suffrage*.

90. Pintado de Rahn, "Grace Abbott, Maestra."

91. Whalen and Vázquez-Hernández, *The Puerto Rican Diaspora*, 2.

92. For more on Puerto Rican migration during this period, see Thomas, *Puerto Rican Citizen*; Chenault, *The Puerto Rican Migrant in New York City*.

93. Thomas, *Puerto Rican Citizen*.

94. Chenault, *The Puerto Rican Migrant in New York City*, 75.

95. On Puerto Ricans and relief, see Thomas, "'How They Ignore Our Rights as American Citizens.'"

96. These agencies claimed that resettlement occurred only in rare cases when migrants were defined as "at risk of becoming permanent 'public charges'" and when social workers could determine that the migrant had access to family support back home. The question of becoming public charges also surfaced in earlier discussions of Puerto Ricans' citizenship and mobility. Erman, "Meanings of Citizenship in the US Empire"; Findlay, "Dangerous Dependence or Productive Masculinity?"

97. On Lassalle's life and work and the history of Puerto Rican social work, see chapter 1 of this book; Amador, "Welfare Is Work."

98. Hall and her husband, Robert A. Hall, kept a journal about their experiences in Puerto Rico, and she published articles about her work for the Puerto Rican government. Hall and Hall, *Puerto Rican Journal (1937–1939)*; Hall, "The Problem of the Migration of Indigent Puerto Ricans to and from New York City"; Hall, "Social and Economic Conditions in Puerto Rico."

99. Hall, "The Problem of the Migration of Indigent Puerto Ricans to and from New York City."

100. See Marcantonio, *I Vote My Conscience*; Meyer, *Vito Marcantonio Radical Politician, 1902–1954*.

101. Thomas, "Resisting the Racial Binary?"; Thomas, "'How They Ignore Our Rights as American Citizens.'"

102. Geraldine Froscher to Vito Marcantonio, February 8, 1936, Vito Marcantonio Papers, box 5, reel 4, New York Public Library Manuscripts and Archives Collection. Froscher had long worked on behalf of Puerto Rican women. In 1917, she petitioned the National Woman Suffrage Association (NWSA) to help support Puerto Rican organizations. She worked closely with Puerto Rican suffrage leader Ana Roqué de Duprey and served alongside her as the English editor of *El Heraldo de la Mujer* (The woman's herald). For more information, see Harper, *History of Woman Suffrage, 1900–1920*, 724.

103. Froscher to Marcantonio, February 8, 1936.

104. Gerald Meyer has written about how Vito Marcantonio served as an advocate for Puerto Ricans from both the United States and the archipelago by developing a particular political platform that responded to the needs of his supporters. In addition, Meyer notes that the extension of Social Security to Puerto Rico was one of Marcantonio's biggest political victories, although he offers little information about how the inclusion of Puerto Rico was negotiated or discussed. Meyer, *Vito Marcantonio*, 156.

105. Meyer notes that on June 6, 1939, Marcantonio wrote a letter to the editor of *El Mundo*, one of the main newspapers on the archipelago, to discuss his support for extending the Social Security Act to Puerto Rico. Meyer, *Vito Marcantonio*, 156.

106. On the 1939 amendments to the Social Security Act, see "Children's Bureau Expands Its Work," *New York Times*, January 30, 1939. The partial coverage of Puerto Rico is noted in United States Children's Bureau, *Maternal and Child-Health Services under the Social Security Act, Title V, Part 1*.

107. On the Children's Bureau of the US Department of Labor, see chapter 1 of this book; Lindenmeyer, *A Right to Childhood*.

108. On the role of the Children's Bureau abroad and in Puerto Rico, see Bullard, "Children's Future, Nation's Future."

109. On populism and "social justice" in Puerto Rico under the PPD, see Findlay, *We Are Left without a Father Here*.

110. Villaronga, *Toward a Discourse of Consent*, 53.

111. Committee on Ways and Means, *Social Security: Hearings Relative to the Social Security Act Amendments of 1939*, 76th Cong., 1st sess., H.R. 728, 1595-1596 (2 June 1939).

112. Committee on Ways and Means, *Social Security: Hearings Relative to the Social Security Act Amendments of 1939*, at 1601 (2 June 1939).

113. Committee on Ways and Means, *Social Security: Hearing Relative to the Social Security Amendments of 1939*, at 1602–9 (2 June 1939). See also, Bullard, "Children's Future, Nation's Future."

114. Committee on Ways and Means, *Social Security: Hearings Relative to the Social Security Act Amendments of 1939*, at 1607 (2 June 1939).

115. Literature on the history of US empire and gender has highlighted this connection. See, for example, Findlay, *Imposing Decency*; Briggs, *Reproducing Empire*.

116. On US empire and eugenics, see Stern, *Eugenic Nation*.

117. Gordon, *Pitied but Not Entitled*.

118. Findlay, *We Are Left without a Father Here*.

CHAPTER 3. WORKING-CLASS WOMEN, CLAIMS FOR BENEFITS,
AND THE POLITICS OF DESERVINGNESS UNDER THE PUERTO
RICAN POPULIST STATE

1. In this chapter, I examine numerous social work case files that are part of the collections of the Archivo General de Puerto Rico, located in Puerta de Tierra, San Juan (cited hereafter as AGPR). The majority of these records are archived in the Fondo Departamento de Salud, which houses the records of the Department of Health of Puerto Rico and the social welfare agencies that were a part of it, such as the Departamento de Bienestar Público (Department of Social Welfare).

Throughout the chapter I have created pseudonyms for social welfare clients whose records are discussed instead of using their real names. However, I provide the location of the case files where the information about the clients is recorded, which generally includes the numbers of boxes, files, and case files in these archives. In each instance where a pseudonym is used, I have noted that "the name has been changed." In some other cases where I reference the file and omit a name entirely, I have noted simply that the information is from a "Client Record."

My reading and interpretation of case files has been shaped by my participation in discussions about microhistory and archival reading practices with historians Rebecca Scott, Jean Hébrard, and Jesse Hoffnung-Garskof. For more on these and similar methods, see Scott, "Reclaiming Gregoria's Mule"; Putnam, "To Study the Fragments/Whole"; Scott and Hébrard, *Freedom Papers*; Putnam, *Radical Moves*; Hoffnung-Garskof, *Racial Migrations*.

In the first case discussed, the name "Camila Pérez" is a pseudonym. See Client Record, file 3967, box 151-A, tarea 65-101, Fondo Departamento de Salud, AGPR.

2. Client Record, file 3967, box 151-A, tarea 65-101, Fondo Departamento de Salud, AGPR. Pérez was born in the town of Camuy and later migrated to the urban area around San Juan. She is listed as "white" alongside her family members on various census records from the period. The records note that her mother and the women in her extended family were needleworkers who worked in the home doing piecework. She also mentioned that her mother was also a care worker who completed washing, ironing, and other domestic tasks for wages. Her parents passed away when she was young, and that is when she became a child servant.

3. For more on the creation of social welfare programs under the PPD, see Morrissey, "The Making of a Colonial Welfare State"; Angueira, *Mujeres puertorriqueñas, "Welfare" y globalización*. For a discussion of sexuality and social work during this period, see Córdova, "Setting them Straight." Historian Solsiree del Moral also provides an important examination of the racial politics of social welfare work in Puerto Rico through her microhistorical examination of social workers interventions in the life of a Black Puerto Rican child in 1950s Puerto Rico. See Del Moral, "'Una niña humilde y de color.'"

4. On the history of the PPD during his period, see Villaronga, *Toward a Discourse of Consent*; Alvarez-Curbelo and Rodríguez Castro, *Del nacionalismo al populismo*; Findlay, *We Are Left without a Father Here*; Flores Ramos, *Mujer, familia, y prostitución*; Ayala and Bernabe, *Puerto Rico in the American Century*.

5. For more on the history of gender and labor politics in the years leading up to the PPD victory and afterward, see Baerga, *Género y trabajo*.

6. For more on the regulation of Puerto Rican women's bodies and reproduction during the PPD years and more generally, see Briggs, *Reproducing Empire*; Córdova, *Pushing in Silence*.

7. For an examination of the negotiation of factory employment, reproductive labor, and work in home industries, see Whalen, *From Puerto Rico to Philadelphia*; Boris, *Home to Work*.

8. Del Moral, "'Una niña humilde y de color.'"

9. Briggs, *Reproducing Empire*.

10. The studies I focus on are Oscar Lewis's *La Vida: A Puerto Rican Family in the Culture of Poverty—San Juan and New York* (1966), supplemented by his *A Study of Slum Culture: Backgrounds for La Vida* (1968), and Helen Safa's *The Urban Poor of Puerto Rico: A Study in Development and Inequality* (1974).

11. For an overview of social welfare programs developed during this period, see Morrissey, "Making of a Colonial Welfare State."

12. For a discussion of the history of populism and political mobilization in Puerto Rico during this period, see Alvarez-Curbelo and Rodríguez Castro, *Del nacionalismo al populismo*; Findlay, *We Are Left without a Father Here*.

13. On the history of social reform, and especially the history of prostitution and regulation of sex work in Puerto Rico while the PPD was in power, see Briggs, *Reproducing Empire*; Flores Ramos, *Mujer, familia, y prostitución*.

14. Scholars have examined how ideas about gender and masculinity shaped political rights during this formative moment in Puerto Rican history, and how working-class people and women fought for representation through party politics. Examples include Findlay, *We Are Left without A Father Here*; Gallart, "Political Empowerment of Puerto Rican Women."

15. For an examination of the production of the Puerto Rican *jíbaro* as cultural and political figure, see Guerra, *Popular Expression and National Identity in Puerto Rico*.

16. Findlay, *We Are Left without a Father Here*.

17. Briggs, *Reproducing Empire*.

18. Flores Ramos, *Mujer, familia, y prostitución*.

19. For more on the history of eugenics, sterilizatio3n, and birth control in Puerto Rico, see, for example, Briggs, *Reproducing Empire*; López, *Matters of Choice*; Córdova, *Pushing in Silence*.

20. Morrissey, "The Making of a Colonial Welfare State."

21. Zalduondo, "El programa de asistencia pública de estado libre asociado de Puerto Rico," 2. For more about the passage of the Ley de Bienestar Público and the creation of social welfare programs in Puerto Rico, see Departamento de Salud, *La división de Bienestar Público en su quinto aniversario*.

22. Departamento de Salud, *La división de Bienestar Público en su quinto aniversario*, 3.

23. "Estado Libre Asociado de Personal, San Juan, Puerto Rico: 20 plazas vacantes de Trabajador de Bienestar del Niño en adiestramiento para los siguientes pueblos: Corozol, Aibonito, Utuado, Yabucoa, Caguas, Barranquitas, Patillas, Comerío, Juncos,

Santa Isabel, Luquillo, Dorado, Isabela, Arecibo, Jayuya, Mayagüez, Coamo, Aguadilla, Quebradillas, Añasco," *El Imparcial*, April 30, 1953.

24. "Acabo Curso Trabajadores de Asistencia: Grupo de 80 Laborara en Oficina Bienestar; Mayoría Eran Maestros," *El Mundo*, April 25, 1953.

25. For more on the idea of the "family wage" in US history, see Fraser, "After the Family Wage"; Gordon, *Pitied but Not Entitled*.

26. Scholarship on gender, race, and US social welfare programs in the United States has explored these dynamics. See, for example, Gordon, *Pitied but Not Entitled*; Abramovitz, *Regulating the Lives of Women*; Mink, *The Wages of Motherhood*.

27. For more on the law in general, see Iglesias, "Como se emplean los $7.50?" The program is also discussed in Angueira, *Mujeres puertorriqueñas, "Welfare," y globalización*, 34; Díaz González, "Metas de asistencia pública y servicios sociales a la familia puertorriqueña," 2.

28. Zalduondo, "El programa de asistencia pública de estado libre asociado de Puerto Rico," 2.

29. Iglesias, "Como se emplean los $7.50?," 10.

30. Iglesias, "Como se emplean los $7.50?," 10.

31. In 1950, Titles I, IV, X, and XIV of the Social Security Act were extended to Puerto Rico. See Díaz Gonzáles, "Metas de asistencia pública."

32. Departmento de Salud, *La división de Bienestar Público en su quinto aniversario*, 13.

33. The case file records of the Department of Public Welfare from this period can be found in the Archivo General de Puerto Rico, Departamento de Salud, Departamento de Bienestar Público.

34. See, for example, Glenn, *Forced to Care*.

35. See, for example, Whalen, *From Puerto Rico to Philadelphia*.

36. Matos Rodríguez, *Women and Urban Change in San Juan, Puerto Rico, 1820–1868*; Crespo, "Domestic Work and Racial Divisions in Women's Employment in Puerto Rico, 1899–1930."

37. Del Moral, "'Una niña humilde y de color,'" 199.

38. Client Record, file 1264, box 152-A, tarea 65-101, Fondo Departamento de Salud, AGPR. Within the case files, various usages of descriptive racial terminology appear that aim to locate clients within societal and state understandings of racial hierarchies. These include numerous skin and hair color descriptions like the ones in this case. For more on the use of racial terminology in Puerto Rico to signify African descent and Blackness, see Godreau, "Slippery Semantics"; Godreau, *Scripts of Blackness*; Quiñones Rivera, "From Trigueñita to Afro-Puerto Rican."

39. See for example, Client Record, file 8343, box 42-58, tarea 64-1. Fondo Departamento de Salud, AGPR. See also Client Record, file 3803029040, box 80-15, tarea 80-52. Fondo Departamento de Salud, AGPR.

40. The client's name has been changed. Client Record, file D3033, folder 6977, box 151-A, tarea 65-101, Fondo Departamento de Salud, AGPR.

41. Client Record, file 1264, box 152-A, tarea 65-101, Fondo Departamento de Salud, AGPR.

42. The client's name has been changed. Client Record, file [missing], tarea 80-64, lista 80-24, Departmento de Servicio Social, Fondo Departamento de Salud, AGPR.

43. The client's name has been changed. Client Record, file A-2211, box 151-A, tarea 65-101, Departamento de Bienestar Público, Fondo Departamento de Salud, AGPR.

44. In addition to her report of having been enslaved, her name and that of her mother and grandmother are listed on historical records in the AGPR. She was born in Guayama, Puerto Rico, in 1868 and her grandmother was born in Africa in 1813. She was listed in US federal census records over the course of her life as "negra," "mulatta," and "blanca." For more on the history of slavery and transition to freedom in Guayama, see Figueroa, *Sugar, Slavery, and Freedom in Nineteenth-Century Puerto Rico*.

45. Client Record, File A-2211, Box 151-A, tarea 65-101, Departamento de Bienestar Público, Fondo Departamento de Salud, AGPR.

46. Client Record, file D-6977, box 151-A, tarea 65-101, Fondo Departamento de Salud, AGPR.

47. Client Record, file D-6977, box 151-A, tarea 65-101, Fondo Departamento de Salud, AGPR.

48. Vélez de Pérez, "Consideraciones en torno a los servicios de 'hogares de crianza' y 'amas de llaves,'; Villarini, "Visitando un ama de llaves."

49. Departmento de Salud, *La división de Bienestar Público en su quinto aniversario*, 19.

50. Boris and Klein, *Caring for America*. For more on the history of housekeeper and homemaker service programs, see Morlock, *Supervised Homemaker Services*; Morlock, *Homemaker Services*.

51. Villarini, "Visitando un ama de llaves."

52. Villarini, "Visitando un ama de llaves."

53. Villarini, "Visitando un ama de llaves."

54. The client's name has been changed. Client Record, file 3626, box 152-A, tarea 65-101, Fondo de Departamento de Salud, AGPR.

55. The name of the housekeeper has also been changed. Client Record, file 3626, box 152-A, tarea 65-101, Fondo de Departamento de Salud, AGPR.

56. The client's name has been changed. Client Record, file 3967, box 151-A, tarea 65-101, Fondo Departamento de Salud, AGPR.

57. Client Record, file 3967, box 151-A, tarea 65-101, Fondo Departamento de Salud, AGPR.

58. The client's name has been changed, Client Record, file 1963, box 151-A, tarea 65-101, Fondo de Departamento de Salud, AGPR.

59. Client Record, file 1963, box 151-A, tarea 65-101, Fondo de Departamento de Salud, AGPR.

60. Client Record, file 1963, box 151-A, tarea 65-101, Fondo de Departamento de Salud, AGPR.

61. For another example of women moving between work in factories and domestic work, see: Client Record, file D19372, box 151-A, tarea 65-101, Fondo de Departamento de Salud, AGPR.

62. Frank, "El centro de cuidado diurno de la escuela José Gautier Benítez." See also Blanch, "Las escuelas maternales del programa de emergencia de guerra."

63. See, for example, Lapp, "The Rise and Fall of Puerto Rico as a Social Laboratory."

64. Lewis, *La Vida*. See also Lewis, *A Study of Slum Culture*.

65. Safa, *The Urban Poor of Puerto Rico*.

66. Duany, "Anthropology in a Postcolonial Colony."

67. Briggs, *Reproducing Empire*.

68. Briggs, "La Vida, Moynihan, and Other Libels." On the historical construction of the welfare queen, see Nadasen, "From Widow to 'Welfare Queen'"; Boris, "On Cowboys and Welfare Queens."

69. For more on the welfare queen trope, see Hancock, *The Politics of Disgust*. On Latinos and the "racial script" of welfare cheating and dependency, see Molina, *How Race Is Made in America*.

70. Kornbluh, *The Battle for Welfare Rights*; Sheehan, *A Welfare Mother*.

71. Méndez, *Las ciencias sociales y el proceso político puertorriqueño*. These studies included numerous investigations of the impact of rural-to-urban migration and the development of new housing projects. See, for example, Back, *Slums, Projects, People*.

72. O'Conner, *Poverty Knowledge*; Goldstein, *Poverty in Common*.

73. Goldstein, *Poverty in Common*.

74. For the Bournes' New Deal activities, see chapter 2.

75. Bourne and Bourne, *Thirty Years of Change in Puerto Rico*. The study followed up on Bourne and Ramos, *Rural Life in Puerto Rico*.

76. For more on Lewis, see Rigdon, *The Culture Facade*; Rosemblatt, "Other Americas"; Dike, "La vida en la colonia."

77. Rosa Celeste Marín was the first Puerto Rican woman to receive a doctoral degree in social work. She received her degree from the University of Pittsburgh in 1953. "Agasajan doctora en trabajo social," *El Mundo*, April 23, 1953; "Colegio trabajadores sociales da homenaje a Dra. Rosa Marin," *El Mundo*, April 7, 1953; Rosa Celeste Marín, "La interpretacion de las funciones del trabajador social," *Revista de Servicio Social*, April 1957.

78. Rigdon, *The Culture Facade*, 74; Marín, *A Cross-Cultural Approach to Measurement of Family Functioning in Multi-Problem Families*; Marín, "Familias menesterosas con problemas múltiples en Puerto Rico."

79. Rigdon, *The Culture Facade*, 74–75.

80. Rigdon, *The Culture Facade*. One example of this collaboration is noted in an article that discusses a visit Lewis made to the University of Puerto Rico after being invited by Marín. See "En conferencia ofreció aqui: Antropólogo Oscar Lewis analiza aspectos del estudio realizó entre boricuas de NY," *El Mundo*, February 26, 1965.

81. Francisca Muriente's work is discussed in Rigdon, *The Culture Facade*; Briggs, *Reproducing Empire*. More details about her life are to be found in González, "Trabajo de campo en 'La Vida,'" which she wrote under the pseudonym Lewis gave her, Rosa González.

82. Rigdon, *The Culture Facade*, 74.

83. Lewis, *La Vida*.

84. González, "Trabajo de campo en 'La Vida,'" 9.

85. González, "Trabajo de campo en 'La Vida,'" 10.

86. González, "Trabajo de campo en 'La Vida,'" 12.

87. González, "Trabajo de campo en 'La Vida,'" 14.

88. González, "Trabajo de campo en 'La Vida.'"

89. Rigdon, *The Culture Facade*.

90. Briggs, "La Vida, Moynihan, and Other Libels"; Briggs, *Reproducing Empire*; Dike, "La vida en la colonia."

91. Rigdon, *The Culture Facade*, 81, 248.

92. See, for example, Dena Motley, "The Culture of Poverty in Puerto Rico and New York," *Social Security Bulletin*, September 1967, 18–23. Lewis received a grant from the Social Security Administration and the Welfare Administration to produce a book about the research process he employed in writing *La Vida*. This was published as *A Study of Slum Culture*.

93. For a life history of Helen Safa, see Yelvington, "The Making of a Marxist-Feminist-Latin Americanist Anthropologist."

94. Duany, "Anthropology in a Postcolonial Colony."

95. Duany, "Anthropology in a Postcolonial Colony."

96. For more on the history of the development of public housing in Puerto Rico and the racial legacies of these projects, see Dinzey-Flores, *Locked In, Locked Out*; LeBrón, *Policing Life and Death*; Tyrrell, *Colonizing Citizens*.

97. For example, while conducting the original research, she was assisted by Sila Nazario de Ferrer, who later became a politician, as well as by Carlos Chardón. Safa, *The Urban Poor of Puerto Rico*, ix. Safa's graduate student Carmen Pérez-Herráns worked with her on numerous studies and conducted the interviews that were used for her research in Puerto Rico in the 1980s. Pérez-Herráns went on to become an anthropologist who wrote about Puerto Rican women, labor, and social reproduction. See Pérez-Herráns, "Our Two Full Time Jobs."

98. Safa, *The Urban Poor of Puerto Rico*.

99. Safa, *The Urban Poor of Puerto Rico*.

100. Duany, "Anthropology in a Postcolonial Colony."

101. Safa, *The Urban Poor of Puerto Rico*, 109.

102. Safa notes in the preface to her book that James Weber was "a young photographer whom I met in Puerto Rico and who has come to love the Puerto Rican people as much as I do." Safa, *The Urban Poor of Puerto Rico*, x.

103. Safa, *The Urban Poor of Puerto Rico*.

104. Safa, *The Urban Poor of Puerto Rico*, 33.

105. Safa, *The Urban Poor of Puerto Rico*, 46.

106. Safa, *The Urban Poor of Puerto Rico*, 33.

107. Safa, *The Urban Poor of Puerto Rico*, 46.

108. Pérez-Herráns, "Our Two Full Time Jobs." See also Duany, "Anthropology in a Postcolonial Colony."

109. Briggs, "La Vida, Moynihan, and Other Libels"; Briggs, *Reproducing Empire*; Dike, "La vida en la colonia."

110. Kornbluh and Mink, *Ensuring Poverty*.

111. Warren et al., *Estirando el peso*.

CHAPTER 4. CARE WORKERS, HOUSEHOLD LABOR ORGANIZING, AND PUERTO RICAN MIGRATION AFTER 1944

Portions of this chapter were previously published in "Organizing Puerto Rican Domestics: Resistance and Household Labor Reform in the Puerto Rican Diaspora after 1930," *ILWCH: International Labor and Working-Class History* 8 (Winter 2015). I am very grateful to Eileen Boris and Premilla Nadasen for their comments.

1. This article builds on a rich tradition of Puerto Rican labor histories that have explored Puerto Rican migration, the central role of Puerto Rican women as founders of Puerto Rican migrant communities, and the important role that care workers and domestic workers played in this history. See, for example, Toro-Morn, "Gender, Class, Family, and Migration"; Toro-Morn, "Género, trabajo y migración"; Toro-Morn, "Yo era muy arriesgada"; Alicea, "'A Chambered Nautilus'"; Whalen, *From Puerto Rico to Philadelphia*; Ramos-Zayas, *National Performances*; Pérez, *The Near Northwest Side Story*; Rúa, *Latino Urban Ethnography and the Work of Elena Padilla*; Rúa, *A Grounded Identidad*; Fernández, *Brown in the Windy City*.

2. For more on the migration of the private labor agency, see, for example, Toro-Morn, "Gender, Class, Family, and Migration"; Toro-Morn, "Yo era muy arriesgada"; Toro-Morn, "Género, trabajo y migración"; Rúa, *Latino Urban Ethnography*; Rúa, *A Grounded Identidad*.

3. For more on gender and Puerto Rican labor migrations during this period, see Whalen, *From Puerto Rico to Philadelphia*; Findlay, *We Are Left without a Father Here*; Meléndez, *Sponsored Migration*; García-Colón, *Colonial Migrants at the Heart of Empire*; Loiselle, *Beyond Norma Rae*.

4. For an overview of this history in Chicago, see Mérida M. Rúa's history of the Puerto Rican diaspora in Chicago. Rúa, *A Grounded Identidad*.

5. On the history of Puerto Rican struggles over citizenship and links to migration to the United States, see Venator-Santiago, *Puerto Rico and the Origins of U.S. Global Empire*; McGreevey, *Borderline Citizens*; Erman, *Almost Citizens*.

6. For more on the history of household workers and care workers and their political organizing in the United States, see, for example, Hunter, *To 'Joy My Freedom*; Romero, *Maid in the U.S.A.*; Nadasen, *Household Workers Unite*; Ervin, *Gateway to Equality*; May, *Unprotected Labor*; Urban, *Brokering Servitude*; Boris, *Caring for America*; Boris and Salazar-Parreñas, *Intimate Labors*; Francisco-Menchavez, *The Labor of Care*.

7. Nadasen, *Household Workers Unite*. See also Ervin, *Gateway to Equality*; Ervin, "Breaking the 'Harness of Household Slavery.'"

8. Rúa, *A Grounded Identidad*.

9. Whalen, *From Puerto Rico to Philadelphia*; Findlay, *We Are Left without a Father Here*.

10. Findlay, *We Are Left without a Father Here*.

11. For more on Operation Bootstrap, see Dietz, *Economic History of Puerto Rico*. On migration policy, see Meléndez, *Sponsored Migration*.

12. Lapp, *Managing Migration*; Lapp, "The Rise and Fall of Puerto Rico as a Social Laboratory, 1945–1965"; Lauria-Perricelli, "A Study in Historical and Critical Anthropology."

13. Briggs, *Reproducing Empire*.

14. Baerga, *Género y trabajo*; Boris, *Home to Work*.

15. Whalen and Vázquez-Hernández, *The Puerto Rican Diaspora*; Maldonado, "Contract Labor and the Origins of Puerto Rican Communities in the United States"; Mills, Senior, and Kohn Goldsen, *The Puerto Rican Journey*; City University of New York, Centro de Estudios Puertorriqueños, and History Task Force, *Labor Migration under Capitalism*.

16. Senior, *Puerto Rican Emigration*; Ayala and Bernabe, *Puerto Rico in the American Century*; Whalen, *From Puerto Rico to Philadelphia*; Lapp, *Managing Migration*, 37.

17. Whalen, *From Puerto Rico to Philadelphia*, 52.

18. Studies of the contract labor program include Maldonado, "Contract Labor and the Origins of Puerto Rican Communities in the United States"; City University of New York, Centro de Estudios Puertorriqueños, and History Task Force, *Labor Migration under Capitalism*; Duany, *Blurred Borders*; Whalen, *From Puerto Rico to Philadelphia*; Rúa, *A Grounded Identidad*.

19. Lawrence R. Chenault wrote one of the most comprehensive sociological studies of Puerto Rican migration during the 1930s and documented the formation of the Puerto Rican Employment Agency. Chenault noted that "[to] the Puerto Rican this office is much more than just an employment agency. It may help him collect his wages, advise him about a pension, assist him with a problem or relief, or perform any of various other necessary services for him." Chenault, *The Puerto Rican Migrant in New York City*, 75. The history of these employment agencies is also described in Thomas, *Puerto Rican Citizen*; Duany, *Blurred Borders*.

20. Lorrin Thomas discusses the way that Puerto Rican government officials in the Bureau of Employment and Identification constructed and deployed racial categories within the employment agency, particularly in the creation of identification documents issued by the agency. Thomas, *Puerto Rican Citizen*. For more on the history of Puerto Ricans and racial formation, see Carlo-Beccera, "Which Is 'White' and Which Is 'Colored'?"

21. Between 1930 and 1936 the agency placed 1,537 women as domestic workers, a number equivalent to those placed as needleworkers and hand sewers (699) and garment workers (694) combined. Moreover, overall far more women were placed (3,641) than men (1,977). Chenault, *The Puerto Rican Migrant in New York City*, 74.

22. For more on gender, race, and the construction of the Puerto Rican as "other" in the United States, see Briggs, "La Vida, Moynihan, and Other Libels"; Findlay, "Dangerous Dependence or Productive Masculinity?"; Thomas, *Puerto Rican Citizen*; Thomas and Lauria-Santiago, *Rethinking the Struggle for Puerto Rican Rights*.

23. On Puerto Ricans and race in the United States, see Rodríguez, *Puerto Ricans*; Rodríguez, *Changing Race*; Duany, *The Puerto Rican Nation on the Move*; Duany, "The Rough Edges of Puerto Rican Identities"; Flores, *The Diaspora Strikes Back*.

24. Thomas, *Puerto Rican Citizen*.

25. Meléndez, "Vito Marcantonio, Puerto Rican Migration, and the 1949 Mayoral Election in New York City"; Meyer, *Vito Marcantonio*.

26. Thomas, *Puerto Rican Citizen.*

27. On the history of employment agencies placing domestic workers, see Palmer, *Domesticity and Dirt*; May, *Unprotected Labor*; Coble, *Cleaning Up.*

28. May, *Unprotected Labor*; Coble, *Cleaning Up.*

29. Chenault, *The Puerto Rican Migrant*, 79.

30. For more on the raced and gendered history of care and domestic work, see Glenn, *Unequal Freedom*; Boris and Salazar Parreñas, *Intimate Labors.*

31. Chenault, *The Puerto Rican Migrant*, 77.

32. For more on the history of Americanization and home economics in the Puerto Rican public education system, see Negrón de Montilla, *Americanization in Puerto Rico and the Public-School System, 1900–1930*; Navarro, *Creating Tropical Yankees.*

33. See Palmer, *Domesticity and Dirt*, 102. The Works Progress Administration trained African American women in household work. Wolcott, *Remaking Respectability*, 226–29; Jones, *Labor of Love, Labor of Sorrow*, 181–85.

34. For more on Casita María, see Sánchez Korrol, "The Forgotten Migrant." See also "Open House Held by Casita Maria," *New York Times*, November 20, 1939, 16.

35. Clark-Lewis, *Living In, Living Out*; Hunter, *To 'Joy My Freedom.*

36. On the PPD modernization programs, see Ayala and Bernabe, *Puerto Rico in the American Century*; Duany, *Blurred Borders.*

37. For more on how working-class Puerto Rican women became the subjects of state-sponsored social reform projects that rested on discourses about overpopulation, see Briggs, *Reproducing Empire.*

38. Dietz, *Economic History of Puerto Rico.*

39. On the contract labor program, see Maldonado, "Contract Labor and the Origins of Puerto Rican Communities in the United States"; City University of New York, Centro de Estudios Puertorriqueños, and History Task Force, *Labor Migration under Capitalism*; Duany, *Blurred Borders*; Whalen, *From Puerto Rico to Philadelphia.*

40. Whalen, *From Puerto Rico to Philadelphia.*

41. For more on the migration of domestic workers to Chicago, see, for example, Toro-Morn, "Gender, Class, Family, and Migration"; Toro-Morn, "Yo era muy arriesgada"; Toro-Morn, "Género, trabajo y migración"; Rúa, *Latino Urban Ethnography*; Rúa, *A Grounded Identidad.*

42. Rúa, *Latino Urban Ethnography.*

43. Toro-Morn, "Género, trabajo y migración."

44. Mérida M. Rúa notes that the racialization of the workers was one of the central concerns of Puerto Rican anthropologist Elena Padilla's thesis on Puerto Rican workers. Rúa, *Latino Urban Ethnography*, 135–37. See also Padilla, "Puerto Rican Immigrants in New York and Chicago."

45. "60 Puerto Ricans Picked up by Vice Squads," *Chicago Daily Tribune*, March 5, 1947. Employers also threatened some domestic workers with "deportation" if they left their jobs. Rúa, *A Grounded Identidad*, 8.

46. De Genova, "'White' Puerto Rican Migrants, the Mexican Colony, 'Americanization,' and Latino History."

47. De Genova, "'White' Puerto Rican Migrants, the Mexican Colony, 'Americanization,' and Latino History."

48. Palmer, *Domesticity and Dirt*.

49. Rúa, *A Grounded Identidad*, 7.

50. Muna Muñoz Lee would later go on to work as a translator for US anthropologist Oscar Lewis on the research that would result in the publication of his book *La Vida*, discussed here in chapter 3. Merida Rúa has documented the network of professional Puerto Rican women and students at the University of Chicago who allied themselves with the Puerto Rican domestic workers. Rúa, *Latino Urban Ethnography*.

51. According to Rúa, a group of more than fifty domestic workers held a protest on Thanksgiving Day where they "refused to work or speak English," and the protest was also attended by "members of the United States Progressives and the Worker's Defense League." Rúa, *A Grounded Identidad*, 11–13.

52. Rúa, *A Grounded Identidad*, 11–13.

53. Isales's full maiden name was Carmen Isales Hernández; after marrying Fred Wale, she often went by her married name, Carmen Wale. Cros and Quintero, "Entrevista a Carmen Isales."

54. Wale and Isales, *The Meaning of Community Development*. For more on the history of the Puerto Rican Division of Community Education (DIVEDCO), see Marsh Kennerly, *Negociaciones culturales*.

55. Cros and Quintero, "Entrevista a Carmen Isales."

56. Cros and Quintero, "Entrevista a Carmen Isales."

57. Rúa, *A Grounded Identidad*.

58. Isales was later hired by the Puerto Rican government to study and write about Puerto Rican migration. Senior and Isales, *The Puerto Ricans of New York City*.

59. Merida Rúa references Isales's report. Carmen Isales, "Report on Cases of Puerto Rican Laborers Brought to Chicago to Work as Domestics and Foundry Workers under Contract with Castle, Barton and Associates, Inc" (Confidential), March 22, 1947, sec. 4, series 2, subseries 9B, folder 277, Fundación Luis Muñoz Marín, San Juan, Puerto Rico; Rúa, *A Grounded Identidad*, 159.

60. Puerto Rican government representative Vicente Giégel-Polanco traveled to Chicago to investigate the case and stated that he "would recommend better contracts for the Puerto Rican workers who come to the United States in groups." See "Puerto Rican Senator Here to Aid Natives," *Chicago Daily Tribune*, January 10, 1947, 26; Whalen, *From Puerto Rico to Philadelphia*, 58.

61. For example, this question was raised during congressional hearings on the Federal Security Appropriations Bill in 1948, within which field agents of the Women's Bureau discussed their role intervening in the domestic work scandal in Chicago. See *Supplemental Hearing on Labor-Federal Security Appropriation Bill for 1949: Hearings before the Subcommittee of the Committee on Appropriations, United States Senate, Construction of Research Facilities*, 81st Cong., 2d Sess. (1948) (testimony of Miss Freida S. Miller, Director of the Women's Bureau, US Department of Labor), at 138–46. The original transcription of Frieda S. Miller's testimony is located in Frieda S. Miller Papers, box 8, folder 168, Schlesinger Library, Radcliffe Institute of Advanced Study, Harvard University.

62. Testimony of Miss Frieda S. Miller, *Supplemental Hearing on Labor-Federal Security Appropriation Bill for 1949*, at 135 (1948).

63. See García-Colón, "Claiming Equality." On the Migration Division, see Lapp, *Managing Migration*.

64. This project would take shape as DIVEDCO, a program that Carmen Isales helped create and direct with her husband Fred Wale. Marsh Kennerly, *Negociaciones culturales*.

65. The article that Isales published, "Welfare Facilities on the Island," included some material previously presented by social worker Celestina Zalduondo Goodsaid. It is included in Senior and Isales, *The Puerto Ricans of New York City*, 84–102.

66. Lapp, *Managing Migration*; Maldonado, "Contract Labor and the Origins of Puerto Rican Communities in the United States"; Duany, "A Transnational Colonial Migration"; Duany, *Blurred Borders*.

67. The African American press published a number of articles about Frances Phillips's departure to Puerto Rico. "Frances Phillips Leaves for Post," *Amsterdam News* (New York), August 28, 1948, 30; "Honored on Eve of Leaving for Assignment in Puerto Rico," *Afro-American* (Baltimore), August 28, 1948, 1; "Fete Gotham Expert Who Takes Puerto Rican Post," *Chicago Defender*, September 4, 1949.

68. On home economics in Puerto Rico, see Flores Ramos, *Mujer, familia y prostitución*.

69. Flores Ramos, *Mujer, familia, y prostitución*.

70. "Fete Gotham Expert Who Takes Puerto Rican Post," 17.

71. "Puerto Ricans Train for U.S. Domestic Jobs," *Chicago Daily Tribune*, August 8, 1947, 15.

72. "Household Workers from Puerto Rico Arrive in New York: First Group in Island Government's Project Go to Scarsdale," *Labor Information Bulletin*, May 1948. For more on this program, see Whalen, *From Puerto Rico to Philadelphia*, 59. For more on the role of these reformers in the creation of the Migration Division, see Lapp, *Managing Migration*.

73. "Household Workers from Puerto Rico Arrive in New York."

74. Whalen, *From Puerto Rico to Philadelphia*.

75. For a history of African American women's struggle to move away from live-in domestic work, see Clark-Lewis, *Living In, Living Out*.

76. On alternative forms of labor resistance developed by African American women domestic workers, see Hunter, *To 'Joy My Freedom*.

77. Petroamérica Pagán de Colón was a social worker, labor reformer, and Migration Division agent. See Lapp, *Managing Migration*.

CHAPTER 5. WOMEN'S LEADERSHIP IN STRUGGLES OVER
WELFARE, CITIZENSHIP RIGHTS, AND DECOLONIZATION IN THE
PUERTO RICAN DIASPORA

1. The article was published in *Bienestar Público*, a journal that was published by the Puerto Rican Department of Public Welfare and that featured articles by Puerto Rican social workers. Piñeiro, "Migrantes puertorriqueños en Nueva York y Santa Cruz." Flor M. Piñeiro (de Rivera) was a social worker who later became a librarian, expert in children's literature, author, and professor at the University of Puerto Rico, Río Piedras. Piñeiro received graduate training in social work from Columbia University

in New York City and graduate training in library sciences from the University of Kentucky. She wrote a book on the history of Puerto Rican children's literature as well as a book about the life and work of Afro-Puerto Rican intellectual Arturo Alfonso Schomburg. For more on her life and work see Gloria Borrás, "Publica libro sobre literatura infantil en PR," *El Mundo*, February 11, 1979, 16C.

2. Piñeiro, "Migrantes puertorriqueños en Nueva York y Santa Cruz."

3. For more on the history of Puerto Ricans, migration, and struggles for Puerto Rican rights in the United States, see, for example, Thomas, *Puerto Rican Citizen*; Findlay, *We Are Left without a Father Here*; Meléndez, *Sponsored Migration*; Thomas and Lauria-Santiago, *Rethinking the Puerto Rican Struggle for Rights*; Duany, *Blurred Borders*.

4. While the majority of studies on migration during this period have not focused on women's leadership, historian Virginia Sánchez Korrol has highlighted the importance of professional women within migrant networks in her scholarship. See, for example, Sánchez Korrol, "The Forgotten Migrant"; Sánchez Korrol, "In Search of Unconventional Women."

5. Chapter 4 of this book explored how social workers in Puerto Rico had been creating forms of casework that addressed migration to the United States since the 1920s and how this work intensified during and after the 1940s.

6. The Migration Division replaced the Puerto Rican Department of Labor's Bureau of Employment and Identification in New York City. As discussed in chapter 2, this agency was established in 1930 and helped provide migrants with identification documents to prove US citizenship and thus more easily obtain employment and social services. The Migration Division continued this work but was completely reimagined and reworked within the newly formed Employment and Migration Bureau. For more on the development of these government agencies, see Thomas, *Puerto Rican Citizen*; Meléndez, *Sponsored Migration*; García-Colón, *Colonial Migrants at the Heart of Empire*; Duany, *Blurred Borders*; Duany, "A Transnational Colonial Migration"; Whalen and Vázquez-Hernández, *The Puerto Rican Diaspora*; Lapp, *Managing Migration*; Cruz, *Puerto Rican Identity, Political Development, and Democracy in New York*

7. Meléndez, *Sponsored Migration*, 204–6.

8. "Informe Annual 1953–1954, División de Migración, Negociado Libre Asociado de Puerto Rico," CENTRO, Migrant Farm Labor in New York and New Jersey, the Puerto Rican Experience, 1948–1993, Offices of the Government of Puerto Rico in the United States, Archives of the Puerto Rican Diaspora, Center for Puerto Rican Studies, Hunter College, City University of New York, reel 52, box 2733, folder 1, box 2734. Hereafter the Offices of the Government of Puerto Rico in the United States collection is cited as OGPRUS.

9. See chapter 3 for a discussion of the creation of the Department of Public Welfare in Puerto Rico during this period. The rapid expansion of social welfare programs is discussed in Departamento de Salud, *La división de Bienestar Público en su quinto aniversario*.

10. Iglesias de Jesús and de Rodríguez, "Las problemas de los Puertorriqueños en Nueva York a traves de los casos referidos a la Unidad de Servicios Interagenciales de la División de Bienestar Público."

11. For a discussion of the increasingly expansive reach of the Puerto Rican government in the United States during this period, see Duany, *Blurred Borders*; Findlay, *We Are Left without a Father Here*; Meléndez, *Sponsored Migration*.

12. Manuel Cabranes was a social worker from Puerto Rico who had participated in the early formation of social work practice on the island, and he was one of the first twenty-five social workers to receive a social work license from the Board of Examiners of Social Workers in Puerto Rico. He also served as a member and secretary of this board. Cabranes received his social work training at Fordham University and worked at Melrose Settlement House in New York City before taking up his post in the Employment and Migration Bureau. "Primeras 25 licencias de trabajadores sociales," *Revista de Servicio Social*, July 1950, 64; "La junta examinadora de trabjadoras sociales tomo posesion," *El Mundo*, October 29, 1934, 1; Lapp, *Managing Migration*.

13. Male leadership in the field of social work was a pattern not only in the US offices but also in Puerto Rico. Many of the agencies on the archipelago were composed largely of women yet had male managers and directors. For example, Antonio Fernós Isern oversaw the Department of Health and therefore all social welfare activities.

14. Petroamérica Pagán de Colón taught in a Second Unit Rural school in Unibón de Cidra and worked for the Vocational Rehabilitation program of the Department of Public Instruction in Puerto Rico before she began working for the Puerto Rican government as a migration specialist. This background made her an ideal collaborator on questions of migrant labor and integration in the United States. She received her BA and social work certificate at the University of Puerto Rico, Río Piedras. Krüger Torres, *Enciclopedia grandes mujeres de Puerto Rico*, 115–16; Marina L. Molina, "Nuestras mujeres: Petroamérica Pagán de Colón," *El Mundo*, November 25, 1961, 2; "Petroamérica Pagán de Cólon Dicta Charla Sobre problemas de los Puertorriqueños en Nueva York," *El Mundo*, March 7, 1960, 9.

15. Mary Antoinette Cannon graduated from Bryn Mawr College in 1907 and received an MA in 1916 from the New York School of Social Work. She was well known in the field for having coauthored numerous publications on the practice of social casework that were used in schools throughout the United States. While in Puerto Rico, Cannon was hired to rework the entire curriculum for the School of Social Work. For more on Cannon's life and work, see Burgos Ortiz, *Pioneras de la profesión de trabajo social*; Pastor, "Antoinette Cannon"; Cannon, "Courses in Social Work at the University of Puerto Rico"; Lapp, *Managing Migration*; Sánchez, *Boricua Power*; Columbia University, School of Social Work, *Social Case Work*.

16. Francisca Bou was trained in medical social work at the School of Social Work at Tulane University and at Johns Hopkins University before working for PRERA and PRRA. Bou traveled to Germany after World War II and worked for the United Nations Relief and Rehabilitation Administration. She later worked in various positions for the Migration Division in New York. "Trabajadoras sociales de la isla están en Europa," *El Mundo*, September 18, 1945, 15. She was hired by the Puerto Rican Department of Labor to work with Puerto Rican domestic workers who were placed in White Plains, New York, as a part of early sponsored labor migration. See "Domesticas hallan idioma es obstaculo," *El Mundo*, March 3, 1948, 3; José Prados Herrero, "Nombran

dama para ayudante de Monserrat," *El Mundo*, December 5, 1956, 2; Lapp, *Managing Migration*, 122.

17. Matilde Pérez de Silva had worked as a medical social worker in Puerto Rico, and part of that work was managing programs for children with tuberculosis. Angela Negrón Mūnoz, "En las oficinas de la comisión para evitar la tuberculosis en los niños de edad escolar," *El Mundo*, April 2, 1939, 9; Pérez de Silva, "Rol del gobierno de Puerto Rico en la migración de Puertorriqueños a Estados Unidos"; Lapp, *Managing Migration*, 131.

18. "Informe Anual 1954–1955, Division de Migración, Negociado Libre Asociado de Puerto Rico," CENTRO, Migrant Farm Labor in New York and New Jersey, the Puerto Rican Experience, 1948–1993, OGPRUS, reel 52, box 2733, folder 2.

19. Aurora Garriga de Baralt studied social work at the University of Puerto Rico and then began working for the Department of Social Welfare, after which she became the director of the Interagency Services Bureau. For biographical details, see de Baralt, "Funciones y logros en los programas de Servicios Interagenciales."

20. For more about interagency services during the period, see, for example, de Baralt, "Se presto atención inmediata a 9,295 casos de naturaleza urgente referidos por agencias sociales del extranjero y del país"; de Baralt, "Se ofrecieron servicios múltiples al migrante Puertorriqueño"; de Baralt, "Un total de 14,246 casos se atendieron y se resolvieron durante el año, y los cuales recibieron 19,721 diferentes clases de servicios"; de Baralt, "La Oficina de Servicios Interagenciales y sus servicios a los niños de Puerto Rico."

21. The client's name has been changed here and a pseudonym is used. Social Service Records of the Migration Division, Archives of the Puerto Rican Diaspora, OGPRUS, box 2265, folder 1, case file 2525. Hereafter cited as María Cruz case file.

22. María Cruz case file.

23. The social services records of the Migration Division reveal the ways that migrant clients faced a variety of challenges as they sought to establish themselves in New York. For more on the history of client experiences applying for benefits from the social services section of the Migration Division of the Puerto Rican Department of Labor, see Amador, "Linked Histories of Welfare, Labor, and Puerto Rican Migration"; Amador, "Unruly Domestics."

24. For more on Puerto Rican arrival in New York and discrimination seeking social services, see Thomas, *Puerto Rican Citizen*; Sánchez Korrol, *From Colonia to Community*.

25. For more on single women and the history of welfare in the United States, see Gordon, *Pitied but Not Entitled*; Mink, *The Wages of Motherhood*.

26. There were numerous other women during the period who sought assistance from the social services section, particularly because they were seeking help to get access to social welfare benefits. In one case, an elder was seeking help when applying for old age assistance benefits. OGPRUS, box 2288, folder F6. In another case, a grandmother sought custody of her grandchild and dealt with a case that required correspondence between the Migration Division and offices in Puerto Rico. OGPRUS, box 2250, folder 3.

27. For more on the portrayal of Puerto Rican migrants as potential dependents on social welfare in the United States, see, for example, Briggs, "La Vida, Moynihan, and Other Libals"; Findlay, "Dangerous Dependence or Productive Masculinity?"

28. Natalia Molina has examined how Black and Latinx people have been understood to be welfare dependent as a part of what she describes as "racial scripts" that circulate in the United States. Molina, *How Race Is Made in America*. For more on the history of race and social welfare programs in the United States, see, for example, Quadagno, *The Color of Welfare*.

29. See Morales, *Puerto Rican Poverty and Migration*.

30. OGPRUS, box 2250, folder 1.

31. In one case, which began in June 1948, a woman dealt specifically with trying to apply for old age assistance and dealing with non–Puerto Rican social workers who sent her to the "Immigration and Naturalization Office" because of questions about her legal status. She had been born before the United States colonized Puerto Rico "but was a citizen." The Migration Division social worker ended up going with her to the social welfare office. OGPRUS, box 2247, folder 3.

32. For more on identification documents, see Thomas, *Puerto Rican Citizen*.

33. For more on residency requirements, access to social rights, and Puerto Ricans, see Rúa, *A Grounded Identidad*, 43. For the impact of residency requirements for social welfare benefits in New York City during the period, see Reese, *Backlash against Welfare Mothers*.

34. For example, in many cases, there were lengthy descriptions of "information for the purpose of determining residence," which might include information like the date of the first trip to the United States, time in Puerto Rico before departure, other trips to Puerto Rico, and the last trip. The social workers often tracked many dates and times people had moved between the United States. For one example, see OGPRUS, box 2360, folder F6.

35. There were numerous cases where Migration Division social workers corresponded with Puerto Rican officials about the "advisability of return to Puerto Rico," and they collected in particular information about the "ability of relatives to give assistance." In these cases, they would keep track of how much money different people in the family were making and what public assistance payment in Puerto Rico they would have access to would be. In some cases, the agencies would also request certified letters and documents that might include birth, death, marriage, or divorce certificates.

36. In one case, a man came to the Migration Division offices to seek assistance getting funds to return to Puerto Rico. According to the file, the social worker "explained that this office has no funds with which to pay his return fare to the island but suggested that to get in touch with the Transportation Unit of the Non-Resident Welfare Center." They suggested specific people for the man to speak with so that he could try to navigate his way back to Puerto Rico. OGPRUS, box 2250, folder 2.

37. In another case, a widow with seven children visited and corresponded with the Migration Division agents about returning to Puerto Rico, and there were numerous documents pertaining to the correspondence between the Department of Welfare and

the Migration Division that were kept in the case file. OGPRUS, box 2248, folder 06, case file 0325.

38. Within the social work case files, the social workers kept track of their correspondence with social welfare agencies on behalf of clients and also recorded in their notes various interactions with social welfare officials. They also listed the names of social work officials who were collaborators or who might be helpful to Puerto Ricans. In the cases they often referred clients to specific officials at social welfare agencies in New York who spoke Spanish or who were more likely to be helpful and nondiscriminatory to Puerto Rican clients.

39. See Lasch-Quinn, *Black Neighbors*. For more on Puerto Ricans and the history of settlement houses, see Lee, *Building a Latino Civil Rights Movement*.

40. Casita María was a Catholic organization that served the Puerto Rican community in New York City; it was founded by a Puerto Rican nun, Carmela Zapata Bonilla Marrero, who was known as "Sister Carmelita." Sánchez Korrol, *From Colonia to Community*; Sánchez Korrol, "In Search of Unconventional Women."

41. For more on Puerto Rican representation in the press during this period, see Findlay, "Dangerous Dependence or Productive Masculinity?"

42. O'Connor, *Poverty Knowledge*.

43. Welfare Council of New York City and the Committee on Puerto Ricans in New York City, *Puerto Ricans in New York City*.

44. Sánchez, *Boricua Power*. According to historian Lorrin Thomas, fifteen out of forty-six members of the committee were Puerto Rican, and it was rumored that Manuel Cabranes was in charge of determining who would be in the group. Thomas, *Puerto Rican Citizen*, 153. While the agency drew criticism for not going far enough to create social change in Puerto Rican communities, its results did challenge the US public and social service agencies to reassess their understandings of Puerto Ricans and welfare.

45. Welfare Council of New York City and the Committee on Puerto Ricans in New York City, *Puerto Ricans in New York City*.

46. Sonia Lee notes that there was only a 10 percent participation rate according to Raymond Hilliard, compared to 4.2 percent of the total population. Lee, *Building a Latino Civil Rights Movement*, 56; Hilliard and Department of Welfare, *The "Puerto Rican Problem" of the City of New York Department of Welfare*.

47. *Extension of Social Security to Puerto Rico and the Virgin Islands: Hearings before a Subcommittee of the Committee on Ways and Means, House of Representatives*, 81st Cong., 1st Sess. (1950).

48. "2 Groups to Study Islands' Problems: House Ways and Means Committee to PR and Virgin Islands," *New York Times*, November 11, 1949. The social work journal *Bienestar Público* published an edition that largely focused on questions surrounding the extension of the Social Security Act to Puerto Rico in March 1949. Included in this issue are reprints of the testimony provided at the House of Representatives in favor of broader coverage to Puerto Rico by Antonio Fernós Isern (resident commissioner of Puerto Rico in Washington) and Celestina Zalduondo Goodsaid (director of the Division of *Bienestar Público*). It also included an essay by Belén Milagros Serra outlining how the Social Security Act had been gradually, provisionally, and partially

extended to Puerto Rico over the years. Serra, "La ley de Seguridad Social vigente y los proyectos H.R. 2645 y H.R. 2892 de la Cámara de Representantes, Congreso Federal No. 81."

49. Social workers reported upon their progress in advocating social policies in Puerto Rico and for the extension of broader coverage under the Social Security Act in their writings from the period. They would also include outlines and overviews of the forms of social legislation that they promoted or introduced in social work journals. See, for example, "Legislación social propulsada por el Colegio de Trabajadores Sociales." For more on the lobbying efforts of Puerto Rican social workers and politicians and how they sought better coverage under the Social Security Act, see Pagán Torres, "Actividades de la Comisión en Washington."

50. Pintado de Rahn, "The People of the Caribbean."

51. Matilde Pérez de Silva in particular oversaw visits of groups from the United States that traveled to Puerto Rico during this period. Lapp, *Managing Migration.*

52. *Extension of Social Security to Puerto Rico and the Virgin Islands: Hearings before a Subcommittee of the Committee on Ways and Means, House of Representatives,* 81st Cong., 1st Sess. (1950).

53. See, for example, "Puerto Rico Left Out," *New York Times,* July 18, 1950; "Puerto Rican Security," *Washington Post,* July 18, 1950.

54. See, for example, Grosfoguel, *Colonial Subjects.* In the press, see "Social Work Held Key to Democracy: Aim to Trained Group Is Sole Way to Ease Problems of Needy People, Class Hears: Point 4 Program Hailed," *New York Times,* October 5, 1950.

55. On the history of Puerto Rico as a "social laboratory," see Lapp, "The Rise and Fall of Puerto Rico as a Social Laboratory"; Briggs, *Reproducing Empire;* Goldstein, *Poverty in Common.*

56. "Ewing Off to Map Puerto Rican Aid: Administrators to Plan Island's Social Security as Congress Approval Is Awaited," *New York Times,* April 25, 1950, 19. See also Grosfougel, *Colonial Subjects,* 108.

57. For more on Matilde Pérez de Silva and other Migration Division representatives taking US government workers and officials to Puerto Rico, see Lapp, *Managing Migration.*

58. See material about earlier conferences referenced in Commonwealth of Puerto Rico, Department of Labor, *Conclusions of the Migration Conference Held in San Juan, Puerto Rico, March 1–7, 1953.*

59. A 1949 issue of *Bienestar Público* was dedicated to articles about the need to extend the Social Security Act. They included some of the arguments that social workers and social reformers made during this period. See, for example, Descartes, "Capacidad economica de Puerto Rico para la seguridad social"; Muñoz, "Instrumentación de los Seguros Sociales en Puerto Rico."

60. These city officials also believed that by traveling to Puerto Rico they could inform those on the archipelago that they would still face hard conditions in the United States and therefore should not migrate. See, for example, "City No Bonanza—Hilliard Warns: Welfare Chief, in Puerto Rico, Declares New York Streets 'Are Not Paved in Gold,'" *New York Times,* August 11, 1950.

61. "Services Extended for Puerto Ricans: City Departments Announce More Aid at Meeting of Mayor's Committee," *New York Times*, October 5, 1949.

62. "Puerto Rican Help Urged by O'Dwyer: Telegrams to Congress Group Call for Social Security Aid for People of Puerto Rico," *New York Times*, July 12, 1950, 27.

63. On the history of the Jayuya Uprising as a part of nationalist organizing led by a Puerto Rican independence leader, see Ayala and Bernable, *Puerto Rico in the American Century*, 167; Wagenheim, *Nationalist Heroines*; Power, *Solidarity across the Americas*.

64. For more on the life of Blanca Canales, see Canales, *La constitución es la revolución*; Wagenheim, *Nationalist Heroines*, 51–90; Burgos Ortiz, *Pioneras de la profesión de trabajo social en Puerto Rico*.

65. There is growing literature on the history of Puerto Rican women's participation in the Puerto Rican movement for independence. This research is rewriting the history of Puerto Rican independence leaders with a focus on the forms of solidarity, resistance, and global connections that were forged during this period. See, for example, Wagenheim, *Nationalist Heroines*; Power, *Solidarity across the Americas*; Plácido, "A Global Vision"; Materson, "Gender, Generation, and Women's Independence Organizing in Puerto Rico"; Power, "Puerto Rican Women Nationalists vs. U.S. Colonialism"; Jiménez, "Puerto Rico under the Colonial Gaze."

66. For more on the lives and political engagement of these social workers, see Burgos Ortiz, *Pioneras de la profesión de trabajo social*; Rivera de Alvarado, *Lucha y visión de Puerto Rico libre*; Canales, *La constitución es la revolución*; Wagenheim, *Nationalist Heroines*.

67. Canales, *La constitución es la revolución*.

68. Canales, *La constitución es la revolución*, 12–23.

69. For more on the history of the nationalist movement and Canales activism during this period, see Wagenheim, *Nationalist Heroines*; Power, *Solidarity across the Americas*.

70. While Blanca Canales was imprisoned in the United States, she befriended African American communist organizer Claudia Jones; for more on this history, see Boyce Davies, *Left of Karl Marx*.

71. The leadership of Puerto Rican women who supported Puerto Rican independence in activism for the expansion of the Social Security Act is one example of this, and Carmen Rivera de Alavardo wrote extensively about this. Rivara de Alvarado, *Lucha y visión de Puerto Rico libre*.

72. Burgos Ortiz, *Pioneras de la profesión de trabajo social*; Rivera de Alvarado, *Lucha y visión de Puerto Rico libre*; Canales, *La constitución es la revolución*.

73. Power, *Solidarity across the Americas*.

74. Rivera de Alvarado, *Lucha y visión de Puerto Rico libre*.

75. Seda Rodríguez, "Legado de Carmen Rivera de Alvarado a la profesion de trabajo social en Puerto Rico"; Rivera de Alvarado, *Lucha y visión de Puerto Rico libre*.

76. Rivera de Alvarado, *Lucha y visión de Puerto Rico libre*, 97. For more of Rivera de Alvarado's writings on the history of social work, see Rivera de Alvarado, Torres

Rivera, and Rivera de Ríos, *Puerto Rico*; Trina Rivera de Ríos, Awilda Paláu de López, Candi Crespo, and Carmen Rivera de Alvarado, *Hacia un Trabaja Social Puertor-riqueño, Accion Social Puertorriqueña: Transcripción de Cuatro Conferencia sobre Trabajo Social en Puerto Rico*, Edición de Haynán Vázquez, April 25, 1970, Colección Puertorriqueña, Universidad de Puerto Rico (UPR), Río Piedras.

77. Rivera de Alvarado, *Lucha y visión de Puerto Rico libre*, 159; Rivera de Alvarado, *Lucha y visión de Puerto Rico libre*, 97.

78. Lapp, *Managing Migration*; Meléndez, *Sponsored Migration*.

79. Senior, *The Puerto Ricans*.

80. Cabranes was initially transferred to the New York branch of the agency, but, frustrated with the demotion, he left the Migration Division for the New York Department of Welfare in 1951. He would continue to hold different public service positions working with Puerto Rican communities in the United States throughout his long career.

81. Joseph Monserrat came to the United States when he was three years old and was raised in a foster home in New York City. As a young man, he studied social science at Columbia University before working as a social worker at Madison House in Manhattan, Melrose House in the Bronx, and the Good Neighbor Federation Settlement. In 1954, he declined a position on the MACPRA in order to focus his efforts on the Migration Division's community work. There is a short biographical essay about Monserrat in his archived personal papers. See Joseph Monserrat Papers, Archives of the Puerto Rican Diaspora, Center for Puerto Rican Studies, Hunter College, City University of New York, box 1, folder 4. See also Wolfgang Saxon, "Joseph Monserrat, 84, Leader in Efforts to Unify Latinos," *New York Times*, November, 19, 2005; Lapp, *Managing Migration*.

82. For more on the history of Puerto Ricans and the politics of social citizenship in particular, see Thomas, *Puerto Rican Citizen*; Lee, *Building a Latino Civil Rights Movement*; Thomas and Lauria-Santiago, *Rethinking the Struggle for Puerto Rican Rights*.

83. In her memoir, Antonia Pantoja discusses how her relationship with Matilde Pérez de Silva helped her win the scholarship. Pérez de Silva had been a medical social worker in Puerto Rico and helped Pantoja when she was treated for tuberculosis at a school sanatorium. Pantoja, *Memoir of a Visionary*.

84. Lapp, *Managing Migration*; Meléndez, *Sponsored Migration*.

85. Lee, *Building a Latino Civil Rights Movement*.

CHAPTER 6. COMMUNITY ORGANIZERS, CIVIL RIGHTS ACTIVISM, AND DEMANDS FOR CARE IN PUERTO RICAN COMMUNITIES IN THE UNITED STATES

1. Antonia Pantoja, "Voces de Mujeres: Puerto Rican Women and Community Development in New York City," unpublished manuscript of a speech delivered at the Bella Abzug Conference Series, Hunter College, May 2, 1989. Antonia Pantoja Papers, box 24, folder 2, Archives of the Puerto Rican Diaspora, Center for Puerto Rican Studies, Hunter College, City University of New York. For more on the life and work of Pantoja, see Pantoja, *Memoir of a Visionary*.

2. Pantoja, "Voces de Mujeres."

3. In "Voces de Mujeres," Pantoja gave an example of this erasure within contemporary narratives of the history of ASPIRA, the educational organization she helped found in New York City, noting that histories of the group had omitted women's leadership in the organization. She described how these histories had described ASPIRA as a group developed by male elites interested in grooming another elite generation of male leaders to follow in their footsteps. For Pantoja, the history of the organization was different and represented and revealed the effectiveness of women's political organization for educational reform and social change. She believed many previous narratives deliberately silenced women's contributions, and this could only be rectified by recovering and documenting the central role that women had played as political actors in New York.

4. For more on the life and work of Pantoja, see Pantoja, *Memoir of a Visionary*; Sánchez Korrol, "Antonia Pantoja and the Power of Community Action"; Jiménez, *Antonia Pantoja*.

5. Pantoja, *Memoir of a Visionary*, 78.

6. For more on the history of Black Puerto Rican and Afro-Puerto Rican activism in the United States, see, for example, Denis-Rosario, *Drops of Inclusivity*; Lee, *Building a Latino Civil Rights Movement*; Hoffnung-Garksof, *Racial Migrations*.

7. For more on Puerto Rican participation in the US civil rights movement, see Lee, *Building a Latino Civil Rights Movement*; Thomas, *Puerto Rican Citizen*; Cruz, *Puerto Rican Identity, Political Development, and Democracy in New York, 1960–1990*; Thomas and Lauria-Santiago, *Rethinking the Struggle for Puerto Rican Rights*; Fernández, *The Young Lords*.

8. Recent studies on Puerto Rican activism have highlighted activists' organizing around health care, public health, social services, and reproductive health justice and rights. In addition, studies of health care and social service activism in New York have also shown the centrality of Puerto Rican activists in these struggles. See, for example, Fernández, *The Young Lords*; Muzio, *Radical Imagination, Radical Humanity*; Carroll, *Mobilizing New York*; Kornbluh, *A Woman's Life Is a Human Life*.

9. Pantoja, *Memoir of a Visionary*, 193.

10. Pantoja, *Memoir of a Visionary*, 84.

11. Pantoja, *Memoir of a Visionary*, 5–13

12. For more on the history of labor and tobacco in Puerto Rico, see Levy, *Puerto Ricans in the Empire*. On Afro-Latino History, see Román and Flores, *The Afro-Latin@ Reader*.

13. Pantoja discusses her identity as a Black Puerto Rican woman in Perry, "Memorias de una vida de obra (Memories of a Life of Work)."

14. For more on PRRA, see Mathews, *Puerto Rican Politics and the New Deal*; Rodríguez, *A New Deal for the Tropics*.

15. Pantoja, *Memoir of a Visionary*, 30.

16. Pantoja, *Memoir of a Visionary*, 33.

17. For more on the Segundas Unidades Rurales, see chapter 2 of this book. See also Vizcarrondo, *Second-Unit Rural Schools of Porto Rico*.

18. Jiménez, *Antonia Pantoja*. In this documentary film, Pantoja discusses the racial and gender restrictions she faced as a young woman in Puerto Rico and how this impacted her desire to migrate.

19. For more on the history of Puerto Rican queer migrations to the United States, see La Fountain-Stokes, *Queer Ricans*. On the life of Antonia Pantoja, see Torres, "Boricua Lesbians"; Torres, "Queering Puerto Rican Women's Narratives"; Negrón-Muntaner, "Can You Imagine?"

20. See Torres, "Boricua Lesbians." In the conclusion of her memoir, Pantoja writes, "Although I have not discussed directly my sexuality, I am also at peace with this part of me. I have decided not to discuss it in this book because I have always drawn a line between my private and public life. However, I wish to eliminate the possibility of being misinterpreted and described as secretive about this matter. I claim it at various points throughout the book." Pantoja, *Memoir of a Visionary*, 197.

21. The Jefferson School was run by the Communist Party of the United States and operated in New York City providing classes to adults.

22. Pantoja, *Memoir of a Visionary*, 69.

23. Pantoja, *Memoir of a Visionary*, 69–70.

24. Pantoja, *Memoir of a Visionary*, 68.

25. Pantoja, *Memoir of a Visionary*, 70.

26. Marta Valle was a Puerto Rican social worker who was born in Harlem and who worked for the Human Resources Administration in New York. In an interview in 1967, she said this about her career trajectory: "After graduating from college in 1954, I became a social investigator with the Welfare Department. I was 20 years old at the time. After a year and a half there, I went to work in an East Harlem settlement house, then went back to school for a year, had a baby (during a short-lived marriage), went back to school to get my master's degree in social work, then worked in the Lower East Side community organizing for years." May Okon, "Little Lady—Big Job: Marta Valle Helps Get to the Roots of the Problems in Her Native Spanish Harlem," *Daily News* (New York), July 2, 1967, 152.

27. For more on the history of social work in the United States, see Walkowitz, *Working with Class*; Gordon, *Pitied but Not Entitled*.

28. Pantoja, *Memoir of a Visionary*, 74.

29. Pantoja and Martell, "Mi Gente." For more on the history of Puerto Rican women in New York during the period, see Sánchez Korrol, "Survival of Puerto Rican Women in New York before World War II."

30. For more on the war on poverty and women's grassroots organizing, see Orleck and Hazirjian, *The War on Poverty*. Also see Back, "Parent Power"; Carrol, *Mobilizing New York*.

31. Lee, *Building a Latino Civil Rights Movement*.

32. For example, as described in the introduction to this book, Yolanda Sánchez was an Afro-Puerto Rican social worker and grassroots organizer with a long political legacy in New York. She began her work as a caseworker with the Department of Welfare and later worked as one of the staff members of both ASPIRA and PRACA. She went on to be president of the East Harlem Council for Human Services, as well as a

director of the Office of Puerto Rican Programs at the City University of New York. For a brief obituary, see González, "East Harlem's Trailblazer Yolanda Sánchez Leaves a Legacy (1932–2012)."

33. Duany, *Blurred Borders*; Meléndez, *Sponsored Migration*.

34. Over time the work of the agency had focused on the discrimination that Puerto Ricans faced, and social workers took up the role of advocates on behalf of migration. See chapter 5 of this book. Also see Lapp, *Managing Migration*.

35. The members included Puerto Rican activists such as Alice Cardona, Josephine Nieves, Yolanda Sánchez, Luis Nuñez, and Eddie González.

36. Pantoja later wrote that "the leadership of the office [the Migration Division] espoused integration and assimilation, but I knew that only those of us who were white-skinned had any hope of this kind of acceptance." Pantoja, *Memoir of a Visionary*, 77.

37. See Cannon, "Courses in Social Work at the University of Puerto Rico"; Lapp, *Managing Migration*.

38. Lapp, *Managing Migration*.

39. These scholarships were the results of earlier organizing and demands for the Puerto Rican social workers in previous years, and one major scholarship fund was organized by Manuel Cabranes, the former director of the Migration Division. Cabranes oversaw the distribution of aid to Puerto Rican students, many of whom went to school for social work. Manuel Cabranes, Scholarship Fund Papers, New York Public Library Archive and Manuscripts Division.

40. Pantoja, *Memoir of a Visionary*.

41. Pantoja, *Memoir of a Visionary*, 84.

42. Lee, *Building a Latino Civil Rights Movement*, 97.

43. For more on the political legacy and work of Manny Díaz, see Lee and Díaz, "'I Was the One Percenter.'" See also Lee, *Building a Latino Civil Rights Movement*. Historian Sonia Lee notes that Díaz was an Afro-Puerto Rican activist who began working at the Union Settlement House when he was a teenager, and after serving in World War II he became a social worker. Like Pantoja he attended Columbia University's School of Social Work.

44. On changes in the settlement house movement, see Lasch-Quinn, *Black Neighbors*. On Puerto Ricans and the settlement house movement, see Lee, *Building a Latino Civil Rights Movement*.

45. Lee, *Building a Latino Civil Rights Movement*. Also see Bell, *The Black Power Movement and American Social Work*.

46. For more on the history of the Commission of Intergroup Relation, see Marta Varela, who notes, "The creation of the Commission on Intergroup Relations in 1955 was an attempt to create an institutionalized mechanism to address the individual problems of discrimination forcefully and systematically." Varela, "The First Forty Years of the Commission on Human Rights," 9.

47. Frank Horne was an African American educator and poet who worked in the 1930s for President Franklin Delano Roosevelt as assistant director of the Division of Negro Affairs, National Youth Administration. He later worked for the US Hous-

ing Authority and various government institutions. For his obituary, see "Frank S. Horne, First Director of City Rights Panel, Dies at 75," *New York Times*, September 8, 1973, 57.

48. In Lillian Jiménez's pathbreaking documentary about the life and legacy of Antonia Pantoja, Pantoja discusses race and describes the majority of Puerto Ricans as a people of color. Jiménez, *Antonia Pantoja ¡Presente!* On racial silencing in Puerto Rican history, see Rodríguez-Silva, *Silencing Race.*

49. The project was first named the Puerto Rican-Hispanic Leadership Forum and then the Puerto Rican Leadership Forum before it was given the name the Puerto Rican Forum. See Sánchez Korrol, *From Colonia to Community*, 225–26.

50. Puerto Rican Forum, *A Study of Poverty Conditions in the Puerto Rican New York Community*; Puerto Rican Forum, *The Puerto Rican Community Development Project.*

51. For more on PRACA, see Sánchez, *Boricua Power.*

52. Pantoja, *Memoir of a Visionary*; ASPIRA, *National Conference.*

53. See Nieto, *Puerto Rican Students in U.S. Schools.*

54. Lee, *Building a Latino Civil Rights Movement*, 114.

55. On queer history and African Americans in the civil rights movement, see Emilio, *Lost Prophet*; Mumford, *Not Straight, Not White.*

56. Pantoja, *Memoir of a Visionary.*

57. Torres, "Queering Puerto Rican Women's Narratives," 104. Torres notes that the silencing of sexuality in Pantoja's memoir highlights "the weight of public secrets and shame" and illuminates how Puerto Rican women managed "negotiating multiple identities in public and private contexts." See also Torres, "Boricua Lesbians"; Negrón-Muntaner, "'Can You Imagine?'"

58. Jiménez, *Antonia Pantoja ¡Presente!*

59. Martell, "'In the Belly of the Beast.'"

60. Martell, "'In the Belly of the Best.'" This story is similar to many others told by women who participated in movements of the time, including that of Iris Morales. See, for example, Morales, "¡Palante, Siempre Palante!"; Morales, *Through the Eyes of Rebel Women.*

61. Pantoja and Martell, "Mi Gente." For more on the Latin Women's Collective, see Muzio, *Radical Imagination, Radical Humanity.*

62. For a history of Puerto Rican activism and leftist politics during this period in the United States, see Torres and Velázquez, *The Puerto Rican Movement.*

63. Torres and Velázquez, *The Puerto Rican Movement.*

64. Fernández, "Between Social Service Reform and Revolutionary Politics."

65. See, for example, the story of Carmen Vivian Rivera who was a member of ASPIRA and later joined the Young Lords. Torres and Velázquez, *The Puerto Rican Movement*, 192. Pantoja reflects on this with pride in the documentary film *Antonia Pantoja¡Presente!*

66. On connections between the Young Lords and other social movements of the period, see Enck-Wanzer, *The New York Young Lords and the Struggle for Liberation*; Ogbar, "Puerto Rico en mi corazón."

67. For example, the Puerto Rican Socialist Party organized in New York during this period. It was first known as the Movimiento Pro-Independencia (MPI), and later as the Partido Socialista Puertorriqueño. For more on this, see Torres and Velázquez, *The Puerto Rican Movement*.

68. For a more complete history of El Comité and its intersection with other groups, see Muzio, *Radical Imagination, Radical Humanity*. Also see "Another West Side Story: An Interview with Members of El Comité-MINP," in Torres and Velázquez, *The Puerto Rican Movement*, 88–106.

69. Martell, "'In the Belly of the Beast'"; Pantoja and Martell, "Mi Gente." A two-part oral history interview with Esperanza Martell conducted by Andrew Viñales is located in the CENTRO: 100 Puerto Ricans Oral History Project, in the Archives of the Puerto Rican Diaspora, Center for Puerto Rican Studies, Hunter College, City University of New York (hereafter CENTRO 100): Esperanza Martell Interview, April 25, 2018, and May 23, 2018.

70. El Comité was also not just composed of Puerto Rican members; it was also composed of members from a variety of backgrounds, including Dominican, African American, and white members.

71. For more on history of the Black Panthers social service and public health activism, see Nelson, *Body and Soul*; Bell, *The Black Power Movement and American Social Work*.

72. Juan González, as cited by historian Carmen Theresa Whalen in "Bridging Homeland and Barrio Politics: The Young Lords in Philadelphia," in Torres and Velázquez, *The Puerto Rican Movement*, 114.

73. In Chicago the group had begun with organizing childcare services for "welfare mothers" so that they could work. Fernández, "Between Social Service Reform and Revolutionary Politics." See also Morales, *Through the Eyes of Rebel Women*.

74. Historian Sonia Lee discusses the connection between radical and reformist perspectives toward community organizing and social work in her work on Puerto Rican civil rights organizing in New York City. Lee, *Building a Latino Civil Rights Movement*.

75. Martell, "'In the Belly of the Beast,'" 173.

76. Carmen Vivan Vivera, "Our Movement: The Women's Story," cited in Torres and Velázquez, *The Puerto Rican Movement*, 192.

77. Martell, "'In the Belly of the Beast,'" 173.

78. See "The Young Lords: Ten Point Health Program," originally published in the newspaper *Young Lords Organization*, January 1970, and republished in Enck-Wanzer, *The Young Lords*, 188–89. For more on the health activism involving Lincoln Hospital, see Chowkwanyun, "Biocitizenship on the Ground."

79. Historians Eileen Boris and Jennifer Klein have traced the development of health care aid training programs. They show how these training programs targeted poor women and women of color who were seen as being potential dependents on welfare or the state to be trained in these low-paying jobs. These women were trained to take care of other poor people through their work in low-waged employment in the health care professions. Boris and Klein, *Caring for America*.

80. This movement would end up becoming even larger as it encompassed other institutions and also began to shed light on the eugenics and sterilization efforts that had been a part of the history of US intervention and colonization in Puerto Rico. For more on the history of sterilization of Puerto Rican women and struggles for reproductive justice in Puerto Rico and the Puerto Rican diaspora, see Nelson, *Women of Color and the Reproductive Rights Movement*; Briggs, *Reproducing Empire*; López, *Matters of Choice*; Kornbluh, *A Woman's Life Is a Human Life*.

81. Nelson, *Women of Color and the Reproductive Rights Movement*, 131.

82. Torres and Velázquez, *The Puerto Rican Movement*, 97.

83. Morales, *Through the Eyes of Rebel Women*, 72.

84. Morales, *Through the Eyes of Rebel Women*.

85. For more on the history of Puerto Rican women in the struggle for Puerto Rican independence, see Wagenheim, *Nationalist Heroines*.

86. "An Interview with Blanca Canales," originally published in the newspaper *Palante*, September 25, 1970, and republished in Eck-Wanzer, *The Young Lords*, 167–69. See also Canales, *La constitución es la revolución*.

87. Rivera de Alvarado, *Lucha y visión de Puerto Rico libre*. For an overview of her life and work, see Seda Rodríguez, "Legado de Carmen Rivera de Alvarado a la profesion de trabajo social en Puerto Rico."

88. Torres and Velázquez, *The Puerto Rican Movement*.

89. While Carmen Rivera de Alvarado was in New York for this trip, she also participated in making a presentation to the United Nations about the colonial status of Puerto Rico. Seda Rodríguez, "Legado de Carmen Rivera de Alvarado a la profesion de trabajo social en Puerto Rico," 25.

90. Rivera de Alvarado, *Lucha y visión de Puerto Rico libre*.

91. The devastating impact of US government-sponsored surveillance and counterintelligence tactics used against the Young Lords during the period have been well documented by scholars. This literature has particularly emphasized the impact of COINTELPRO, the counterintelligence program of the FBI. Gautier-Mayoral and Blanco-Stahl, "COINTELPRO en Puerto Rico." Historian Johanna Fernández has also shed new light on the significant surveillance of the Young Lords and other leftist organizations of the period by COINTELPRO as well as by the New York police. See, for example, Fernández, *The Young Lords*; Joseph Goldstein, "Old Surveillance Is Found, Forcing Big Brother Out of Hiding," *New York Times*, June 16, 2016.

92. Morales, *Through the Eyes of Rebel Women*, 144.

93. Morales, *Through the Eyes of Rebel Women*, 147.

94. Esperanza Martell Interview, April 25, 2018, and May 23, 2018, CENTRO 100.

95. Perry, "Memorias de una vida de obra (Memories of a Life of Work)," 256.

96. Perry, "Memorias de una vida de obra (Memories of a Life of Work)," 254; Pantoja and Martell, "Mi Gente."

97. Pantoja, *Memoir of a Visionary*.

98. Pantoja, *Memoir of a Visionary*; Olivares, "LGBT Activist Wilhelmina Perry Remembers Her Partner, Antonia Pantoja."

99. Pantoja and Blourock, "Cultural Pluralism Redefined," 7.

100. Pantoja and Blourock, "Cultural Pluralism Redfined," 8.

101. Pantoja and Blourock, "Cultural Pluralism Redfined," 20.

102. Rivera de Alvarado, *Lucha y visión de Puerto Rico libre*.

103. Rivera de Alvarado, "Trabajo social, vocación de libertad," in *Lucha y visión de Puerto Rico libre*, 99. Also see Seda Rodríguez, "Legado Carmen Rivera de Alvarado a la profesion de trabajo social en Puerto Rico." For more on the history of social workers and nationalism in Puerto Rico, see Burgos Ortiz, *Pioneras de la profesión de trabajo social.*

104. Cotté Morales et al., *Trabajo comunitario y decolonización*.

105. Pantoja and Blourock, "Cultural Pluralism Redefined," 255.

106. Pantoja and Perry, "Community Development and Restoration," 221.

107. Pantoja, *Memoir of a Visionary*, 193.

108. For more on Nieves and her cohort of activists, see, for example, Nieto, *Puerto Rican Students in U.S. Schools;* Lee, *Building a Latino Civil Rights Movement;* Cruz, *Puerto Rican Identity, Political Development and Democracy in New York, 1960–1990*.

109. Nieves and Martínez, "Puerto Rican Women in Higher Education in the United States."

110. Nieves et al., "Puerto Rican Studies," 5.

111. Nieves et al., "Puerto Rican Studies," 10.

112. During this period, Nieves said, "Cutbacks to social welfare programs will put the nation on a course for economic and demographic self-destruction. . . . The market economy makes it crucial that we must demonstrate that social work is effective." Walter Griffin, "Future of Social Work Discussed—Ethical Questions Remain a Challenge," *Bangor Daily News*, April 17, 1998.

EPILOGUE. ENVISIONING CARING FUTURES

1. For more on the political mobilization of women around care within social movements, see, for example, Nadasen, *Care;* Nadasen, *Household Workers Unite;* Wilkerson, *To Live Here, You Have to Fight;* Francisco-Menchavez, *The Labor of Care;* Tungohan, *Care Activism*. For more on the history of care labor and social reproduction more broadly, see, for example, Boris and Klein, *Caring for America;* Glenn, *Forced to Care;* Duffy, *Making Care Count*.

2. For more on the welfare rights movement in the United States, see Orleck, *Storming Caesar's Palace;* Nadasen, *Welfare Warriors;* Kornbluh, *The Battle for Welfare Rights*. There has been little written about Puerto Rican women's participation in this movement, but see Amador, "Collective Care Is Essential."

3. Dietz, *Economic History of Puerto Rico*, 229; Ayala and Barnable, *Puerto Rico in the American Century*, 267.

4. On the impact of welfare reform in the United States, see Kornbluh and Mink, *Ensuring Poverty;* Hays, *Flat Broke with Children*. On Puerto Rico, see Angueira, *Mujeres puertorriqueñas, "Welfare" y globalización*.

5. Ramírez, "Welfare Reform Implementation in Puerto Rico."

6. Cabán, "PROMESA, Puerto Rico and the American Empire"; Meléndez and Hinojosa, "Research Brief."

7. For more on PROMESA, see Cabán, "PROMESA, Puerto Rico and the American Empire"; Bonilla and LeBrón, *Aftershocks of Disaster.*

8. For more on the FEMA response to Hurricane Maria, see Molinari, "Authentication Loss and Contesting Recovery." Also see Frances Robles, "FEMA Was Sorely Unprepared for Puerto Rico Hurricane, Report Says," *New York Times*, July 12, 2018; Arelis R. Hernández, "FEMA Admits Failures in Puerto Rico Disaster Response, in After-Action Report," *Washington Post*, July 12, 2018.

9. For more, see Yarimar Bonilla, "The Leaked Texts at the Heart of Puerto Rico's Mass Protests," *Nation*, July 22, 2019; Ed Morales, "Why Half a Million Puerto Ricans Are Protesting in the Streets," *Nation*, July 19, 2019.

10. Cyndi Suarez, "After Deposing the Governor Puerto Ricans Shift Attention to Popular Democracy," *NonProfit Quarterley*, September 11, 2019; Villarrubia-Mendoza and Vélez-Vélez, "Puerto Rican People's Assemblies Shift from Protest to Proposal."

11. Hinojosa, "Two Sides of the Coin of Puerto Rican Migration."

12. Meléndez and Hinojosa, "Research Brief."

13. Silver and Vélez, "'Let Me Go Check Out Florida.'"

14. For more on *auto-gestión*, see Garriga-López, "Puerto Rico." In this article, Garriga-López translates the term as "autonomous organizing," and she argues, "*Auto-gestión* was about more than just physical recovery activities, however, as different structures and modalities of care were created out of an awareness of the manifold needs of the community" (180–81).

15. Molinari, "Authentication Loss and Contesting Recovery"; Lloréns, *Making Livable Worlds.*

16. For an overview of contemporary environmental struggles and political action in Puerto Rico, see Lloréns and Stanchich, "Water Is Life, but the Colony Is a Necropolis." For more on environmental activism, see Lloréns, "The Making of a Community Activist"; Lloréns, *Making Livable Worlds.*

17. Cándida Cotto, "Taller Salud = activism y educación," *Claridad*, December 10, 2019; Toro, *Un cuerpo propio.*

18. Santiago Ortiz, "La Colectiva Feminista en Construcción Are Leading the Puerto Rican Resistance."

19. Guzmán, "Meet the Women Leading Puerto Rico's Feminist Revolution."

20. United Nations General Assembly, "Special Committee on the Situation with Regard to the Implementation of the Declaration of the Granting of Independence to Colonial Countries and Peoples.".

21. See, for example, "Los trabajadores sociales de Pueto Rico rechazan junta de control fiscal," *San Diego Union-Tribune*, September 21, 2016. In the statement, board representative Alicea Rodríguez says that colonialism violates nations' rights and is "incompatible with the principles of citizenship, social justice, and democracy promoted by the social work profession."

Bibliography

ARCHIVES

Puerto Rico
  Archivo General de Puerto Rico (AGPR), Puerta de Tierra
  Biblioteca José M. Lázaro, Universidad de Puerto Rico (UPR), Río Piedras
  Colección Puertorriqueña, Universidad de Puerto Rico (UPR), Río Piedras
  Fundación Luis Muñoz Marín, Trujillo Alto

United States
  Archives of the Puerto Rican Diaspora, Center for Puerto Rican Studies, Hunter
    College, City University of New York
      Offices of the Government of Puerto Rico in the United States Records
        (OGPRUS)
          Social Service Program Records (OGPRUS-SSP)
      CENTRO: 100 Puerto Ricans Oral History Project (CENTRO 100)
      Michael Lapp Migration Division Oral History Collection
      Joseph Monserrat Papers
      Antonia Pantoja Papers
  Brooklyn Historical Society, Brooklyn, New York
  Columbia University Library and Manuscripts, New York
  Library of Congress, Washington, DC
  New York Public Library, Manuscripts and Archives Division, New York
  Schlesinger Library, Radcliffe Institute of Advanced Study, Harvard University,
    Cambridge, Massachusetts
  University of Chicago Library, Chicago

US Federal Census Records (Consulted on Ancestry.com)
  1910 Federal Population Census
  1920 Federal Population Census
  1930 Federal Population Census
  1940 Federal Population Census
  1935–1936, Puerto Rico Social and Population Schedules

NEWSPAPERS, MAGAZINES, AND PERIODICALS

Puerto Rico
  Claridad
  El Diario de Puerto Rico
  El Imparcial
  El Mundo
  El Nuevo Día
  Porto Rico Health Review
  Porto Rico School Review
  Puerto Rico Ilustrado
  San Juan Star

United States
  Afro-American (Baltimore)
  Amsterdam News (New York)
  Atlantic Monthly
  Bangor Daily News
  Chicago Daily Tribune
  Chicago Defender
  Daily Mirror (New York)
  Daily News (New York)
  El Diario de Nueva York
  The Nation
  New York Times
  San Diego Union-Tribune
  The Survey
  Washington Post

BOOKS, ARTICLES, AND OTHER SOURCES

Abramovitz, Mimi. *Regulating the Lives of Women: Social Welfare Policy from Colonial Times to the Present*. Boston: South End Press, 1996.

Acosta-Belén, Edna, and Elia Hidalgo Christensen. *The Puerto Rican Woman*. New York: Praeger, 1979.

Agnew, Elizabeth N. *From Charity to Social Work: Mary E. Richmond and the Creation of an American Profession*. Urbana: University of Illinois Press, 2003.

Alamo-Pastrana, Carlos. *Seams of Empire: Race and Radicalism in Puerto Rico and the United States*. Gainesville: University Press of Florida, 2016.

Alberto Maldonado, Adál. *Portraits of the Puerto Rican Experience*. Edited by Louis Reyes Rivera and Julio Rodríguez. New York: IPRUS Institute, 1984.

Alegría Ortega, Ida E., and Palmira N. Ríos González. *Contrapunto de género y raza en Puerto Rico*. Centro de Investigaciones Sociales, Universidad de Puerto Rico, Recinto de Río Piedras, 2005.

Alicea, Marixsa. "'A Chambered Nautilus': The Contradictory Nature of Puerto Rican Women's Role in the Social Construction of a Transnational Community." *Gender and Society* 11, no. 5 (October 1997): 597–626.

Alvarez-Curbelo, Silvia, and María Elena Rodríguez Castro, eds. *Del nacionalismo al populismo: Cultura y política en Puerto Rico*. Rio Pedras: Ediciones Huracan, 1993.

Amador, Emma. "Collective Care Is Essential: Puerto Rican Feminist Activists and Welfare Rights Organizing." Unpublished ms.

Amador, Emma. "Linked Histories of Welfare, Labor, and Puerto Rican Migration." Forum: Puerto Rico and the United States at Critical Junctures. *Modern American History* 2 (Fall 2019): 165–68.

Amador, Emma. "Organizing Puerto Rican Domestics: Resistance and Household Labor Reform in the Puerto Rican Diaspora after 1930." *ILWCH: International Labor and Working-Class History*, no. 8 (Fall 2015): 67–86.

Amador, Emma. "Unruly Domestics: Puerto Rican Women Care Workers, Reproductive Labor, and Feminist Political Organizing in the United States." Unpublished ms.

Amador, Emma. "Welfare Is Work: Social Welfare, Migration, and Women's Activism in Puerto Rican Communities after 1917." PhD diss., University of Michigan, 2015.

Amador, Emma. "'Women Ask Relief for Puerto Ricans': Social Workers, the Social Security Act and Puerto Rican Communities, 1933–1943." *LABOR: Studies in Working-Class History of the Americas* 12, no. 3 (December 2016): 105–29.

Amador, José. *Medicine and Nation Building in the Americas, 1890–1940*. Nashville: Vanderbilt University Press, 2015.

American Junior Red Cross. *A Program of Junior Red Cross Service, Outlined in Proceedings of the Educational Conference, January 7, 1918*. New York: University Printing Office, Columbia University, 1918.

Anderson, Warwick. *Colonial Pathologies: American Tropical Medicine, Race, and Hygiene in the Philippines*. Durham, NC: Duke University Press, 2006.

Angelis, María Luisa de. *Mujeres puertorriqueñas: que se han distinguido en el cultivo de las ciencias, las letras y las artes desde el siglo XVII hasta nuestros días*. San Juan: Tip. del Boletín Mercantil, 1908.

Angueira, Luisa Hernández. *Mujeres puertorriqueñas, "Welfare" y globalización: Desconstruyendo el estigma*. Hato Rey: Publicaciones Puertorriqueñas, 2001.

Aruzza, Ciniza, Tithi Bhattacharya, and Nancy Fraser. *Feminism for the 99%: A Manifesto*, New York: Verso, 2019.

ASPIRA. *National Conference: Meeting the Special Educational Needs of Urban Puerto Rican Youth*. Washington, DC: US Department of Health, Education, and Welfare, Office of Education, Bureau of Research, 1968.

Ayala, César J., and Rafael Bernabe. *Puerto Rico in the American Century: A History since 1898*. Chapel Hill: University of North Carolina Press, 2007.

Azize Vargas, Yamila. *La mujer en la lucha*. Río Piedras: Editorial Cultural, 1985.

Back, Adina. "Parent Power: Evelina López Antonetty, the United Bronx Parents, and the War on Poverty." In *The War on Poverty: A New Grassroots History, 1964–1980*, edited by Annelise Orleck and Lisa Gayle Hazirjian, 184–208. Athens: University of Georgia Press, 2011.

Back, Kurt W. *Slums, Projects, and People: Social Psychological Problems of Relocation in Puerto Rico*. Durham, NC: Duke University Press, 1962.

Baerga, María del Carmen. *Género y trabajo: la industria de la aguja en Puerto Rico y el Caribe hispánico*. San Juan: Editorial de la Universidad de Puerto Rico, 1993.

Baerga, María del Carmen. *Negociaciones de sangre: dinámicas racializantes en el Puerto Rico decimonónico*. Madrid: Iberomaericana Editorial Vervuert: 2015.

Baerga, María del Carmen. "Puerto Rico: From Colony to Colony." In *Creating and Transforming Households: The Constraints of the World-Economy*, edited by Joan Smith and Immanuel Wallerstein, 121–42. Cambridge: Cambridge University Press, 1992.

Baerga, María del Carmen. "Routes to Whiteness, or How to Scrub Off the Stain: Hegemonic Masculinity and Racialization in Nineteenth-Century Puerto Rico." *Translating the Americas* 3 (2015).

Bailkin, Jordanna. *The Afterlife of Empire*. Berkeley: University of California Press, 2012.

Barceló Miller, María de Fátima. "Halfhearted Solidarity: Women Workers and the Women's Suffrage Movement in Puerto Rico during the 1920s." In *Puerto Rican Women's History: New Perspectives*, edited by Felix Matos Rodríguez and Linda Delgado, 126–42. New York: Routledge, 1998.

Barceló Miller, María de Fátima. *La lucha por el sufragio femenino en Puerto Rico, 1896–1935*. Río Piedras: Centro de Investigaciones Sociales, Ediciones Huracán, 1997.

Bary, Helen Valeska, and the Children's Bureau, United States Department of Labor. *Child Welfare in the Insular Possessions of the United States, Part I*. Washington, DC: US Government Printing Office, 1923.

Bary, Helen Valeska, Jacqueline K. Parker, and James R. W. Leiby. *Labor Administration and Social Security: A Woman's Life*. Berkeley, CA: Regional Oral History Office, 1972.

Bell, Christopher. *East Harlem Remembered: Oral Histories of Community and Diversity*. Jefferson, NC: McFarland, 2013.

Bell, Joyce M. *The Black Power Movement and American Social Work*. New York: Columbia University Press, 2014.

Benmayor, Rina, Ana Juarbe, Blanca Vásquez Erazo, and Celia Álvarez. *Stories to Live By: Continuity and Change in Three Generations of Puerto Rican Women*. Centro de Estudios Puertorriqueños, Hunter College of the City University of New York, 1987.

Berengarten, Sidney, Columbia University School of Social Work, and cussw Alumni Association Committee on School History, eds. *The Columbia University School of Social Work: A History of Social Pioneering: Proceedings of the First Oral History Day for Entering Students, September 18, 1986*. New York: Columbia University School of Social Work, 1987.

Bernstein, Robin. *Racial Innocence: Performing American Childhood from Slavery to Civil Rights*. New York: New York University Press, 2011.

Bhattacharya, Tithi, ed. *Social Reproduction Theory: Remapping Class, Recentering Oppression*. London: Pluto Press, 2017.

Blain, Keisha. *Set the World on Fire: Black Nationalist Women and the Global Struggle for Freedom*. Philadelphia: University of Pennsylvania Press, 2019.

Blanch, Luisa O. "Las escuelas maternales del programa de emergencia de guerra." *Bienestar Público* 3, no. 12 (June 1948): 7–8.

Blum, Ann Shelby. *Domestic Economies: Family, Work, and Welfare in Mexico City, 1884–1943*. Lincoln: University of Nebraska Press, 2009.

Bonilla, Yarimar, and Marisol LeBrón. *Aftershocks of Disaster: Puerto Rico before and after the Storm*. Chicago: Haymarket Books, 2019.

Boria, Felicia. *Cuidado diurno para niños de madres que trabajan: Establecimientos de casas cunas en Puerto Rico*. San Juan: Gobierno de Puerto Rico, Departamento del Trabajo, 1942.

Boris, Eileen. "Force and the Shadow of Precarity: Racialized Bodies and State Power." *Kalfou: A Journal of Comparative and Relational Ethnic Studies* 2, no. 2, (2015): 307.

Boris, Eileen. *Home to Work: Motherhood and the Politics of Industrial Homework in the United States*. Cambridge: Cambridge University Press, 1994.

Boris, Eileen. *Making the Woman Worker: Precarious Labor and the Fight for Global Labor Standards, 1919-2019*. New York: Oxford University Press, 2019.

Boris, Eileen. "On Cowboys and Welfare Queens." *Journal of American Studies* 41 (2007): 599–621.

Boris, Eileen. "The Racialized Gendered State: Constructions of Citizenship in the United States." *Social Politics: International Studies in Gender, State and Society* 2, no. 2 (1995): 160–80.

Boris, Eileen, and Jennifer Klein. *Caring for America: Home Health Workers in the Shadow of the Welfare State*. New York: Oxford University Press, 2012.

Boris, Eileen, and Rhacel Salazar Parreñas. *Intimate Labors: Cultures, Technologies, and the Politics of Care*. Stanford, CA: Stanford University Press, 2010.

Bourne, Dorothy Dulles. *Professional Training for Social Work in Puerto Rico*. San Juan: University of Puerto Rico, 1935.

Bourne, Dorothy Dulles. "Puerto Rico's Predicament." *The Survey* 25, no 7 (July 1936): 200–203.

Bourne, Dorothy Dulles, and James Russell Bourne. *Thirty Years of Change in Puerto Rico: A Case Study of Ten Selected Rural Areas*. New York: F. A. Praeger, 1966.

Bourne, Dorothy Dulles, and Luz M. Ramos. *Rural Life in Puerto Rico*. San Juan: Department of Education, 1933.

Boyce Davies, Carole. *Left of Karl Marx: The Political Life of Black Communist Claudia Jones*. Durham, NC: Duke University Press, 2007.

Briggs, Laura. *How All Politics Became Reproductive Politics: From Welfare Reform to Trump*. Berkeley: University of California Press, 2017.

Briggs, Laura. "La Vida, Moynihan, and Other Libels: Migration, Social Science, and the Making of the Puerto Rican Welfare Queen." *Centro Journal* 14, no. 1 (2002): 75–101.

Briggs, Laura. *Reproducing Empire: Race, Sex, Science, and U.S. Imperialism in Puerto Rico*. Berkeley: University of California Press, 2002.

Bronfman, Alejandra, *Measures of Equality: Social Science, Citizenship, and Race in Cuba, 1902–1940*. Chapel Hill: University of North Carolina Press, 2004.

Bullard, Katharine S. "Children's Future, Nation's Future: Race, Citizenship, and the United States Children's Bureau." In *Raising Citizens in the "Century of the Child": The United States and German Central Europe in Comparative Perspective*, edited by Dirk Schumann, 53–67. New York: Berghahn Books, 2010.

Bullard, Katharine S. *Civilizing the Child: Discourses of Race, Nation, and Child Welfare in America*. Plymouth: Lexington Books, 2013.

Burgos Ortiz, Nilsa M. *Pioneras de la profesión de trabajo social en Puerto Rico*. Hato Rey: Publicaciones Puertorriqueñas, 1997.

Burnett, Christina Duffy, and Burke Marshall. *Foreign in a Domestic Sense: Puerto Rico, American Expansion, and the Constitution*. Durham, NC: Duke University Press, 2001.

Cabán, Pedro A. *Constructing a Colonial People: Puerto Rico and the United States, 1898–1932*. New York: Routledge, 2018.

Cabán, Pedro A. "PROMESA, Puerto Rico and the American Empire." *Latino Studies* 16 (2018): 161–84.

Cabranes, José. *A Study of Federal Public Assistance Payments to Puerto Rico*. Washington, DC: Office of the Commonwealth of Puerto Rico in Washington, D.C., 1974.

Cabranes, Manuel. "El trabajo social en las Segundas Unidades Rurales." *Revista de Servicio Social* 1, no. 4 (September 1939): 8–10.

Canales, Blanca. *La constitución es la revolución*. San Juan: Comité de Estudios, Congreso Nacional Hostosiano, 1997.

Cannon, Mary Antoinette. "Courses in Social Work at the University of Puerto Rico." *Revista de Servicio Social* 3, no. 1 (November 1941): 9.

Carlo-Becerra, Peter. "Which Is 'White' and Which Is 'Colored'? Notes on Race and/or Color among Puerto Ricans in Interwar New York City." PhD diss., State University of New York at Binghamton, 2012.

Carrasquillo, Rosa E. *Our Landless Patria: Marginal Citizenship and Race in Caguas, Puerto Rico, 1880–1910*. Lincoln: University of Nebraska Press, 2006.

Carroll, Tamar. *Mobilizing New York: AIDS, Antipoverty, and Feminist Action*. Chapel Hill: University of North Carolina Press, 2015.

Chaney, Elsa, Mary Garcia Castro, and Margo L. Smith. *Muchachas No More: Household Workers in Latin America and the Caribbean*. Philadelphia: Temple University Press, 1989.

Chenault, Lawrence R. *The Puerto Rican Migrant in New York City*. New York: Columbia University Press, 1938.

Chowkwanyun, Merlin. "Biocitizenship on the Ground: Health Activism and the Medical Governance Revolution." In *Biocitizenship: The Politics of Bodies, Governance, and Power*, edited by Kelly E. Happe, Jenell Johnson, and Marina Levina, 178–203. New York: New York University Press, 2018.

Choy, Catherine Ceniza. *Empire of Care: Nursing and Migration in Filipino American History*. Durham, NC: Duke University Press, 2003.

City University of New York, Centro de Estudios Puertorriqueños, and History Task Force. *Labor Migration under Capitalism: The Puerto Rican Experience*. New York: Monthly Review Press, 1979.

Clark-Lewis, Elizabeth. *Living In, Living Out: African American Domestics in Washington, D.C., 1910–1940*. Washington, DC: Smithsonian Institution Press, 1994.

Cobble, Dorothy Sue. *The Other Women's Movement: Workplace Justice and Social Rights in Modern America*. Princeton, NJ: Princeton University Press, 2004.

Coble, Alana Erickson. *Cleaning Up: The Transformation of Domestic Service in Twentieth-Century New York City*. New York: Routledge, 2006.

Collins, Susan, Barry P. Bosworth, and Miguel A. Soto-Class. *The Economy of Puerto Rico: Restoring Growth*. Washington, DC: Brookings Institution, 2006.

Colón, Alice, Margarita Mergal, and Nilsa Torres. *Participación de la mujer en la historia de Puerto Rico: Las primeras décadas del siglo veinte*. New Brunswick: Rutgers, 1986.

Colón, Jesús. *A Puerto Rican in New York, and Other Sketches*. New York: International Publishers, 1982.

Columbia University, School of Social Work. *Social Case Work: An Outline for Teaching with Annotated Case Records and Sample Course Syllabi*. Edited by Mary Antoinette Cannon and Philip Klein. New York: Columbia University Press, 1933.

Commonwealth of Puerto Rico, Department of Labor. *Conclusions of the Migration Conference Held in San Juan, Puerto Rico, March 1–7, 1953*. New York: Migration Division.

Córdova, Isabel M. *Pushing in Silence: Modernizing Puerto Rico and the Medicalization of Childbirth*. Austin: University of Texas Press, 2018.

Córdova, Isabel M. "Setting them Straight: Social Services, Youth, Sexuality, and Modernization in Postwar Puerto Rico." *Centro Journal* 19, no. 1 (2007).

Costin, Lela. *Two Sisters for Social Justice: A Biography of Grace and Edith Abbott*. Urbana: University of Illinois Press, 1983.

Cotera, María Eugenia. *Native Speakers: Ella Deloria, Zora Neale Hurston, Jovita González, and the Poetics of Culture*. Austin: University of Texas Press, 2008.

Cotté Morales, Alejandro, Magda Orfila Barreto, Doris Pizarro Claudio, Wilfredo Quiñones Sierra, Raquel Seda de Calderón, and Luz A. Vega Rodríguez. *Trabajo comunitario y decolonización*. Puerto Rico: Fundación Francisco Manrique Cabrera, 2012.

Crespo, Elizabeth. "Domestic Work and Racial Divisions in Women's Employment in Puerto Rico, 1899–1930." *Centro Journal* 8, no. 1–2 (1996): 30–41.

Crocker, Ruth. *Social Work and Social Order: The Settlement Movement in Two Industrial Cities, 1889–1930*. Urbana: University of Illinois Press, 1992.

Cros, Fernando, and Ana Helvia Quintero. "Entrevista a Carmen Isales." *Revista del Consejo General de Educación* 1, no. 1 (1993), 34.

Cruz, José E. *Puerto Rican Identity, Political Development, and Democracy in New York, 1960–1990*. Lanham, MD: Lexington Books, 2017.

D'Antonio, Patricia. *American Nursing: A History of Knowledge, Authority, and the Meaning of Work*. Baltimore: Johns Hopkins University Press, 2010.

De Genova, Nicholas. "'White' Puerto Rican Migrants, the Mexican Colony, 'Americanization,' and Latino History." In *Latino Urban Ethnography and the Work of Elena Padilla*, edited by Mérida M. Rúa, 157–77. Urbana: University of Illinois Press, 2010.

de Goenaga, Francisco. "Desarrollo historico del asilo de beneficencia de Puerto Rico." *Bienestar Público* 1, no. 1 (September 1945): 36–39.

Del Moral, Solsiree. *Negotiating Empire: The Cultural Politics of Schools in Puerto Rico, 1898–1952*. Madison: University of Wisconsin Press, 2013.

Del Moral, Solsiree. "Rescuing the *Jíbaro*: Renewing the Puerto Rican *Patria* through School Reform." *Caribbean Studies* 41 (July-December 2013): 91–135.

Del Moral, Solsiree. "'Una niña humilde y de color': Sources for the History of an Afro-Puerto Rican Childhood." *Journal of Caribbean History* 53, no. 2 (December 2019): 192–222.

Denis-Rosario, Milagros. *Drops of Inclusivity: Racial Formations and Meanings in Puerto Rican Society, 1898–1965*. Albany: State University of New York Press, 2022.

Denoyers, Julia. "Servir, divisa de una vida: Entrevista con Beatriz Lassalle." *Revista de Servicio Social* 7, no. 4 (1946): 114–21.

de Pagán, Clara Igualdad Iglesias. *El obrerismo en Puerto Rico: Época de Santiago Iglesias, 1896–1905*. San Juan: Ediciones Juan Ponce de León, 1973.

Departamento de Salud (Puerto Rico). *La división de Bienestar Público en su quinto aniversario*. San Juan: Departamento de Salud, 1948.

Descartes, Sol Luis. "Capacidad economica de Puerto Rico para la seguridad social." *Bienestar Público* 4, no. 16 (June 1949): 2.

Díaz González, Elisa. "Metas de asistencia pública y servicios sociales a la familia puertorriqueña," *Bienestar Público* 17, no. 68 (June 1962): 2–16.

Dietz, James L. *Economic History of Puerto Rico: Institutional Change and Capitalist Development*. Princeton, NJ: Princeton University Press, 1986.

Dietz, James L. *Negotiating Development and Change*. Boulder, CO: Lynne Reinner, 2003.

Dike, Steven. "La vida en la colonia: Oscar Lewis, the Culture of Poverty, and the Struggle for the Meaning of the Puerto Rican Nation." CENTRO: *Journal of the Center for Puerto Rican Studies* 26, no. 1 (Spring 2014).

Dinzey-Flores, Zaire. *Locked In, Locked Out: Gated Communities in a Puerto Rican City*. Philadelphia: University of Pennsylvania Press, 2013.

Dock, Lavinia L., Sarah Elizabeth Pickett, and Clara D. Noyes. *History of American Red Cross Nursing*. New York: Macmillan, 1922.

Dore, Elizabeth, and Maxine Molyneux. *Hidden Histories of Gender and the State in Latin America*. Durham, NC: Duke University Press, 2000.

Dorsey, Joseph C. *Slave Traffic in the Age of Abolition: Puerto Rico, West Africa, and the Non-Hispanic Caribbean, 1815–1859*. Gainesville: University Press of Florida, 2003.

Dowden-White, Priscilla A. *Groping toward Democracy: African American Social Welfare Reform in St. Louis, 1910–1949*. Columbia: University of Missouri Press, 2011.

Duany, Jorge. "Anthropology in a Postcolonial Colony: Helen I. Safa's Contribution to Puerto Rican Ethnography." *Caribbean Studies* 38, no. 2 (2010): 33–57.

Duany, Jorge. *Blurred Borders: Transnational Migration between the Hispanic Caribbean and the United States*. Chapel Hill: University of North Carolina Press, 2011.

Duany, Jorge. *The Puerto Rican Nation on the Move: Identities on the Island and in the United States*. Chapel Hill: University of North Carolina Press, 2002.

Duany, Jorge. "The Rough Edges of Puerto Rican Identities: Race, Gender, and Transnationalism." *Latin American Research Review* 40, no. 3 (2005): 177–90.

Duany, Jorge. "A Transnational Colonial Migration: Puerto Rico's Farm Labor Program." *New West Indian Guide/Nieuwe West-Indische Gids* 84, no. 3–4 (January 1, 2010): 225–51.

Duffy, Mignon. *Making Care Count: A Century of Gender, Race, and Paid Care Work.* New Brunswick, NJ: Rutgers University Press, 2011.

Emilio, John D. *Lost Prophet: The Life and Times of Bayard Rustin.* New York: Free Press, 2003.

Enck-Wanzer, Darrel. *The New York Young Lords and the Struggle for Liberation.* Philadelphia: Temple University Press, 2015.

Enck-Wanzer, Darrel, ed. *The Young Lords: A Reader.* New York: New York University Press, 2010.

Enríquez Seiders, Sandra A. *Ricarda López de Ramos Casellas: Tizas, conciencia y sufragio.* Colombia: Ediciones Callejón, 2006.

Erman, Sam. *Almost Citizens: Puerto Rico, the U.S. Constitution, and Empire.* Cambridge: Cambridge University Press, 2019.

Erman, Sam. "Meanings of Citizenship in the US Empire: Puerto Rico, Isabel González, and the Supreme Court, 1898 to 1905." *Journal of American Ethnic History* (2008): 5–33.

Ervin, Keona. "Breaking the 'Harness of Household Slavery': Domestic Workers, the Women's Division of the St. Louis Urban League, and the Politics of Labor Reform during the Great Depression." *ILWCH: International Labor and Working-Class History*, no. 88 (Fall 2015): 49–66.

Ervin, Keona. *Gateway to Equality: Black Women and the Struggle for Economic Justice in St. Louis.* Lexington: University Press of Kentucky, 2017.

Espino, Rafaela. "Trabajo social dentro de un programa de reconstrucíon." *Revista de Servicio Social* 5 (1939): 23–26.

Esterrich, Carmelo. *Concrete and Countryside: The Urban and Rural in 1950s Puerto Rican Culture.* Pittsburgh: University of Pittsburgh Press, 2018.

Feldman, Ronald A., and Sheila B. Kamerman. *The Columbia University School of Social Work: A Centennial Celebration.* New York: Columbia University Press, 2001.

Ferguson, Grace J. *Home Making and Home Keeping: A Text Book for the First Two Years' Work in Home Economics in the Public Schools of Porto Rico.* San Juan: Bureau of Supplies, Printing, and Transportation, 1915.

Ferguson, Susan. *Women and Work: Feminism, Labour, and Social Reproduction.* London: Pluto Press, 2019.

Fernández, Johanna. "Between Social Service Reform and Revolutionary Politics: The Young Lords, Late Sixties Radicalism, and Community Organizing in New York City." In *Freedom North: Black Freedom Struggles Outside the South, 1940–1980*, edited by Jeanne F. Theoharis and Komozi Woodard, 255–85. New York: Palgrave Macmillan, 2003.

Fernández, Johanna. *The Young Lords: A Radical History.* Chapel Hill: University of North Carolina Press, 2020.

Fernández, Lilia. *Brown in the Windy City: Mexicans and Puerto Ricans in Postwar Chicago*. Chicago: University of Chicago Press, 2012.

Figueroa, Luis A. *Sugar, Slavery, and Freedom in Nineteenth-Century Puerto Rico*. Chapel Hill: University of North Carolina Press, 2005.

Figueroa-Vásquez, Yomaira C. "Afro-Boricua Archives: Paperless People and Photo/ Poetics as Resistance." *Post45*, January 21, 2020. http://post45.org/2020/01/afro -boricua-archives-paperless-people-and-photo-poetics-as-resistance/.

Findlay, Eileen. "Dangerous Dependence or Productive Masculinity? Gendered Representations of Puerto Ricans in the US Press, 1940–1950." *Radical History Review* 2017, no. 128 (2017): 173–98.

Findlay, Eileen. *Imposing Decency: The Politics of Sexuality and Race in Puerto Rico, 1870–1920*. Durham, NC: Duke University Press, 1999.

Findlay, Eileen. "Love in the Tropics: Marriage, Divorce, and Benevolent Colonialism in Puerto Rico, 1898–1910." In *Close Encounters of Empire: Writing the Cultural History of U.S.-Latin American Relations*, edited by Gilbert M. Joseph, Catherine LeGrand and Ricardo D. Salvatore, 139–72. Durham, NC: Duke University Press, 1998.

Findlay, Eileen. *We Are Left without a Father Here: Masculinity, Domesticity, and Migration in Postwar Puerto Rico*. Durham, NC: Duke University Press, 2014.

Flores, Juan. *The Diaspora Strikes Back: Caribeño Tales of Learning and Turning*. New York: Routledge, 2010.

Flores Ramos, José. *Eugenesia, higiene pública y alcanfor para las pasiones: La prostitución en San Juan de Puerto Rico, 1876–1919*. Hato Rey: Publicaciones Puertorriqueñas, 2006.

Flores Ramos, José. *Mujer, familia y prostitución: La construcción del género bajo la hegemonía del Partido Popular Democrático, 1940–1968*. San Juan: Oficina de la Procuradora de las Mujeres, 2007.

Fox, Cybelle. *Three Worlds of Relief: Race, Immigration, and the American Welfare State from the Progressive Era to the New Deal*. Princeton, NJ: Princeton University Press, 2012.

Francisco-Menchavez, Valerie. *The Labor of Care: Filipina Migrants and Transnational Families in the Digital Age*. Urbana: University of Illinois Press, 2018.

Frank, Idida. "El centro de cuidado diurno de la escuela José Gautier Benítez." *Bienestar Público* 3, no. 12 (June 1948): 31–36.

Fraser, Nancy. "After the Family Wage: Gender Equity and the Welfare State." *Political Theory* 22, no. 4 (November 1994): 591–618.

Fraser, Nancy. *Fortunes of Feminism: From State-Managed Capitalism to Neoliberal Crisis*. New York: Verso, 2020.

French, John D., and Daniel James. *The Gendered Worlds of Latin American Women Workers: From Household and Factory to the Union Hall and Ballot Box*. Durham, NC: Duke University Press, 1997.

Gallart, Mary Frances. "Political Empowerment of Puerto Rican Women, 1952–1956." In *Puerto Rican Women's History: New Perspectives*, edited by Feilx Matos Rodríguez and Linda Delgado, 227–52. New York: Routledge, 1998.

García-Colón, Ismael. "Claiming Equality: Puerto Rican Farmworkers in Western New York." *Latino Studies* 6, no. 3 (2008): 269–89.

García-Colón, Ismael. *Colonial Migrants at the Heart of Empire: Puerto Rican Workers on U.S. Farms*. Berkeley: University of California Press, 2020.

García-Colón, Ismael. *Land Reform in Puerto Rico: Modernizing the Colonial State, 1941–1969*. Gainesville: University Press of Florida, 2009.

Garriga de Baralt, Aurora. "Funciones y logros en los programas de Servicios Inter-agenciales." *Bienestar Público* 15, no. 59 (January–March 1960): 33–34.

Garriga de Baralt, Aurora. "La Oficina de Servicios Interagenciales y sus servicios a los niños de Puerto Rico." *Bienestar Público* 13, no. 51 (1958): 30.

Garriga de Baralt, Aurora. "Se ofrecieron servicios múltiples al migrante Puertor-riqueño." *Bienestar Público* 16, no. 61–62 (July–December 1960): 25–26.

Garriga de Baralt, Aurora. "Se presto atención inmediata a 9,295 casos de naturaleza urgente referidos por agencias sociales del extranjero y del país." *Bienestar Público* 13, no. 54 (October–December 1958): 25–27.

Garriga de Baralt, Aurora. "Un total de 14,246 casos se atendieron y se resolvieron durante el año, y los cuales recibieron 19,721 diferentes clases de servicios." *Bienestar Público* 15, no. 58 (October–December 1959): 25–27.

Garriga-López, Adriana. "Puerto Rico: The Future is the Question." *Shima* 13, no. 2 (2019): 174–92.

Gautier-Mayoral, Carmen, and Teresa Blanco-Stahl. "COINTELPRO en Puerto Rico: Documentos secretos del FBI (1960–1971)." In *Las Carpetas: Persecucion politica y derechos civiles en Puerto Rico*, edited by Ramón Bosque Pérez and José Javier Colón Morera, 255–97. Honduras: Centro para la Investigacion y Promocion de los Derechos Civiles, 1997.

Glasser, Ruth. *My Music Is My Flag: Puerto Rican Musicians and Their New York Com-munities, 1917–1940*. Berkeley: University of California Press, 1997.

Glenn, Evelyn Nakano. *Forced to Care: Coercion and Caregiving in America*. Cam-bridge, MA: Harvard University Press, 2010.

Glenn, Evelyn Nakano. *Unequal Freedom: How Race and Gender Shaped American Citizenship and Labor*. Cambridge, MA: Harvard University Press, 2012.

Go, Julian. *American Empire and the Politics of Meaning: Elite Political Cultures in the Philippines and Puerto Rico during U.S. Colonialism*. Durham, NC: Duke University Press, 2008.

Godreau, Isar. *Scripts of Blackness: Race, Cultural Nationalism, and US Colonialism in Puerto Rico*. Urbana: University of Illinois Press, 2015.

Godreau, Isar. "Slippery Semantics: Race Talk and Everyday Uses of Racial Terminol-ogy in Puerto Rico." *Centro Journal* 20, no. 2 (Fall 2008): 5–33.

Gold, Roberta. *When Tenants Claimed the City: The Struggle for Citizenship in New York City*. Urbana: University of Illinois Press, 2014.

Goldstein, Alyosha. *Poverty in Common: The Politics of Community Action during the American Century*. Durham, NC: Duke University Press, 2012.

González, Clarisel. "East Harlem's Trailblazer Yolanda Sánchez Leaves a Legacy (1932–2012)." Center for Puerto Rican Studies, Hunter College, City University of New York, accessed May 24, 2014. http://centroweb.hunter.cuny.edu/about/centro-news/east-harlem%E2%80%99s-trailblazer-yolanda-s%C3%A1nchez-leaves-legacy.

González, Elise M. "Nurturing the Citizens of the Future: Milk Stations and Child Nutrition in Puerto Rico, 1929-60." *Medical History* 59, no 2 (April 2015): 177–98.

González, Rosa. "Trabajo de campo en 'La Vida.'" *Humanidad* 1, no. 1 (December 1967): 9–14.

González García, Lydia Milagros. *Una puntada en el tiempo: La industria de la aguja en Puerto Rico (1900–1920)*. Santo Domingo: Editorial Universidad, 1990.

Gordon, Linda. *Heroes of Their Own Lives: The Politics and History of Family Violence: Boston, 1880–1960*. Urbana: University of Illinois Press, 2002.

Gordon, Linda. *Pitied but Not Entitled: Single Mothers and the History of Welfare, 1890–1935*. Cambridge, MA: Harvard University Press, 1995.

Gordon, Linda. *Women, the State, and Welfare*. Madison: University of Wisconsin Press, 1990.

Grosfoguel, Ramón. *Colonial Subjects: Puerto Ricans in a Global Perspective*. Berkeley: University of California Press, 2003.

Guardiola Ortiz, Dagmar. *El trabajo social en Puerto Rico: Asistencia, desarrollo o transformación?* Río Piedras: Decandto de Estudios Gruaduados e Investigaciones, Recinto de Río Piedras, 1998.

Guerra, Lillian. *Popular Expression and National Identity in Puerto Rico: The Struggle for Self, Community, and Nation*. Gainesville: University Press of Florida, 1998.

Guridy, Frank Andre. *Forging Diaspora: Afro-Cubans and African Americans in a World of Empire and Jim Crow*. Chapel Hill: University of North Carolina Press, 2010.

Guy, Donna J. *White Slavery and Mothers Alive and Dead: The Troubled Meeting of Sex, Gender, Public Health, and Progress in Latin America*. Lincoln: University of Nebraska Press, 2000.

Guy, Donna J. *Women Build the Welfare State: Performing Charity and Creating Rights in Argentina, 1880–1955*. Durham, NC: Duke University Press, 2009.

Guzmán, Sandra. "Meet the Women Leading Puerto Rico's Feminist Revolution." Shondaland, August 9, 2019. https://www.shondaland.com/change-makers /a28653844/puerto-rico-protests-feminist-revolution/.

Hall, Frances Adkins. "The Problem of the Migration of Indigent Puerto Ricans to and from New York City." *Puerto Rico Health Bulletin* 3, no. 12 (n.d.): 495.

Hall, Frances Adkins. "Social and Economic Conditions in Puerto Rico." *Puerto Rico Health Bulletin* 3, no. 7 (July 1939) 496–504.

Hall, Frances Adkins, and Robert A. Hall. *Puerto Rican Journal (1937–1939)*. Ithaca, NY: Unknown, 1979.

Hancock, Angie-Marie. *The Politics of Disgust: The Public Identity of the Welfare Queen*. New York: New York University Press, 2004.

Hanson, Earl Parker. *Puerto Rico, Land of Wonders*. New York: Knopf, 1960.

Hanson, Earl Parker. *Transformation: The Story of Modern Puerto Rico*. New York: Simon and Schuster, 1955.

Harper, Ida Husted. *The History of Woman Suffrage, 1900–1920*. Vol. 6. New York: J. J. Little & Ives, 1922.

Hays, Sharon. *Flat Broke with Children: Women in the Age of Welfare Reform*. Oxford: Oxford University Press, 2004.

Hicks, Anasa. *Hierarchies at Home: Domestic Service in Cuba from Abolition to Revolution*. Cambridge: Cambridge University Press, 2022.

Hill, Reuben. *The Family and Population Control: A Puerto Rican Experiment in Social Change*. Chapel Hill: University of North Carolina Press, 1959.

Hilliard, Raymond, and Department of Welfare. *The "Puerto Rican Problem" of the City of New York Department of Welfare*. New York: Department of Welfare, 1949.

Hine, Darlene Clark. *Black Women in White: Racial Conflict and Cooperation in the Nursing Profession, 1890–1950*. Bloomington: Indiana University Press, 1989.

Hinojosa, Jennifer. "Two Sides of the Coin of Puerto Rican Migration: Depopulation in Puerto Rico and the Redefinition of the Diaspora." CENTRO *Journal* 30, no. 3 (2018): 230–53.

Hoffnung-Garskof, Jesse. "The Migrations of Arturo Schomburg: On Being Antillano, Negro, and Puerto Rican in New York 1891–1938." *Journal of American Ethnic History* 21, no. 1 (2001): 3–49.

Hoffnung-Garskof, Jesse. *Racial Migrations: New York City and the Revolutionary Politics of the Spanish Caribbean, 1850–1902*. Princeton, NJ: Princeton University Press, 2019.

Hoffnung-Garskof, Jesse. *A Tale of Two Cities: Santo Domingo and New York after 1950*. Princeton, NJ: Princeton University Press, 2008.

Hoffnung-Garskof, Jesse. "To Abolish the Law of Castes: Merit, Manhood and the Problem of Colour in the Puerto Rican Liberal Movement, 1873–92." *Social History* 36, no. 3 (2011): 312–42.

Hunter, Tera W. *To 'Joy My Freedom: Southern Black Women's Lives and Labors after the Civil War*. Cambridge, MA: Harvard University Press, 1997.

Iglesias, Luisa V. "Como se empean los $7.50?" *Bienestar Público* 1, no. 3 (1946): 10–16.

Iglesias de Jesús, Luisa, and Rosario Neveres de Rodríguez. "Las problemas de los Puertorriqueños en Nueva York a traves de los casos referidos a la Unidad de Servicios Interagenciales de la División de Bienestar Público." *Bienestar Público* 2, no. 6 (December 1946): 17–22.

Irwin, Julia. *Making the World Safe: The American Red Cross and a Nation's Humanitarian Awakening*. Oxford: Oxford University Press, 2013.

Jiménez, Lillian, dir. *Antonia Pantoja ¡Presente!* Los Angeles: Latino Public Broadcasting, 2009.

Jiménez, Mónica, A. "Puerto Rico under the Colonial Gaze: Oppression, Resistance and the Myth of the Nationalist Enemy." *Latino Studies* 18, no. 1 (January 2020): 27–44.

Jiménez-Muñoz, Gladys M. "'A Storm Dressed in Skirts': Ambivalence in the Debate on Women's Suffrage in Puerto Rico, 1927–1929." PhD diss., State University of New York at Binghamton, 1994.

Jones, Jacqueline. *Labor of Love, Labor of Sorrow: Black Women, Work, and the Family from Slavery to the Present*. New York: Basic Books, 1985.

Jones, Marian Moser. *The American Red Cross from Clara Barton to the New Deal*. Baltimore: Johns Hopkins University Press, 2013.

Joseph, Gilbert M., Catherine C. LeGrand, and Ricardo D. Salvatore. *Close Encounters of Empire: Writing the Cultural History of U.S.-Latin American Relations*. Durham, NC: Duke University Press, 1998.

Junior Red Cross. *The Junior Red Cross: A Program*. Washington, DC: American Red Cross, 1921.

Katz, Michael B. *In the Shadow of the Poorhouse: A Social History of Welfare in America*. New York: Basic Books, 1986.

Klein, Marian van der, Rebecca Jo Plant, Nichole Sanders, and Lori R. Weintrob. *Maternalism Reconsidered: Motherhood, Welfare and Social Policy in the Twentieth Century*. New York: Berghahn Books, 2012.

Kornbluh, Felicia. *The Battle for Welfare Rights: Politics and Poverty in Modern America*. Philadelphia: University of Pennsylvania Press, 2007.

Kornbluh, Felicia. *A Woman's Life Is a Human Life: My Mother, Our Neighbor, and the Journey from Reproductive Rights to Reproductive Justice*. New York: Grove Press, 2023.

Kornbluh, Felicia, and Gwendolyn Mink. *Ensuring Poverty: Welfare Reform in Feminist Perspective*. Philadelphia: University of Pennsylvania Press, 2019.

Koven, Seth, and Sonya Michel. *Mothers of a New World: Maternalist Politics and the Origins of Welfare States*. New York: Routledge, 1993.

Krüger Torres, Lola. *Enciclopedia grandes mujeres de Puerto Rico*. Hato Rey: Ramallo Brothers Printing, 1975.

Kunzel, Regina G. *Fallen Women, Problem Girls: Unmarried Mothers and the Professionalization of Social Work, 1890–1945*. New Haven, CT: Yale University Press, 1993.

Ladd-Taylor, Molly. *Mother-Work: Women, Child Welfare, and the State, 1890–1930*. Urbana: University of Illinois Press, 1995.

La Fountain-Stokes, Lawrence. *Queer Ricans: Cultures and Sexualities in the Diaspora*. Minneapolis: University of Minnesota Press, 2009.

Lane, Sarah. "Educational Activities of the Department of Health of Porto Rico." *Porto Rico Journal of Tropical Medicine* (October 1924): 5–8.

Lapp, Michael. "Managing Migration: The Migration Division of Puerto Rico and Puerto Ricans in New York City, 1948–1968." PhD diss., Johns Hopkins University, 1990.

Lapp, Michael. "The Rise and Fall of Puerto Rico as a Social Laboratory, 1945–1965." *Social Science History* 19, no. 2 (1995): 169–99.

Lasch-Quinn, Elisabeth. *Black Neighbors: Race and the Limits of Reform in the American Settlement House Movement, 1890–1945*. Chapel Hill: University of North Carolina Press, 1993.

Lassalle, Beatriz. "Breves palabras." *Revista de Servicio Social* 8, no. 1 (January 1947): 3–6.

Lassalle, Beatriz. *Cuentos mitológicos: Narrados para los niños de habla española*. New York: Rand McNally, 1925.

Lassalle, Beatriz. "El año del los niños: Influencia del año de los niños en la desarrollo del trabajo social en Puerto Rico." *Bienestar Público* 4, no. 17 (September 1949): 7–13.

Lassalle, Beatriz. "Mi sentir sobre Celestina Zalduondo." *Bienestar Público* 14, no. 53 (July–September 1958): 19–20.

Lassalle, Beatriz. "Veinticinco años de servicios sociales públicos en Puerto Rico." *Bienestar Público* 4, no. 17 (September 1949): 16–19.

Lauria-Perricelli, Antonio. "A Study in Historical and Critical Anthropology: The Making of the People of Puerto Rico." PhD diss., New School for Social Research, 1989.

Lee, Sonia Song-Ha. *Building a Latino Civil Rights Movement: Puerto Ricans, African Americans, and the Pursuit of Racial Justice in New York City.* Chapel Hill: University of North Carolina Press, 2014.

Lee, Sonia Song-Ha, and Ande Diaz. "'I Was the One Percenter': Manny Diaz and the Beginnings of Black–Puerto Rican Coalition." *Journal of American Ethnic History* 26, no. 3 (Spring 2007): 52–80.

LeBrón, Marisol. *Policing Life and Death: Race, Violence, and Resistance in Puerto Rico.* Berkeley: University of California Press, 2019.

"Legislación social propulsada por el Colegio de Trabajadores Sociales." *Revista de Servicio Social* 3, no. 3–4 (March 1942), 33–43.

Levy, Teresita A. *Puerto Ricans in the Empire: Tobacco Growers and U.S. Colonialism.* New Brunswick, NJ: Rutgers University Press, 2015.

Lewis, Gordon K. *Puerto Rico: Freedom and Power in the Caribbean.* New York: Monthly Review Press, 1963.

Lewis, Oscar. *La Vida: A Puerto Rican Family in the Culture of Poverty—San Juan and New York.* New York: Random House, 1966.

Lewis, Oscar. *A Study of Slum Culture: Backgrounds for La Vida.* New York: Random House, 1968.

Lindenmeyer, Kriste. *A Right to Childhood: The U.S. Children's Bureau and Child Welfare, 1912–46.* Urbana: University of Illinois Press, 1997.

Lindsay, Samuel McCune. "The United States and Porto Rico." *Proceedings of the Academy of Political Science in the City of New York* 7, no. 2 (1917): 245–49.

Lloréns, Hilda. *Imaging the Great Puerto Rican Family: Framing Nation, Race, and Gender during the American Century.* Lanham, MD: Rowman and Littlefield, 2014.

Lloréns, Hilda. *Making Livable Worlds: Afro-Puerto Rican Women Building Environmental Justice.* Seattle: University of Washington Press, 2021.

Lloréns, Hilda. "The Making of a Community Activist." *Sapiens,* May 5, 2017. https://www.sapiens.org/culture/jobos-bay-community-activist/.

Lloréns, Hilda, and Martiza Stanchich. "Water Is Life, but the Colony Is a Necropolis: Environmental Terrains of Struggle in Puerto Rico." *Cultural Dynamics* 31, no. 1–2 (2019): 81–101.

Loiselle, Aimee. *Beyond Norma Rae: How Puerto Rican and Southern White Women Fought for a Place in the American Working Class.* Chapel Hill: University of North Carolina Press, 2023.

López, Iris O. *Matters of Choice: Puerto Rican Women's Struggle for Reproductive Freedom.* New Brunswick, NJ: Rutgers University Press, 2008.

Macpherson, Anne. "Citizens vs. Clients: Workingwomen and Colonial Reform in Puerto Rico and Belize, 1932–1945." *Journal of Latin American Studies* 35, no. 2 (May 2003): 279–310.

Macpherson, Anne. "Doing Comparative Caribbean (Gender) History: Puerto Rican and Belizean Working-Class Women, 1830s–1930s." *Small Axe: A Journal of Caribbean Criticism* 43 (March 2014): 72–86.

Macpherson, Anne. *From Colony to Nation: Women Activists and the Gendering of Politics in Belize, 1912–82.* Lincoln: University of Nebraska Press, 2007.

Maldonado, Edwin. "Contract Labor and the Origins of Puerto Rican Communities in the United States." *International Migration Review* (1979): 103–21.

Marcantonio, Vito. *I Vote My Conscience: Debates, Speeches and Writings of Vito Marcantonio, 1935–1950*. New York: Vito Marcantonio Memorial, 1956.

Marín, Rosa Celeste. *A Cross-Cultural Approach to Measurement of Family Functioning in Multi-Problem Families*. Río Piedras: School of Social Work, University of Puerto Rico, 1964.

Marín, Rosa Celeste. "Familias menesterosas con problemas múltiples en Puerto Rico." *Humanidad* 2, no. 2 (December 1968): 5–14.

Marín, Rosa Celeste. "La interpretación de las funciones del trabajador social." *Revista de Servicio Social* 18, no. 2 (April 1957): 2–8.

Marino, Katherine. *Feminism for the Americas: The Making of an International Human Rights Movement*. Chapel Hill: University of North Carolina Press, 2019.

Marsh Kennerly, Catherine. *Negociaciones culturales: Los intelectuales y el proyecto pedagógico del estado muñocista*. San Juan: Ediciones Callejón, 2008.

Martell, Esperanza. "'In the Belly of the Beast': Beyond Survival." In *The Puerto Rican Movement*, edited by Andrés Torres and José E. Velázquez, 173–91. Philadelphia: Temple University Press, 1998, 173–91.

Martínez-Vergne, Teresita. *Shaping the Discourse on Space: Charity and Its Wards in Nineteenth-Century San Juan, Puerto Rico*. Austin: University of Texas Press, 1999.

Materson, Lisa G. "Gender, Generation, and Women's Independence Organizing in Puerto Rico." *Radical History Review* 128 (2017): 121–46.

Mathews, Thomas G. *Puerto Rican Politics and the New Deal*. Gainesville: University Press of Florida, 1960.

Matos Rodríguez, Félix. *Women and Urban Change in San Juan, Puerto Rico, 1820–1868*. Gainesville: University Press of Florida, 1999.

Matos Rodríguez, Félix, and Linda C. Delgado, eds. *Puerto Rican Women's History: New Perspective*. Armonk, NY: M. E. Sharpe, 1998.

May, Vanessa. *Unprotected Labor: Household Workers, Politics, and Middle-Class Reform in New York, 1870–1940*. Chapel Hill, University of North Carolina Press, 2011.

McCoy, Alfred W., and Francisco A. Scarano. *The Colonial Crucible: Empire in the Making of the Modern American State*. Madison: University of Wisconsin Press, 2009.

McGreevey, Robert C. *Borderline Citizens: The United States, Puerto Rico, and the Politics of Colonial Migration*. Ithaca, NY: Cornell University Press, 2018.

Meier, Elizabeth G. *A History of the New York School of Social Work*. New York: Columbia University Press, 1954.

Meléndez, Edgardo. *Sponsored Migration: The State and Puerto Rican Postwar Migration to the United States*. Columbus: Ohio State University Press, 2017.

Meléndez, Edgardo. "Vito Marcantonio, Puerto Rican Migration, and the 1949 Mayoral Election in New York City." *Centro Journal* 22, no. 2 (2010): 199–233.

Meléndez, Edwin, and Jennifer Hinojosa. "Research Brief: Estimates of Post-Hurricane Maria Exodus from Puerto Rico." Center for Puerto Rican Studies,

October 2017. https://centropr.hunter.cuny.edu/reports/estimates-post-hurricane -maria-exodus-puerto-rico/.

Meléndez-Badillo, Jorell A. "Labor History's Transnational Turn: Rethinking Latin American and Caribbean Migrant Workers." *Latin American Perspectives* 42, no. 4 (July 2015): 117–22.

Meléndez-Badillo, Jorell A. *The Lettered Barriada: Workers, Archival Power, and the Politics of Knowledge in Puerto Rico.* Durham, NC: Duke University Press, 2021.

Meléndez-Badillo, Jorell A. "Mateo and Juana: Racial Silencing, Epistemic Violence, and Counterarchives in Puerto Rican Labor History." *ILWCH: International Labor and Working-Class History* 96 (Fall 2019): 103–21.

Méndez, José Luis. *Las ciencias sociales y el proceso político puertorriqueño.* San Juan: Ediciones Puerto, 2005.

Mendoza Tío, Carlos F. "Beatriz Lassalle del Valle." *Al Margen: Revista Anual de las Artes* 7 (1988): 49–56.

Meyer, Gerald. *Vito Marcantonio: Radical Politician, 1902–1954.* Albany: State University of New York Press, 1989.

Midgley, James, and David Piachaud. *Colonialism and Welfare: Social Policy and the British Imperial Legacy.* Cheltenham and Northampton, MA: Edward Elgar, 2011.

Mills, Charles Wright, Clarence Ollson Senior, and Rose Kohn Goldsen. *The Puerto Rican Journey: New York's Newest Migrants.* New York: Russell and Russell, 1967.

Mink, Gwendolyn. *The Wages of Motherhood: Inequality in the Welfare State, 1917– 1942.* Ithaca, NY: Cornell University Press, 1996.

Mintz, Sidney. *Worker in the Cane: A Puerto Rican Life History.* New Haven, CT: Yale University Press, 1960.

Mixer, Knowlton. *Porto Rico: History and Conditions, Social, Economic and Political.* New York: Macmillan, 1926.

Molina, Natalia. *How Race Is Made in America: Immigration, Citizenship, and the Historical Power of Racial Scripts.* Berkeley: University of California Press, 2014.

Molinari, Sarah. "Authentication Loss and Contesting Recovery: FEMA and the Politics of Colonial Disaster Management." In *Aftershocks of Disaster: Puerto Rico before and after the Storm*, edited by Yarimar Bonilla and Marisol LeBrón, 285–97. Chicago: Haymarket Books, 2019.

Morales, Iris. "¡Palante, Siempre Palante!: The Young Lords." In *The Puerto Rican Movement*, edited by Andrés Torres and José E. Velázquez, 210–27. Philadelphia: Temple University Press, 1998.

Morales, Iris. *Through the Eyes of Rebel Women: The Young Lords, 1969–1976.* New York: Red Sugarcane Press, 2016.

Morales, Julio. *Puerto Rican Poverty and Migration: We Just Had to Try Elsewhere.* Westport, CT: Praeger, 1986.

Moreno Fraginals, Manuel, Frank Moya Pons, and Stanley L. Engerman, eds. *Between Slavery and Free Labor: The Spanish-Speaking Caribbean in the Nineteenth Century.* Baltimore: Johns Hopkins University Press, 1985.

Morlock, Maud. *Homemaker Services: History and Bibliography.* Washington, DC: US Department of Health, Education, and Welfare, 1964.

Morlock, Maud. *Supervised Homemaker Service: A Method of Child Care.* Washington, DC: United States Department of Labor, Children's Bureau, 1943.

Morrissey, Marietta. "The Making of a Colonial Welfare State: U.S. Social Insurance and Public Assistance in Puerto Rico." *Latin American Perspectives* 33, no. 1 (January 2006): 23–41.

Mumford, Kevin. *Not Straight, Not White: Black Gay Men from the March on Washington to the AIDS Crisis.* Chapel Hill: University of North Carolina Press, 2016.

Muncy, Robyn. *Creating a Female Dominion in American Reform, 1890–1935.* Oxford: Oxford University Press, 1991.

Muñiz-Mas, Félix O. "Gender, Work, and Institutional Change in the Early Stage of Industrialization: The Case of the Women's Bureau and the Home Needlework Industry in Puerto Rico 1940–1952." In *Puerto Rican Women's History: New Perspectives,* edited by Felix Matos Rodríguez and Linda Delgado, 181–205. New York: Routledge, 1998.

Muñoz, Raúl. "Instrumentación de los Seguros Sociales en Puerto Rico." *Bienestar Público* 4, no. 15 (March 1949): 30.

Muzio, Rosie. *Radical Imagination, Radical Humanity: Puerto Rican Political Activism in New York.* Albany: State University of New York Press, 2017.

Nadasen, Premilla. *Care: The Highest Stage of Capitalism.* Chicago: Haymarket Books, 2023.

Nadasen, Premilla. "From Widow to 'Welfare Queen': Welfare and the Politics of Race." *Black Women, Gender, and Families* 1, no. 2 (Fall 2007): 52–77.

Nadasen, Premilla. *Household Workers Unite: The Untold Story of African American Women Who Built a Movement.* Boston: Beacon Press, 2016.

Nadasen, Premilla. *Rethinking the Welfare Rights Movement.* New York: Routledge, 2012.

Nadasen, Premilla. *Welfare Warriors: The Welfare Rights Movement in the United States.* New York: Routledge, 2004.

Nasiali, Minayo A. *Native to the Republic: Empire, Social Citizenship, and Everyday Life in Marseille since 1945.* Ithaca, NY: Cornell University Press, 2016.

Navarro, José-Manuel. *Creating Tropical Yankees: Social Science Textbooks and U.S. Ideological Control in Puerto Rico, 1898–1908.* New York: Routledge, 2002.

Navarro-Rivera, Pablo. "Acculturation under Duress: The Puerto Rican Experience at the Carlisle Indian Industrial School, 1898–1918." CENTRO *Journal* 18, no. 1 (2006): 222–29.

Navas Dávila, Gerardo. *Cambio y desarrollo en Puerto Rico: La transformación ideológica del Partido Popular Democrático.* Río Piedras: Editorial Universitaria, Universidad de Puerto Rico, 1977.

Negrón de Montilla, Aida. *Americanization in Puerto Rico and the Public-School System, 1900–1930.* Río Piedras: Editorial Universitaria, Universidad de Puerto Rico, 1975.

Negrón Muñoz, Angela. *Mujeres de Puerto Rico: Desde el período de colonización hasta el primer tercio del siglo XX.* San Juan: Imprenta Venezuela, 1935.

Negrón-Muntaner, Frances. "Can You Imagine?: Puerto Rican Lesbian Activism, 1972–1991." *Centro Journal* 30, no. 2 (2018).

Nelson, Alondra. *Body and Soul: The Black Panther Party and the Fight against Medical Discrimination.* Minneapolis: University of Minnesota Press, 2011.

Nelson, Jennifer. *Women of Color and the Reproductive Rights Movement.* New York: New York University Press, 2003.

Nieto, Sonia, ed. *Puerto Rican Students in U.S. Schools.* New York: Routledge, 2013.

Nieves, Josephine, María Canino, Sherry Gorelick, Hildamar Ortiz, Camilo Rodríguez, and Jesse Vazquez. "Puerto Rican Studies: Roots and Challenges." In *Towards a Renaissance of Puerto Rican Studies,* edited by María Sánchez and Antonio M. Stevens-Arroyo, 3–12. Charlottesville, VA: Atlantic Research and Publications, 1987.

Nieves, Josephine, and M. Martínez. "Puerto Rican Women in Higher Education in the United States." In *Conference on the Educational and Occupational Needs of Hispanic Women.* Washington, DC: US Department of Education, National Institute of Education, 1980.

Ngai, Mae M. *Impossible Subjects: Illegal Aliens and the Making of Modern America.* Princeton, NJ: Princeton University Press, 2004.

O'Connor, Alice. *Poverty Knowledge: Social Science, Social Policy, and the Poor in Twentieth-Century U.S. History.* Princeton, NJ: Princeton University Press, 2000.

Ogbar, Jeffrey O. G. "Puerto Rico en mi corazón: The Young Lords, Black Power, and Puerto Rican Nationalism in the U.S., 1966–1972." *Centro Journal* 18, no. 1 (2006): 148–69.

Olcott, Jocelyn. *Revolutionary Women in Postrevolutionary Mexico.* Durham, NC: Duke University Press, 2005.

Olivares, Samy Nemir. "LGBT Activist Wilhelmina Perry Remembers Her Partner, Antonia Pantoja." NBC News, June 10, 2016. https://www.nbcnews.com/news/latino/lgbt-activist-wilhelmina-perry-remembers-her-partner-antonia-pantoja-n589661.

Orleck, Annelise. *Storming Caesar's Palace: How Black Mothers Fought Their Own War on Poverty.* Boston: Beacon Press, 2006.

Orleck, Annelise, and Lisa Gayle Hazirjian. *The War on Poverty: A New Grassroots History, 1964–1980.* Athens: University of Georgia Press, 2011.

Ortiz, Altagracia, ed. *Puerto Rican Women and Work: Bridges in Transnational Labor.* Philadelphia: Temple University Press, 1996.

Ortiz Díaz, Alberto. *Raising the Living Dead: Rehabilitative Corrections in Puerto Rico and the Caribbean.* Chicago: University of Chicago Press, 2023.

Osuna, Juan José. *A History of Education in Puerto Rico.* New York: Arno Press, 1975.

Osuna, Juan José. "An Indian in Spite of Myself." *Summer School Review* 10, no. 5 (1932): 3.

Padilla, Elena. "Puerto Rican Immigrants in New York and Chicago: A Study in Comparative Assimilation." Master's thesis, University of Chicago, 1947.

Pagán, Aida G. "Celestina Zalduondo: Lo que ella ha significado para la obra de bienestar público en Puerto Rico." *Bienestar Público* 16, no. 53 (June–September 1958): 20–21.

Págan Torres, Santos. "Actividades de la Comisión en Washington." *Bienestar Público* 1, no. 3 (March 1946): 38–40.

Palmer, Phyllis M. *Domesticity and Dirt: Housewives and Domestic Servants in the United States, 1920–1945.* Philadelphia: Temple University Press, 1989.

Pantoja, Antonia. *Memoir of a Visionary: Antonia Pantoja*. Houston: Arte Público Press, 2002.

Pantoja, Antonia, and Barbara Blourock. "Cultural Pluralism Redefined." In *Badges and Indicia of Slavery: Cultural Pluralism Redefined*, edited by Antonia Pantoja, Barbara Blourock, and James Bowman, 2–25. Lincoln: University of Nebraska Press, 1975.

Pantoja, Antonia, and Esperanza Martell. "Mi Gente" *Centro Journal* 2, no. 7 (1989): 48–55.

Pantoja, Antonia, and Wilhelmina Perry. "Community Development and Restoration: A Perspective and Case Study." In *Community Organizing in a Diverse Society*, edited by Felix G. Rivera and John L. Erlich, 220–42. Boston: Allyn and Bacon, 1998.

Paris-Chitanvis, Jacqueline. "Yolanda Sánchez: A New York Activist with a World View." In *Women Making History: Conversations with Fifteen New Yorkers*, edited by Maxine Gold, 91–98. New York: New York City Commission on the Status of Women, 1985.

Parreñas, Rhacel Salazar. *The Force of Domesticity: Filipina Migrants and Globalization*. New York: New York University Press, 2008.

Parreñas, Rhacel Salazar. *Servants of Globalization: Migration and Domestic Work*. 2nd ed. Stanford, CA: Stanford University Press, 2015.

Pastor, Georgina A. "Antoinette Cannon." *Revista de Servicio Social* 3, no. 8 (October 1942): 2–3.

Pastor, Georgina A. "History and Development of the Laws Licensing Social Workers in Puerto Rico." Master's thesis, University of Washington, 1943.

Peel, Mark. *Miss Cutler and the Case of the Resurrected Horse: Social Work and the Story of Poverty in America, Australia, and Britain*. Chicago: University of Chicago Press, 2012.

Pérez, Gina M. *The Near Northwest Side Story: Migration, Displacement, and Puerto Rican Families*. Berkeley: University of California Press, 2004.

Pérez de Silva, Matilde. "Rol del gobierno de Puerto Rico en la migración de Puertorriqueños a Estados Unidos." *Bienestar Público* 13, no. 52 (April–June 1958): 20–25.

Pérez-Herráns, Carmen. "Our Two Full Time Jobs: Women Workers Balance Factory and Domestic Demands." In *Puerto Rican Women and Work: Bridges in Transnational Labor*, edited by Altagracia Ortiz, 139–60. Philadelphia: Temple University Press, 1996.

Pérez Rosario, Vanessa. *Becoming Julia de Burgos: The Making of a Puerto Rican Icon*. Urbana: University of Illinois Press, 2014.

Perry, Wilhelmina. "Memorias de una vida de obra (Memories of a Life of Work): An Interview with Antonia Pantoja." *Harvard Educational Review* 68, no. 2 (Summer 1998): 244–58.

Piñeiro, Flor M. "Migrantes puertorriqueños en Nueva York y Santa Cruz." *Bienestar Público* 3, no. 11 (March 1948): 33–37.

Pintado de Rahn, María. "Grace Abbott, Maestra." *Revista de Servicio Social* 1, no. 3 (June–July 1939): 5–6.

Pintado de Rahn, María. "The People of the Caribbean." *Revista de Servicio Social* 7, no. 3 (July 1947): 83–84.

Plácido, Sandy. "A Global Vision: Dr. Ana Livia Codero and the Puerto Rican Liberation Struggle, 1931–1992." PhD diss., Harvard University, 2017.

Power, Margaret. "Puerto Rican Women Nationalists vs. U.S. Colonialism: An Exploration of Their Conditions and Struggles in Jail and in Court." *Chicago-Kent Law Review* 87, no. 2 (2012): 463–79.

Power, Margaret. *Solidarity across the Americas: The Puerto Rican Nationalist Party and Anti-Imperialism*. Chapel Hill: University of North Carolina Press, 2023.

Poole, Mary. *The Segregated Origins of Social Security: African Americans and the Welfare State*. Chapel Hill: University of North Carolina Press, 2006.

Puerto Rico Emergency Relief Administration. *First Annual Report of the Puerto Rican Emergency Relief Administration from August 19, 1933, to August 31, 1934*. San Juan: Bureau of Supplies, Printing, and Transportation, 1935.

Puerto Rico Emergency Relief Administration. *Second Report of the Puerto Rican Emergency Relief Administration from September 1, 1934, to September 30, 1935, and Report of the Federal Emergency Relief Administration for Puerto Rico from October 1, 1935, to June 30, 1936, in liquidation to October, 1937*. Washington, DC: US Government Printing Office, 1939.

Puerto Rican Forum. *A Study of Poverty Conditions in the Puerto Rican New York Community*. New York: Puerto Rican Forum, 1970.

Puerto Rican Forum. *The Puerto Rican Community Development Project*. 2nd ed. New York: Arno Press, 1964.

Putnam, Lara. "Citizenship from the Margins: Vernacular Theories of Rights and the State in the Interwar Caribbean." *Journal of British Studies* 53, no. 1 (2014): 162–91.

Putnam, Lara. *The Company They Kept: Migrants and the Politics of Gender in Caribbean Costa Rica, 1870–1960*. Chapel Hill: University of North Carolina Press, 2002.

Putnam, Lara. *Radical Moves: Caribbean Migrants and the Politics of Race in the Jazz Age*. Chapel Hill: University of North Carolina Press, 2013.

Putnam, Lara. "To Study the Fragments/Whole: Microhistory and the Atlantic World." *Journal of Social History* 39, no. 3 (2006): 615–30.

Quadagno, Jill. *The Color of Welfare: How Racism Undermined the War on Poverty*. New York: Oxford University Press, 1994.

Quiñones Rivera, Martiza. "From Trigueñita to Afro-Puerto Rican: Intersections of the Racialized, Gendered, and Sexualized Body in Puerto Rico and the Mainland." *Meridians: Feminism, Race, Transnationalism* 7, no. 1 (2006): 162–82.

Ramírez, Norma Boujouen. "Welfare Reform Implementation in Puerto Rico: A Status Report." National Council of La Raza, April 2001.

Ramírez de Arellano, Annette B., and Conrad Seipp. *Colonialism, Catholicism, and Contraception: A History of Birth Control in Puerto Rico*. Chapel Hill: University of North Carolina Press, 1983.

Ramos-Zayas, Ana Y. *National Performances: The Politics of Class, Race, and Space in Puerto Rican Chicago*. Chicago: University of Chicago Press, 2003.

Ramú de Guzmán, Adriana. "Historia de la escuela de trabajo social de la Universidad de Puerto Rico." *Revista de Servicio Social* 10, no. 4 (October 1949): 2–7.

Ransby, Barbara. *Ella Baker and the Black Freedom Movement: A Radical Democratic Vision*. Chapel Hill: University of North Carolina Press, 2003.

Reese, Ellen. *Backlash against Welfare Mothers: Past and Present*. Berkeley: University of California Press, 2005.

Reisch, Michael, and Janice Andrews. *The Road Not Taken: A History of Radical Social Work in the United States*. New York: Routledge, 2002.

Reyes, Linda Colón. *Sobrevivencia, pobreza y "mantengo": La política asistencialista estadounidense en Puerto Rico: El PAN y el TANF*. Puerto Rico: Ediciones Callejón, 2011.

Richardson, Lewis Cutter. *Puerto Rico, Caribbean Crossroads*. Photographs by Charles E. Rotkin. New York: US Camera Publishing and the University of Puerto Rico, 1947.

Richmond, Mary Ellen. *Social Diagnosis*. New York: Russell Sage, 1955.

Rigdon, Susan M. *The Culture Facade: Art, Science, and Politics in the Work of Oscar Lewis*. Urbana: University of Illinois Press, 1988.

Rivera, Louis Reyes, and Julio Rodríguez, eds. *Portraits of the Puerto Rican Experience*. Photographs by Adál Alberto Maldonado. New York: Institute for Puerto Rican Urban Studies–IPRUS, 1984.

Rivera de Alvarado, Carmen. *El trabajo social: Una profesión en la encrucijada*. San Juan: Asociación Nacional de Trabajadores Sociales de Puerto Rico, 1973.

Rivera de Alvarado, Carmen. "La contribución de la mujer al desarrollo de la nacionalidad Puertorriqueña." In *La mujer en la lucha hoy*, edited by Nancy Zayas and Juan A. Silen, 37–47. Venezuela: Ediciones Kikirikí, 1972.

Rivera de Alvarado, Carmen. *Lucha y visión de Puerto Rico libre*. Río Piedras: T. Rivera de Ríos, 1986.

Rivera de Alvarado, Carmen, Francisco Torres Rivera, and Trina Rivera de Ríos. *Puerto Rico: The Look from Within / Puerto Rico: Somos*. [Puerto Rico]: RF Publishing, 1975.

Rodríguez, Antonio. *The Second Unit and the Rural School Problem of Puerto Rico*. San Juan: Imprenta Venezuela, 1945.

Rodríguez, Clara E. *Changing Race: Latinos, the Census, and the History of Ethnicity in the United States*. New York: New York University Press, 2000.

Rodríguez, Clara E. *Puerto Ricans: Born in the U.S.A.* San Francisco: Westview Press, 1989.

Rodríguez, Manuel F. "A Study of the Puerto Ricans in New York and Their Difficulties in Adjusting to Cosmopolitan Life." Master's thesis, New York School of Social Work, 1938.

Rodríguez, Manuel R. *A New Deal for the Tropics: Puerto Rico during the Depression Era, 1932–1935*. Princeton, NJ: Markus Wiener, 2010.

Rodríguez-Silva, Ileana. "Libertos and Libertas in the Construction of the Free Worker in Postemancipation Puerto Rico." In *Gender and Slave Emancipation in the Atlantic World*, edited by Pamella Scully and Diana Paton, 199–222. Durham, NC: Duke University Press, 2005.

Rodríguez-Silva, Ileana. *Silencing Race: Disentangling Blackness, Colonialism, and National Identities in Puerto Rico*. New York: Palgrave Macmillan, 2012.

Rodríguez Pastor, J. "Our Bureau of Social Welfare." *Porto Rico Review of Public Health and Tropical Medicine: Official Bulletin of the Department of Health and the School of Tropical Medicine* 3, no. 3 (September 1927): 108–12.

Román, Miriam Jiménez, and Juan Flores, eds. *The Afro-Latin@ Reader: History and Culture in the United States.* Durham, NC: Duke University Press, 2009.

Romero, Mary. *Maid in the U.S.A.* London: Routledge, 2002.

Romero, Mary, *The Maid's Daughter: Living Inside and Outside the American Dream.* New York: New York University Press, 2011.

Rosado Morales, Isabel. *Mis testimonios.* Río Piedras: Biblioteca Albizu Campos, 2007.

Rosemblatt, Karin Alejandra. *Gendered Compromises: Political Cultures and the State in Chile, 1920–1950.* Chapel Hill: University of North Carolina Press, 2000.

Rosemblatt, Karin Alejandra. "Other Americas: Transnationalism, Scholarship, and the Culture of Poverty in Mexico and the United States." *Hispanic American Historical Review* 89, no. 4 (2009): 603–41.

Roy-Féquiére, Magali. *Women, Creole Identity, and Intellectual Life in Early Twentieth-Century Puerto Rico.* Philadelphia: Temple University Press, 2004.

Rúa, Mérida M. *A Grounded Identidad: Making New Lives in Chicago's Puerto Rican Neighborhoods.* Oxford: Oxford University Press, 2012.

Rúa, Mérida M. *Latino Urban Ethnography and the Work of Elena Padilla.* Urbana: University of Illinois Press, 2010.

Ruiz, Vicki L., and Virginia Sánchez Korrol, eds. *Latina Legacies: Identity, Biography, and Community.* Oxford: Oxford University Press, 2005.

Safa, Helen Icken. *The Myth of the Male Breadwinner: Women and Industrialization in the Caribbean.* New York: Westview Press, 1995.

Safa, Helen Icken. *The Urban Poor of Puerto Rico: A Study in Development and Inequality.* New York: Holt, Rinehart, and Winston, 1974.

Sanabria, Carlos. *Puerto Rican Labor History 1898–1934: Revolutionary Ideals and Reformist Politics.* Lanham, MD: Rowman and Littlefield, 2017.

Sánchez, José Ramón. *Boricua Power: A Political History of Puerto Ricans in the United States.* New York: New York University Press, 2007.

Sánchez Korrol, Virginia. "Antonia Pantoja and the Power of Community Action." In *Latina Legacies: Identity, Biography and Community*, edited by Vicki Ruiz and Virginia Sánchez Korrol, 209–27. Oxford: Oxford University Press, 2005.

Sánchez Korrol, Virginia. "The Forgotten Migrant: Educated Puerto Rican Women in New York City, 1920–1940." In *The Puerto Rican Woman: Perspectives on Culture, History and Society*, edited by Edna Acosta-Belén, 170–79. New York: Praeger, 1986.

Sánchez Korrol, Virginia. *From Colonia to Community: The History of Puerto Ricans in New York City.* Berkeley: University of California Press, 1994.

Sánchez Korrol, Virginia. "In Search of Unconventional Women: Histories of Puerto Rican Women in Religious Vocations before Mid-Century." *Oral History Review* 16, no. 2 (Autumn 1988): 47–63.

Sánchez Korrol, Virginia. "Survival of Puerto Rican Women in New York before World War II." In *Historical Perspectives on Puerto Rican Survival in the US*, edited by Clara E. Rodríguez and Virginia Sánchez Korrol, 55–68. Princeton, NJ: Markus Wiener, 1996.

Sanders, Nichole. *Gender and Welfare in Mexico: The Consolidation of a Post-Revolutionary State*. University Park: Pennsylvania State University Press, 2011.

Santiago Ortiz, Aurora. "La Colectiva Feminista en Construcción Are Leading the Puerto Rican Resistance." *Open Democracy*, January 4, 2020. https://www.opendemocracy.net/en/oureconomy/la-colectiva-feminista-en-construccion-are-leading-the-puerto-rican-resistance/.

Santiago-Valles, Kelvin A. *"Subject People" and Colonial Discourses: Economic Transformation and Social Disorder in Puerto Rico, 1898–1947*. Albany: State University of New York Press, 1994.

Schechter, Patricia A. *Exploring the Decolonial Imaginary: Four Transnational Lives*. New York: Palgrave Macmillan, 2012.

Scott, Rebecca J., and Jean M. Hébrard. *Freedom Papers: An Atlantic Odyssey in the Age of Emancipation*. Cambridge, MA: Harvard University Press, 2012.

Scott, Rebecca J. "Reclaiming Gregoria's Mule: The Meanings of Freedom in the Arimao and Caunao Valleys, Cienfuegos, Cuba, 1880–1899." *Past & Present*, no. 170 (February 1, 2001): 181–216.

Seda Rodríguez, Raquel. "Legado de Carmen Rivera de Alvarado a la profesion de trabajo social en Puerto Rico." *Voces Desde el Trabajo Social: Colegio de Profesionales de Trabajo Social* 1 (2012): 21–29.

Senior, Clarence Ollson. *Puerto Rican Emigration*. Río Piedras: Social Science Research Center, University of Puerto Rico, 1947.

Senior, Clarence Ollson. *The Puerto Ricans: Strangers—Then Neighbors*. Chicago: Anti-Defamation League of B'nai B'rith and Quadrangle Books, 1965.

Senior, Clarence Ollson, and Carmen Isales. *The Puerto Ricans of New York City*. New York: New York Office of Employment and Migration Bureau, Puerto Rico Department of Labor, 1948.

Serbiá, Celina. "Historia de la cruz roja juvenil." *Bienestar Público* 4, no. 21 (September 1950): 12–19.

Serra, Belén Milagros. "Bienestar público en Puerto Rico: Desarrollo historico." *Revista de Servicio Social* 10, no. 1 (January 1949): 16–32.

Serra, Belén Milagros. "La ley de Seguridad Social vigente y los proyectos H.R. 2645 y H.R. 2892 de la Cámara de Representantes, Congreso Federal No. 81." *Bienestar Público* 4, no. 15 (March 1949): 2–8.

Sheehan, Susan. *A Welfare Mother*. New York: New American Library, 1977.

Silva, Antonio R. "Beatriz Lassalle y su obra para la Cruz Roja." *Revista de Servicio Social* 8, no. 4 (October 1946): 125–26.

Silver, Patricia, and William Vélez. "'Let Me Go Check Out Florida:' Rethinking Puerto Rican Diaspora." *CENTRO Journal* (Fall 2017): 98–135.

Silvestrini, Blanca G. "La política de salud pública de los Estados Unidos en Puerto Rico, 1898–1913: Consecuencias de la americanización." In *Politics, Society, and Culture in the Caribbean*, edited by Blanca Silvestrini, 69–83. San Juan: Editorial de la Universidad de Puerto Rico, 1983.

Silvestrini, Blanca G. *Los trabajadores puertorriqueños y el Partido Socialista (1932–1940)*. Río Piedras: Editorial Universitaria, 1979.

Silvestrini, Blanca G. *Women and Resistance: Herstory in Contemporary Caribbean History*. Mona: Department of History, University of the West Indies, 1990.

Silvestrini, Blanca G. "Women as Workers: The Experience of the Puerto Rican Women in the 1930s." In *Cross-Cultural Perspectives on the Women's Movement*, edited by Ruby Leavitt, 247–61. Le Hague: Mouton, 1975.

Sklar, Kathryn Kish. *Florence Kelley and the Nation's Work: The Rise of Women's Political Culture, 1830–1900*. New Haven, CT: Yale University Press, 1995.

Sklar, Kathryn Kish, Anja Schuler, and Susan Strasser. *Social Justice Feminists in the United States and Germany: A Dialogue in Documents, 1885–1933*. Ithaca, NY: Cornell University Press, 2018.

"Social Service Activities of the Department of Health." *Porto Rico Health Review: Official Bulletin of the Department of Health* 1, no. 4 (October 1925): 25–28.

Stepan, Nancy. *The Hour of Eugenics: Race, Gender, and Nation in Latin America*. Ithaca, NY: Cornell University Press, 1991.

Stern, Alexandra. *Eugenic Nation: Faults and Frontiers of Better Breeding in Modern America*. Berkeley: University of California Press, 2005.

Stoler, Ann Laura. *Carnal Knowledge and Imperial Power: Race and the Intimate in Colonial Rule*. Berkeley: University of California Press, 2002.

Stoler, Ann Laura. *Haunted by Empire: Geographies of Intimacy in North American History*. Durham, NC: Duke University Press, 2006.

Swain, Martha H. *Ellen S. Woodward: New Deal Advocate for Women*. Jackson: University Press of Mississippi, 1995.

Taylor, Ula Y. *The Veiled Garvey: The Life and Times of Amy Jacques Garvey*. Chapel Hill: University of North Carolina Press, 2002.

Thomas, Lorrin. "'How They Ignore Our Rights as American Citizens': Puerto Rican Migrants and the Politics of Citizenship in the New Deal Era." *Latino Studies* 2, no. 2 (2004): 140–59.

Thomas, Lorrin. *Puerto Rican Citizen: History and Political Identity in Twentieth-Century New York City*. Chicago: University of Chicago Press, 2010.

Thomas, Lorrin. "Resisting the Racial Binary? Puerto Ricans' Encounter with Race in Depression-Era New York City." *Centro Journal* 21, no. 1 (2009): 5–35.

Thomas, Lorrin, and Aldo Lauria-Santiago. *Rethinking the Struggle for Puerto Rican Rights*. New York: Routledge, 2019.

Threat, Charissa J. *Nursing Civil Rights: Gender and Race in the Army Nurse Corps*. Urbana: University of Illinois Press, 2015.

Tice, Karen Whitney. *Tales of Wayward Girls and Immoral Women: Case Records and the Professionalization of Social Work*. Urbana: University of Illinois Press, 1998.

Tinsman, Heidi. *Partners in Conflict: The Politics of Gender, Sexuality, and Labor in the Chilean Agrarian Reform, 1950–1973*. Durham, NC: Duke University Press, 2002.

Toro, Ana Teresa. *Un cuerpo propio: 40 años de taller salud*. Loíza: Taller Salud, 2019.

Toro-Morn, Maura I. "Gender, Class, Family, and Migration: Puerto Rican Women in Chicago." *Gender and Society* 9, no. 6 (December 1995): 712–26.

Toro-Morn, Maura I. "Género, trabajo y migración: Las empleadas domésticas puertorriqueñas en Chicago." *Revista de Ciencias Sociales* 7 (1999): 102–25.

Toro-Morn, Maura I. "Yo era muy arriesgada: A Historical Overview of the Work Experiences of Puerto Rican Women in Chicago." *Centro Journal* 13, no. 2 (2001): 25–43.

Torres, Andrés, and José E. Velázquez. *The Puerto Rican Movement: Voices from the Diaspora.* Philadelphia: Temple University Press, 1998.

Torres, Lourdes. "Boricua Lesbians: Sexuality, Nationality, and the Politics of Passing." *Centro Journal* 19, no. 1 (2007): 230–49.

Torres, Lourdes. "Queering Puerto Rican Women's Narratives: Gaps and Silences in the Memoirs of Antonia Pantoja and Luisita López Torregrosa." *Meridians* 9, no. 1 (2008): 83–112

Trattner, Walter I. *From Poor Law to Welfare State: A History of Social Welfare in America.* New York: Simon and Schuster, 1999.

Trías Monge, José. *Puerto Rico: The Trials of the Oldest Colony in the World.* New Haven, CT: Yale University Press, 1997.

Tungohan, Ethel. *Care Activism: Migrant Domestic Workers, Movement-Building, and Communities of Care.* Urbana: University of Illinois Press, 2023.

Tyrrell, Ian R. *Woman's World/Woman's Empire: The Woman's Christian Temperance Union in International Perspective, 1880–1930.* Chapel Hill: University of North Carolina Press, 1991.

Tyrrell, Marygrace. "Colonizing Citizens: Housing Puerto Ricans, 1917–1952." PhD diss., Northwestern University, 2009.

Urban, Andrew. *Brokering Servitude: Migration and the Politics of Domestic Labor during the Long Nineteenth Century.* New York: New York University Press, 2018.

United Nations General Assembly. "Special Committee on the Situation with Regard to the Implementation of the Declaration of the Granting of Independence to Colonial Countries and Peoples." Summary of 6th Meeting, Held at Headquarters, New York, June 18, 2018. https://undocs.org/pdf?symbol=en/A/AC.109/2018/SR.6.

United States Department of Labor, Children's Bureau. *Children's Year: A Brief Summary of Work Done and Suggestions for Follow-up Work.* Washington, D.C: US Government Printing Office, 1920.

United States Department of Labor, Children's Bureau. *Maternal and Child-Health Services under the Social Security Act, Title V, Part 1: Development of Program, 1936–1939.* Washington, DC: US Government Printing Office, 1939.

Varela, Marta B. "The First Forty Years of the Commission on Human Rights." *Fordham Urban Law Journal* 23, no. 4 (1996).

Vélez de Pérez, Mercedes. "Consideraciones en torno a los servicios de 'hogares de crianza' y 'amas de llaves." *Bienestar Público* 3, no. 2 (September 1947): 1–3.

Venator-Santiago, Charles R. *Puerto Rico and the Origins of U.S. Global Empire: The Disembodied Shade.* New York: Routledge, 2015.

Villarini, Carmen. "Visitando un ama de llaves." *Bienestar Público* 3, no. 12 (June 1948): 24–27.

Villaronga, Gabriel. *Toward a Discourse of Consent: Mass Mobilization and Colonial Politics in Puerto Rico, 1932–1948.* Westport, CT: Praeger, 2004.

Villarrubia-Mendoza, Jacqueline, and Roberto Vélez-Vélez. "Puerto Rican People's Assemblies Shift from Protest to Proposal." *NACLA: Report on the Americas,*

August 2019. https://nacla.org/news/2019/08/22/puerto-rican-people%E2%80%99s
-assemblies-shift-protest-proposal.

Vizcarrondo, Francisco. *The Second-Unit Rural Schools of Porto Rico: Pre-Vocational Schools for Pupils of Intermediate Grades.* Puerto Rico: Insular Department of Education, 1930.

Wagenheim, Olga Jiménez de. *Puerto Rico's Revolt for Independence: El Grito de Lares.* Boulder: Westview Press, 1985.

Wagenheim, Olga Jiménez de. *Nationalist Heroines: Puerto Rican Women History Forgot, 1930s–1950s.* Princeton, NJ: Markus Wiener, 2016.

Wale, Fred, and Carmen Isales. *The Meaning of Community Development.* A Report from the Division of Community Education. San Juan: Department of Education, 1967.

Walkowitz, Daniel J. *Working with Class: Social Workers and the Politics of Middle-Class Identity.* Chapel Hill: University of North Carolina Press, 1999.

Ward, Deborah E. *The White Welfare State: The Racialization of U.S. Welfare Policy.* Ann Arbor: University of Michigan Press, 2005.

Ward, Geoff K. *The Black Child-Savers: Racial Democracy and Juvenile Justice.* Chicago: University of Chicago Press, 2012.

Ware, Susan. *Beyond Suffrage: Women in the New Deal.* Cambridge, MA: Harvard University Press, 1981.

Warren, Alice E. Colón. "Puerto Rico Feminism and Feminist Studies." *Gender & Society* 17, no. 5 (October 1, 2003): 664–90.

Warren, Alice E. Colón, María Maite Mulero, Luis Santiago, and Nilsa Burgos. *Estirando el peso: Acciones de ajuste y relaciones de género ante el cierre de fábricas en Puerto Rico.* Río Piedras: Centro de Investiaciones Sociales, 2008.

Welfare Council of New York City and the Committee on Puerto Ricans in New York City. *Puerto Ricans in New York City: The Report of the Committee on Puerto Ricans in New York City of the Welfare Council of New York City.* New York: Arno Press, 1975.

Whalen, Carmen Teresa. *From Puerto Rico to Philadelphia: Puerto Rican Workers and Postwar Economies.* Philadelphia: Temple University Press, 2001.

Whalen, Carmen Teresa. "Radical Contexts: Puerto Rican Politics in the 1960s and 1970s and the Center for Puerto Rican Studies." CENTRO: *Journal of the Center for Puerto Rican Studies* 21, no. 2 (Fall 2009): 220–55.

Whalen, Carmen Teresa. "Sweatshops Here and There: The Garment Industry, Latinas, and Labor Migrations." ILWCH: *International Labor and Working-Class History* 61 (Spring 2002): 45–68.

Whalen, Carmen Teresa, and Víctor Vázquez-Hernández. *The Puerto Rican Diaspora: Historical Perspectives.* Philadelphia: Temple University Press, 2005.

Wildenthal, Lora. *German Women for Empire, 1884–1945.* Durham, NC: Duke University Press, 2001.

Wilkerson, Jessica. *To Live Here, You Have to Fight: How Women Led Appalachian Movements for Social Justice.* Urbana: University of Illinois Press, 2019.

Williams, Rhonda Y. *The Politics of Public Housing: Black Women's Struggles against Urban Inequality.* Oxford: Oxford University Press, 2004.

Wilson, Jan Doolittle. *The Women's Joint Congressional Committee and the Politics of Maternalism, 1920–30.* Urbana: University of Illinois Press, 2007.

Wolcott, Victoria W. *Remaking Respectability: African American Women in Interwar Detroit.* Chapel Hill: University of North Carolina Press, 2001.

Yelvington, Kevin A. "The Making of a Marxist-Feminist-Latin Americanist Anthropologist: An Interview with Helen I. Safa." *Caribbean Studies* 38, no. 2 (July-December 2010): 3–23.

Zalduondo, Celestina. "Bienestar de la niñez en Puerto Rico." *Bienestar Público* 10, no. 32 (July-September 1954): 2–4.

Zalduondo, Celestina. "El programa de asistencia pública de estado libre asociado de Puerto Rico." *Bienestar Público*, 8, no. 32 (April–June 1953): 2–4.

Index

Page numbers in italics refer to figures.

Rivera de Alvarado, Carmen, 62, 66–68, 70–71, 80–81, 83, 177, 179–80, 205–7, 209, 234n19, 237n79, 264n89
Rivera Martínez, Prudencio, 70
Robles, Zaida, 219
Rodríguez, Alicea, 266n21
Rodríguez, Gloria M., 206
Rodríguez, Manuel, 236n48
Rodríguez Trías, Helen, 204
Romero, Carolina, 112–14
Roosevelt, Eleanor, 68
Roosevelt, Franklin D., 67, 72, 89, 234n23, 261n47
Roqué de Duprey, Ana, 239n102
Rosado Morales, Isabel, 71, 177, 235n43
Rosello, Ricardo, 217
Rúa, Merida, 248n44, 249nn50–51

Safa, Helen, 97, 121, 245n97; *The Myth of the Male Breadwinner*, 124; *The Urban Poor of Puerto Rico*, 115–16, 122–26, 241n10
Sánchez, Yolanda, 1–5, 13, 22, 26, 188, 193–94, 199, 212, 213, 260n32, 261n35
Sánchez Korrol, Virginia, 251n4
San Diego State University, 208
San German, Puerto Rico, 163
San Juan, Puerto Rico, 37, 40, 56, 107, 119, 131, 226n15, 227n22, 240n2; Children's Bureau census in, 53; El Fanguito, 99, 121; labor in, 47, 54, 97; labor recruitment in, 141; La Perla, 94, 118–20; racialization in, 45; social workers in, 58, 163; social work programs in, 118
Santurce, Puerto Rico, 58, 114
scientific motherhood, 43, 46–47, 151
Segundas Unidades Rurales (SUR), 66–71
Senior, Clarence, 148, 181
Serra, Belén Milagros, 226n15, 255n48
settlement house movement, 41–42, 49, 140, 160, 168, 181, 185, 196–98, 203, 207
sexuality, 36, 51, 55, 98, 101, 191, 199, 207–8, 260n20, 262n57; pathologization of, 120, 127; regulation of, 8, 40, 58, 96, 99–100, 141
sex work, 49; accusations of, 49, 55, 100, 143; campaigns against, 3, 8, 39, 51, 55, 143
Sheppard-Towner Maternity and Infancy Protection Act (1921), 23, 34, 60
Sierra Berdecia, Fernando, 146, 151

Sklar, Kathryn Kish, 39
slavery, 20, 32, 51, 53, 104, 107, 226n15, 243n44
slum clearance programs, 75
Smith College, 83
social insurance provisions, 90–91
socialism, 52, 60–61, 63, 66–67, 70–72, 80, 83, 92, 138, 180, 184, 188, 237n79; feminist, 21, 38–39, 69, 124; US fears of, 117. *See also* Partido Socialista Puertorriqueño
social reproduction, 48, 64, 104, 114–15, 124–27, 133–35, 245n97; and care work, 14–15, 68–69, 214–15, 220; social welfare support for, 34, 47–48, 64
social science, 159, 168–71, 174, 181, 184, 258n81; and colonialism, 32; and PPD, 88, 115–17, 126; and Puerto Rican citizenship, 34; and social welfare, 6, 49, 71; studies of poverty, 96, 115–17, 125–27
Social Security Act (1935), 26, 62, 230n56, 238nn88–89, 256n59, 257n71; and migration, 171–76; Puerto Rican coverage by, 10–11, 13, 23, 62, 64–65, 82–83, 87–93, 102, 157, 171–76, 179, 239nn104–5, 255n48, 256n49; Title V, 89–90; Title VI, 90; and welfare reform, 211
Social Security vs. welfare split, 10, 87–88
social welfare clinics, 32, 100, 102–3, 163
Sociedad Insular de Trabajadores Sociales, 80
Solla, Minerva, 206
Spanish–American War, 36
Spanish colonialism, 8, 48–49, 226n15
spiritual motherhood, 38
statehood, 11, 184
sterilization, forced, 8, 19, 70, 100, 204, 264n80. *See also* eugenics; population control
strikes, 48, 74, 143–44, 147, 190
suffrage movements, 44, 57, 63; Puerto Rican, 35, 37, 79, 239n102; women's, 38, 235n42, 239n102
sugar industry, 36, 77, 107, 223n33
Supreme Court of Puerto Rico, 227n22
surveys, 33, 35, 42, 44, 47, 49, 51–52, 55, 117, 182

Taller Salud group, 218
Thomas, Lorrin, 138, 247n20, 255n44
Torres, Lourdes, 199, 262n57
Torres Zeno, Olimpia, 40
transnationalism, 7, 14, 118–19, 222n17, 223n23

www.ingramcontent.com/pod-product-compliance
Lightning Source LLC
Chambersburg PA
CBHW020826270326
41928CB00006B/450